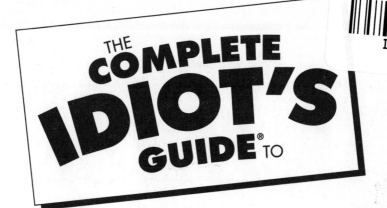

THE COMPLETE IDIOT'S GUIDE® TO

Eating Well After Weight Loss Surgery

by Margaret Furtado, M.S., R.D., L.D.N., R.Y.T.,
and Joseph Ewing

ALPHA

A member of Penguin Group (USA) Inc.

ALPHA BOOKS

Published by the Penguin Group

Penguin Group (USA) Inc., 375 Hudson Street, New York, New York 10014, USA

Penguin Group (Canada), 90 Eglinton Avenue East, Suite 700, Toronto, Ontario M4P 2Y3, Canada (a division of Pearson Penguin Canada Inc.)

Penguin Books Ltd., 80 Strand, London WC2R 0RL, England

Penguin Ireland, 25 St. Stephen's Green, Dublin 2, Ireland (a division of Penguin Books Ltd.)

Penguin Group (Australia), 250 Camberwell Road, Camberwell, Victoria 3124, Australia (a division of Pearson Australia Group Pty. Ltd.)

Penguin Books India Pvt. Ltd., 11 Community Centre, Panchsheel Park, New Delhi—110 017, India

Penguin Group (NZ), 67 Apollo Drive, Rosedale, North Shore, Auckland 1311, New Zealand (a division of Pearson New Zealand Ltd.)

Penguin Books (South Africa) (Pty.) Ltd., 24 Sturdee Avenue, Rosebank, Johannesburg 2196, South Africa

Penguin Books Ltd., Registered Offices: 80 Strand, London WC2R 0RL, England

International Standard Book Number: 978-1-59257-951-8
Library of Congress Catalog Card Number: 2009928403

11   10   09   8   7   6   5   4   3   2   1

Interpretation of the printing code: The rightmost number of the first series of numbers is the year of the book's printing; the rightmost number of the second series of numbers is the number of the book's printing. For example, a printing code of 09-1 shows that the first printing occurred in 2009.

Printed in the United States of America

Note: This publication contains the opinions and ideas of its authors. It is intended to provide helpful and informative material on the subject matter covered. It is sold with the understanding that the authors and publisher are not engaged in rendering professional services in the book. If the reader requires personal assistance or advice, a competent professional should be consulted.

The authors and publisher specifically disclaim any responsibility for any liability, loss, or risk, personal or otherwise, which is incurred as a consequence, directly or indirectly, of the use and application of any of the contents of this book.

Publisher: *Marie Butler-Knight*
Editorial Director: *Mike Sanders*
Senior Managing Editor: *Billy Fields*
Senior Development Editor: *Christy Wagner*
Senior Production Editor: *Megan Douglass*
Copy Editor: *Emily Garner*

Cartoonist: *Richard King*
Cover Designer: *Becky Harmon*
Book Designer: *Trina Wurst*
Indexer: *Johnna Vanhoose Dinse*
Layout: *Ayanna Lacey*
Proofreader: *Laura Caddell*

Contents at a Glance

Contents

Appendixes

Introduction

Whether you're just contemplating having weight loss surgery, or you're reading this in your post-op recovery room, the book you hold in your hands will soon become your best ally in eating well after weight loss surgery.

This book is designed to provide you with state-of-the-art information regarding optimal nutrition and eating after weight loss surgery. Nothing operates in a vacuum, however, so you'll also read about health, wellness, and alternative medicine techniques in the following pages. We feel these approaches can help you not only maximize your weight loss, but potentially significantly improve your chances of *keeping* off the weight—for good.

In addition to the several chapters on nutrition and wellness, we've dedicated nearly half the book to chapters chock full of delicious, delectable, recipes—150 in all! We hope you'll find the recipes as easy to make as they are healthful and satisfying. Our goal is to help you feel like a person instead of a patient and still get the same results as if you had slaved in the kitchen all day!

Come along with us on this journey!

How This Book Is Organized

This book is divided into four parts to help you easily find and access all the information you need:

In **Part 1, "Nutritional Needs After Weight Loss Surgery,"** we cover the nitty-gritty of what your body truly needs post-op, from the various weight loss procedures and how to get the most success out of your chosen bariatric procedure, to all the information you need about carbohydrates, protein, and fats and how they apply to you. You also get the "skinny" on fluids and vitamins and minerals, and how to lift your health and well-being to its utmost potential.

In **Part 2, "Demystifying Food Labels and Nutrition Buzzwords,"** we tackle food labels and give you the low-down on the latest nutrition buzzwords. There are a lot of new and exciting developments within the field of nutrition, and here we bring you some of the highlights of the very best tools to help maximize your health, including the hot topic, antioxidants.

In **Part 3, "Ensuring Your Continued Success,"** we discuss SMART goal setting and strategies to keep the weight off, negotiating the grocery aisles, and making good choices when eating out. We also discuss ways to reduce stress, as well as culinary helpful hints and what to have in your kitchen to make cooking easy and fun.

Finally, we discuss red flags for weight regain and how to get back on track should you find yourself slipping.

In **Part 4, "Recipes for Eating Well After Weight Loss Surgery,"** we've assembled 150 recipes you're sure to love. From soups, salads, and appetizers to decadent desserts, all the recipes in this part are healthful and delicious! We know you're going to have a blast trying all these great new dishes and putting a new, healthful spin on the foods you prepare at home.

After all that, we still have more to give you. In the back of the book you'll find a helpful glossary of terms along with an appendix of resources to help you along your journey of eating well after weight loss surgery.

Extras

Throughout this book, you'll see boxes set apart from the main text. These contain extra jewels of information you won't want to miss:

Cooking Tip
These helpful hints or ideas help you maximize your weight loss success.

Food for Thought
These boxes hold bits of nutrition and/or culinary trivia we feel you'll find helpful.

Post-Op Pitfall
Here we provide information about possible dangers and/or misconceptions.

def•i•ni•tion
Check these boxes for definitions of terms you might not be familiar with.

Acknowledgments

From Margaret: First of all, I'd like to acknowledge my amazing agent, Marilyn Allen, for being so wonderful throughout this whole process. Thank you also to Mike Sanders, Christy Wagner, Megan Douglass, and everyone else at Alpha who helped produce this book. A big thank you to my wonderful technical writer, Laura Frank, Ph.D., R.D., M.P.H., for her expert editing, and a huge thanks to Joe for his expert culinary work and endless energy and creativity.

Thanks so much to all of my wonderful patients, who inspire me each and every day. I thank God that I love what I do so much and pray everyone reading this book will find it helpful.

I want to send a big thank you to my family, parents Ed and Sara, and to Maria, Karen, and Kirby, as well as the rest of my family and friends, who have been so supportive and loving during this whole process.

From Joe: Thank you to all of you who helped me get where I am today. Without your guidance and support, none of this would have been possible. I feel so blessed to be surrounded by such amazing people.

Special Thanks to the Technical Reviewer

The Complete Idiot's Guide to Eating Well After Weight Loss Surgery was reviewed by an expert who double-checked the accuracy of what you'll learn here, to help us ensure that this book gives you everything you need to know about eating well after your weight loss surgery. Special thanks are extended to Laura Lewis Frank.

Trademarks

All terms mentioned in this book that are known to be or are suspected of being trademarks or service marks have been appropriately capitalized. Alpha Books and Penguin Group (USA) Inc. cannot attest to the accuracy of this information. Use of a term in this book should not be regarded as affecting the validity of any trademark or service mark.

Part

Nutritional Needs After Weight Loss Surgery

Congratulations on your weight loss surgery! After your procedure is over, the journey truly begins, and in the following pages, we cover the different weight loss surgeries, including how weight loss happens and what you can do to help maximize your weight loss. We also cover your unique nutritional needs and tolerances post-op so you'll have a good handle on what to expect down the road.

Part 1 is chock full of nutrition information, including carbohydrates, protein, fats, fluids, and vitamins and minerals as they pertain to you and your procedure. So turn the page to begin soaking up the nutrition information that just may help you get to a higher level of weight loss success and vibrant health.

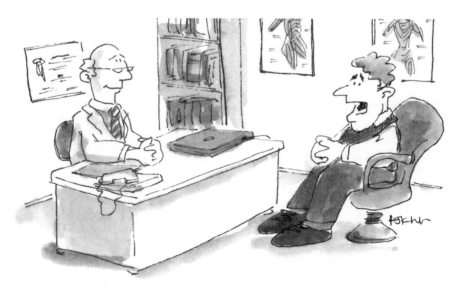

"The surgery was the easy part?"

What to Expect After Surgery

In This Chapter

◆ How weight loss surgeries work

◆ What to expect after various weight loss surgeries

◆ General nutrition goals by procedure

◆ Nutritional challenges to watch out for

The most brilliant physicians and scientists in the world have cited bariatric (a.k.a. weight loss) surgery as cutting-edge treatment for obesity. Although weight loss surgery is certainly not a quick fix or cure-all, it is a great ally in beating your battle with weight for good, and it's a whole new paradigm in weight loss. Weight loss surgery, for sure, can and should change your weight loss results, particularly the metabolic surgeries we talk about in this chapter. The purely restrictive surgeries have yielded great results as well, and in the following pages and chapters, we give you all the weight loss tools you need—and then some—to help ensure your success for a long and healthy lifetime.

This chapter is chock full of the latest information on why and how bariatric surgery works and how you can optimize your results with the right nutrition, so get ready!

Gastric Bypass Surgery

Gastric bypass surgery is one of the *metabolic* surgeries, and it can be a fantastic tool to help you win the weight loss battle. We're sure you researched your gastric bypass surgery at length before you had it, but let's review some key points about how this surgery really works.

> **Food for Thought**
>
> Metabolic surgeries, including gastric bypass surgery and duodenal switch (D/S), are so called because they cause changes in connections between your gastrointestinal tract and brain and help your brain "want" to go to a lower weight. Restrictive surgeries (e.g., gastric banding) are not metabolic because they simply limit the amount of food, particularly solid foods, you can eat, without changing brain connections.

The Honeymoon Period and the Gene Fight

After gastric bypass surgery, you might experience a "honeymoon period" for about 4 to 6 months when you have no real appetite or hunger for food. Why is this? According to research, about eight different metabolic pathways are affected after gastric bypass surgery. Particularly in the first 6 months or so after surgery, hunger hormones such as ghrelin basically shut down the hunger hormone factory. I've had patients forget to eat meals and have to set alarms on their watches or put notes on their fridge to remind them to eat. You also need to get your fluids during this time, so set an alarm if you need to, or never be without a drink in your hand. (More on fluids in Chapter 5.)

> **Food for Thought**
>
> It's believed that one of the metabolic pathways affected by gastric bypass can help fight unfriendly weight genes by giving your brain orders to settle in at a much lower weight.

Research suggests that the main way gastric bypass surgery works is not the small pouch or malabsorption. In essence, gastric bypass results in certain vitamins and minerals not being absorbed as well (more about that in Chapter 6), but otherwise, it's more of a restrictive procedure (e.g., having a stomach reduced to about 1 ounce, called a pouch, limits food you can eat but doesn't cause malabsorption, like you see with duodenal switch [D/S] surgery) with metabolic aspects, which we talk more about in this chapter.

If there were a list of the "top 10 reasons why gastric bypass surgery works long-term," the number-one reason would be because your brain gets a message from your intestinal area that there's too much weight and fat onboard. This occurs thanks to a complicated set of connections and pathways (including leptin and insulin, long-term weight and fat regulators) that help your body release fat. Unlike dieting, these changes cause an *increase* in your metabolism, resulting in long-term weight loss, rather than the short-term type of weight loss you probably experienced over and over with dieting.

The metabolic aspects of gastric bypass essentially help level the playing field against unfriendly weight genes. Therefore, this surgery is one of the best chances for fighting certain mechanisms and higher-weight genes that may have kept you on the dieting and weight roller coaster all your life. The metabolic aspect of this surgery may also give you a significant chance for remission of diseases such as diabetes and sleep apnea.

When counseling patients prior to gastric bypass surgery, I urge them never to diet again after surgery because that can, over time, reverse their lower weight thermostat or set point. I urge patients not to skip meals and deprive themselves when they're truly hungry. I realize it takes a huge leap of faith to never diet again and trust that your new weight set point will be what's healthy for you, even if it's not necessarily what some table in a book says you should weigh.

Where your body settles, weight wise, depends on many factors, including genetics, physical activity, age, muscle mass, gender, and even height. Of course, your daily meal plan can't be underestimated in the weight loss equation. It's important to follow your nutritional guidelines and keep regular appointments with your dietitian and health-care team. Realistic weight goals are key. (We talk more about this in Chapter 9.)

> **Food for Thought**
>
> Your lowest weight after gastric bypass surgery is not typically your new weight set point or thermostat. Research studies involving mice and rats, as well as humans, reveal weight regain of 5 to 15 percent of weight lost is normal as "famine insurance."

The first 6 to 9 months after gastric bypass are like metabolic boot camp. Your body is revved up and burning more calories than ever before. In addition, it's producing all kinds of weight friendly hormones. You can maximize your weight loss results during this time by eating right and exercising regularly.

After the first year or so, studies reveal your calorie burning is closer to normal, and hunger hormones most likely have returned. However, a healthy lifestyle helps maintain most of the weight loss and is priceless toward keeping you healthy and avoiding common pitfalls after surgery (see Chapter 11). It's also important to realize that over time, your gastrointestinal (GI) tract adapts or evolves by increasing its absorption of more nutrients and, therefore, calories.

If you're wondering if you're going to gain back all the weight you've lost, know that statistics are on your side in terms of weight loss success, especially if you're maintaining a healthy lifestyle. Research in the United States reveals that the average gastric bypass patient loses 60 to 70 percent of his or her excess weight after about 2 years (about 65 pounds lost for every 100 pounds overweight). Roughly 5 years post-op, the average person keeps off 50 pounds for every 100 pounds he or she had in excess, or a gain of about 15 pounds from years 2 to 5 post-op, if they had 100 pounds of excess weight before surgery. This may sound a little disappointing, but compare this to the fact that 95 percent of diets fail by causing you to gain back all the weight you lost—and more!

Avoid panicking and overly restricting eating to get back to your lowest weight. Instead, eat a healthful, balanced diet; exercise; keep stress under control; and visit your doctor, dietitian, and the rest of your health-care team on a regular basis. Attending post-op support groups are important as well. If your surgical center is too far away or inconvenient for you to attend support groups, ask for resources in your area, call nearby hospitals, or consider some of the popular patient websites like www. obesityhelp.com for some suggestions on post-op support groups.

Pouch Friends and Foes

Understanding the metabolic part of gastric bypass helps you gain the key to success with long-term weight loss. Another factor in your success is understanding your new anatomy, or your customized stomach pouch.

As you know, your surgeon took your stomach, which was the size of a football, and made it the size of a small egg. Although the metabolic changes after surgery were the real star of the show, your small pouch may help you keep down the volume of food, especially when the hunger starts to creep back in, typically by 6 months post-op.

> **Cooking Tip**
>
> Pouch-friendly foods after gastric bypass, in terms of long-term weight loss success, include foods with protein and fiber, such as high-fiber cereal and skim milk or all-natural peanut butter and an apple. Foods that aren't pouch-friendly but are usually well tolerated include crackers and pretzels.

Simple and processed carbohydrates, typically well tolerated by your pouch, seem to be well absorbed by your new GI tract. If you find yourself mindlessly snacking on these foods, you'll likely gain weight. Instead, stick with protein and fiber at meals and snacks. Also, keep in mind that as you advance your diet, pouch foes will include tough or dry chicken or meats. Other poorly tolerated foods include fruit and vegetable skins, stringy foods like celery, rice, pasta, and doughy breads. These foods tend to get stuck and may cause vomiting and/or a very uncomfortable feeling.

Advancing Your Diet After Surgery

Although each surgical center does things differently, there are some general rules of thumb in terms of advancing your diet after gastric bypass surgery.

First, don't expect to get a tray of liquids the day of your surgery. When you do get liquids to drink in the hospital, many weight loss centers, mine included, give you 1-ounce (30-cc) medicine cups and suggest you drink only 1 medicine cup per hour the first day and 2 medicine cups per hour the following day. Most centers include at least clear liquids like broths, diet gelatin, low-calorie clear drinks, and high-protein beverages. Some may give you full liquids such as skim milk; low-fat, low-sugar strained yogurt; or high-protein drinks the following day. Many people go home on full liquids for a week or two, followed with a few weeks of puréed foods, and then advance to mechanical soft/ground foods. Your meal plan may not include raw fruits and vegetables for at least 6 to 8 weeks post-op, especially if your fluid intake is lower than your dietitian would like it to be.

> **Cooking Tip**
>
> When you go home after surgery, it's critical that you get enough fluids—48 to 64 ounces a day is a common goal—and listen to your body. Sip, don't gulp your fluids to minimize both pain and fear of stretching out your pouch.

Your new feeling of fullness will most likely feel like chest fullness or pressure, so don't expect a Thanksgiving-type fullness. It's very important to avoid drinking with your meals and not drink until 30 minutes after eating to help with tolerance and to decrease the competition between fluids and solids in your pouch. Separating your solids from your liquids can also decrease the risk of *dumping*, which some studies cite anywhere from 15 to 40 percent of post-op gastric bypass patients experience. Some centers may want you to avoid fluids 30 minutes or so before your meals as well.

def•i•ni•tion

Dumping goes something like this: you're a few weeks post-op and mistakenly eat fruit with syrup. When the concentrated syrup reaches your middle intestinal area, the jejunum, it can't handle it the way the first part of your bypassed intestine did. Essentially, there's no more gatekeeper for gastric (stomach) emptying due to the removal of the pyloric sphincter, and water goes rushing in to save the day. Unfortunately, this increase in fluid in your intestines tends to cause a vaso-vagal response, so you may start to feel dizzy, sweaty, nauseous, and just exhausted the rest of the day, with diarrhea a possibility as well.

Don't try to multitask when you're eating because that might increase your risk of vomiting and/or food getting stuck. If food gets stuck, don't try to wash it down with fluids—that's the equivalent of putting more water in a clogged drain without anything to dissolve the clog—and do try to breathe and stay calm. If it doesn't go away or you're feeling something just isn't normal, call your surgical center or go to the emergency department to get it checked out. Better safe than sorry.

If you're anxious or stressed about not tolerating your diet, particularly as you're advancing to solid textures, remember to try only one new food at a time. Stick with your center's nutritional guidelines, and be sure you chew your foods until they're absolutely liquid. Also, when you get to the point where you're ready to add fresh fruits and vegetables, perhaps around 6 to 8 weeks post-op, watch out for tough/stringy foods and avoid skins and seeds. In addition, you probably want to avoid trying foods for the first time when you're dining out.

I also often recommend keeping a food journal to better understand which foods you can tolerate and which situations and/or moods may cause you to overeat. (See samples of logs in Appendix B.) We talk about stress reduction and ways to stay successful in future chapters.

Finally, because the first part of your small intestine, the duodenum, is bypassed, you may have issues with lactose, or milk sugar. Enzymes that break down milk sugar, available in pill form and also in lactose-reduced products, can help alleviate the gas, bloating, and diarrhea often associated with lactose intolerance.

Gastric Banding

You've taken an important step toward getting your weight into a healthy range for good, and no doubt you've done a lot of research on how your band works. Whatever brand name band you have, they all work in similar ways, to restrict the amount of food, particularly solid food, you can take in at one time.

Your band could be likened to a funnel in that it slows the amount of solid food you can get in, especially when you have an adjustment or fill to tighten it. However, keep in mind that liquids and continuous snacking can and often will be absorbed, which can increase weight regain or even cause weight loss failure. Therefore, mindful eating and the avoidance of empty calories such as milkshakes, soda, and high-calorie juice drinks, are recommended.

Now let's talk about the fills and how they can work for you.

To Fill or Not to Fill?

The first couple weeks post-op, you may not feel hungry because it's common for your stomach to swell in response to band placement. However, typically a week or two post-op, the swelling subsides and you may feel hungry. In most surgical centers, the first fill or adjustment happens around 6 weeks after your band is placed. This may leave you feeling anxious and perhaps scared you'll never lose weight. However, all is not lost! Keep in mind that the band surgery is a slower boat when it comes to weight loss.

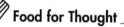 **Food for Thought**

Research studies reveal that hunger hormones such as ghrelin may be increased for as long as 1 year after your band is placed.

Unlike gastric bypass surgery, most band patients don't have a honeymoon period during which they're not hungry for several months. Although I've had band patients who, several weeks post-op, aren't hungry at all, the vast majority note at least some hunger the first few weeks after the band is placed.

Around 6 weeks post-op, you may be offered your first fill or adjustment, when a saline (salt and water) solution is injected into your port (a circular area the size of a quarter or so), which tightens the silicone band around the top of your stomach. The amount of fluid injected depends on at least a few factors, including your level of hunger, weight loss and/or lack thereof, and your surgical center's protocol. Some centers fill the band more aggressively than others. Ultimately, if you feel your band is not giving you restriction and/or a feeling of fullness upon eating, chances are your surgeon will inject at least a small amount of saline into your port to tighten your band. On the other hand, sometimes people's bands are so tight even liquids won't go down, and in that case your surgeon may remove fluid from your band to help with tolerance.

⊘ **Post-Op Pitfall** _____

If you don't chew solid food until it's a liquid consistency, you could increase your risk of food getting stuck and causing a blockage. This rare but painful occurrence may result in persistent vomiting and chest pain. Consult your surgeon immediately if you feel this is happening to you.

Keep in mind that although your stomach hasn't been surgically altered, you're only able to tolerate food particles as narrow as your band opening or stoma.

In my experience working with the band over the past several years, most people need 3 or 4 fills until they get the right level of restriction, or what's called the "sweet spot." This often means that you can get in the recommended protein (e.g., a deck of cards' worth of meat, chicken, fish, or tofu) and some vegetables, but not much more. Inability to get fluids down may be the result of your band being too tight.

If your band feels too loose and you're constantly hungry, you probably need a fill. Poor weight loss and your ability to eat more than a deck of cards' worth of protein is another possible indication. It's important to keep in contact with your surgical team to help ensure long-term weight loss success.

Band-Friendly Eating Strategies

As I mentioned at the start of this section, hunger may be increased for up to a year after your band is placed, so hang in there! I tell my patients the band is kind of like a manual lawn mower: it may feel like you'll never get the lawn mowed, but persistence can help you get there!

Certain foods are more weight friendly than others. For example, protein foods, such as low-fat cottage cheese and low-fat ricotta cheese, may help with your hunger. Furthermore, studies have concluded that calcium, which is found in these dairy foods, may assist your body with weight loss. And certain other foods can really help with weight-friendly hormones. (More on gut hormones in Chapter 9.)

On the other hand, some foods are well tolerated but are not weight friendly. Liquids such as sodas, milkshakes, ice cream, juices, and high-calorie juice drinks go down like a slowly moving drain but don't help you feel full. Instead, you might feel hungry 30 to 60 minutes later and crave more simple sugars.

Even if you're not hungry within the first few weeks, it's key to include high-quality protein supplements at least 3 times a day to help meet your protein needs (see Chapter 3).

Advancing Your Diet After Surgery

Many centers' protocols include full liquids such as skim milk, soy milk, low-fat yogurt, and high-protein supplements for the first week or two. After a couple weeks, you may be advanced to soft or mushy solids, like chopped tuna with light mayo, or at least puréed foods. By 4 weeks post-op, your diet may include soft solids such as tofu, ground chicken, and/or "slow-cooker-consistency" foods. At the 6-week mark, it's common to have your first fill. This typically involves downgrading texture in your diet from soft solids to a liquid or puréed consistency for a day or two. Around 6 to 8 weeks post-op, you may be allowed to increase to a regular texture, including fresh fruits and vegetables and whole grains.

> **Cooking Tip**
>
> Tough skins and fibrous vegetables such as corn are not typically tolerated post-op band. Section grapefruits and oranges to avoid eating the skins and seeds, and always try only one new food at a time. Otherwise, you won't know which food was ill tolerated.

Mindful eating and avoiding multitasking can be key to preventing or minimizing intolerance to your diet. In addition to chewing thoroughly, stop eating when you feel chest fullness or tightness to minimize the risk of discomfort.

Gastric Sleeve

The gastric sleeve is a fairly new weight loss surgery that's having good results so far. Although it's considered a restrictive surgery without any malabsorption, research suggests metabolic effects may, in fact, be involved with the sleeve, which could help with weight loss surgery in more ways than you might have thought. I'm sure you'll want to maximize your success after your sleeve surgery, so let's get started!

How the "Banana Stomach" Works

As you know, your surgeon has removed a good deal of your stomach and left you with a stomach about the size and shape of a banana.

Ghrelin, a major hunger hormone, is made primarily in the fundus, or the top of your stomach, which is largely removed with the sleeve procedure. Therefore, you may have a honeymoon period for several months when you're not hungry—and may even forget to eat!

The sleeve isn't malabsorptive, but because your intestines are intact, it may be maldigestive to some extent since your stomach is a significantly smaller version of the football-size churning and grinding organ it used to be. If you eat too quickly, especially in the first weeks post-op, you may find you have chest pain or pressure and may even vomit. Keep in mind that chronic vomiting is not normal after surgery, so call your surgical team if this occurs.

Why a Banana Is Not Just a Banana

Although the gastric sleeve surgery is a restrictive surgery, it differs from the gastric band, another restrictive surgery. New studies are showing that the sleeve can result in metabolic changes, some of which are similar to those that occur with gastric bypass surgery. Ghrelin production and/or secretion is decreased and your intestines or gut experiences an increase in the influx of weight friendly chemicals. These hormones increase the stimulation of the fullness or satiety receptors in your brain, which aids weight loss (see Chapter 8).

> **Food for Thought**
>
> Research studies on the sleeve indicate that the tensile pressure (or pulling) on the sides of your banana-size stomach induce positive metabolic changes that help increase metabolic rate, change insulin receptors, and increase weight friendly hormones.

Due to metabolic changes, the gastric sleeve is believed to help fight unfriendly weight genes, so it's not just the smaller size of your stomach that causes long-term weight loss. Complicated weight friendly hormones are believed to play a significant role in weight loss post-op. In addition to helping with weight loss, studies reveal that the gastric sleeve can also help with remission of diseases such as diabetes.

Advancing Your Diet After Surgery

Your surgical center will guide you regarding how to advance your diet after your sleeve surgery. However, many centers include full liquids such as skim or soy milk, cottage cheese, and high-protein drinks for the first 2 weeks and puréed foods like baby food, mashed tofu, or puréed meat, chicken, or scrambled eggs during weeks 2 through 4. Your regimen may even include soft solids such as ground meat, chicken, fish, or chili by week 2.

The key when advancing your diet is to try only one new food at a time and avoid liquids with your meals and until 30 minutes after to optimize tolerance. Your center's guidelines may also include avoiding fluid 30 minutes prior to meals. Of course, every center may do things differently, and there's currently no consensus on the "right" way to advance the diet, other than to eat and drink mindfully. That means, for sure, not to gulp your fluids and to chew solid foods thoroughly, until liquid, to minimize the risk of chest pain and vomiting, or food getting stuck. As soon as you feel chest fullness, stop eating or drinking because continuing on could cause severe chest pain and/or vomiting.

By weeks 6 to 8, your diet might be advanced to allow you to add fresh fruits, vegetables, and some starches. However, keep in mind that stringy foods such as corn and celery aren't well tolerated. Also, rice, pasta, and doughy breads typically are a problem for many people after weight loss surgery. When in doubt, try a small amount, only one new food at a time, and when you're eating at home.

Duodenal Switch (D/S)

The biliopancreatic diversion (BPD) is a different surgery from the duodenal switch (D/S) and not done very much in the United States, so we refer strictly to the duodenal switch (D/S) throughout this book. This surgery has the best weight loss results of all the procedures done in the United States. Unlike the other procedures mentioned thus far, the D/S is truly malabsorptive in that your body is incapable of retaining a good deal of the fat (and fat calories) you take in. However, you're also malabsorbing some protein, so you may need to work harder post-op to meet your body's needs.

Although there are possible risks of diarrhea post-op D/S, there's also the potential for greater weight loss than with all the other procedures.

Maximizing the Gene and Disease Fight

The D/S is a malabsorptive procedure. As you most likely learned in your pre-op research, your surgeon first removes about $^2/_3$ to $^3/_4$ of your stomach. This decrease in stomach size helps restrict the amount of food you're able to eat and helps you fill up quicker. However, your pylorus, the valve at the outlet of your stomach, is left intact, which helps reduce, if not obliterate, the risk of dumping.

Your surgeon has divided and rearranged your small intestines to separate food from digestive juices, allowing malabsorption to occur. A portion of your intestine is attached to the first part of your small intestine (the duodenum) and receives food from your stomach. The remainder of the bypassed small intestine is left attached with the ability to carry the digestive enzymes.

Finally, your surgeon attached your small intestines together down near your colon, or large intestine, allowing a 100-centimeter "common channel" for the digestive enzymes and food to combine and absorb nutrients.

Food for Thought

Because the D/S involves removal of a significant amount of your small intestines, studies cite malabsorption of approximately 73 percent of fats and 30 percent of protein. Therefore, your protein needs will be about ⅓ higher than with other procedures.

The D/S restricts the amount of calories, vitamins, and minerals your body can absorb from food and results in significant weight loss, but research studies cite metabolic surgery as the principal reason for long-term weight loss success. As with gastric bypass, it appears that your brain gets a message from your intestinal area to lower your weight thermostat or set point. At the same time, hunger hormones such as ghrelin and other weight friendly hormones like PYY and GLP-1 cause a decrease in appetite. At the same time, your metabolism, your body's calorie-burning furnace, is revved up.

Although no weight loss surgery is a cure-all, the D/S holds the best chance for the remission of not only obesity, but also diabetes, sleep apnea, and many other chronic diseases. According to the latest scientific studies, if you have diabetes, you have about a 98 percent chance of getting it into remission after your D/S, with the best chance if you've had diabetes less than 5 years and have been on insulin less than 4 years. The D/S is truly a wonderful weight loss and health tool.

D/S Challenges and Salvages

Despite fat and protein malabsorption post-op D/S, many people find their body is too carb friendly because foods like pretzels and crackers appear to be well absorbed. D/S research reveals that weight regain is possible with a high-carb diet, particularly simple carbs like pretzels and crackers.

Challenges of the D/S and, therefore, issues to be on the lookout for include greater chance of chronic diarrhea and/or foul-smelling stools and flatulence due to significant fat malabsorption. This malabsorptive component increases the risk for vitamin/mineral absorption, including fat-soluble vitamins A, D, E, and K. This is because bypassing a large section of your small intestines in the D/S results in about 72 percent fat malabsorption, so A, D, E, and K, fat-soluble vitamins, are not as well absorbed. Therefore, aim for about 10 to 15 grams fat (about 3 ounces salmon has 14 grams fat) to help fat-soluble vitamin absorption. Unfortunately for carb-lovers, this component of your diet is generally well tolerated and absorbed, which may increase the risk for weight regain.

Despite the possible risks, there certainly are advantages to the D/S, including the larger stomach capacity that allows you to eat more normally. Many D/S patients like the fact that dumping syndrome, seen with some gastric bypass patients, is rare because your pylorus is still intact. Finally, the D/S has the highest rate of weight loss, at 75 to 80 percent of excess body weight, so it's the best chance for significant, long-lasting weight loss success among all the procedures.

D/S-Friendly Eating Strategies

Recommended D/S eating strategies include protein such as high-quality protein drinks, low-fat, high-protein yogurt at regular intervals, and keeping simple carbs low. You may find, like most D/S patients, that you have no appetite the first several months after your procedure, courtesy of the metabolic changes and temporary hunger hormone shut-down or honeymoon period, and you may need to remind yourself to eat.

At the same time, your protein needs are highest of all the surgeries, especially the first weeks post-op when your body is healing from your procedure. Therefore, it's vital to eat or drink something with high-quality protein (see Chapter 3) every few hours to help meet your body's significant nutritional needs.

You probably want to avoid high-fat foods initially, not only because you may have loose stools, but so you can find a healthy balance between carbs, protein, and fats while keeping in mind higher needs due to malabsorption. Healthy fats, however, are preferable over unhealthy fats (see Chapter 4).

Advancing Your Diet After Surgery

Although surgical centers differ with respect to post-op diet progression, many include 2 weeks of full liquids like skim or 1 percent milk or soy milk, fat-free high-protein yogurt and cottage cheese, and high-protein supplements. Typically, you might be advanced to soft solids or purées at week 2, and many centers allow you to progress to regular textures by weeks 6 to 8, including fresh fruits and vegetables as well as starches. However, you'll probably want to stay away from fibrous vegetables like celery, fruit skins such as those on oranges and grapefruit, and thick-skinned apples, rice, pasta, and doughy breads, to name a few common offenders. The thinner skins like grapes and peaches are usually okay.

Also, try only one new food at a time, preferably at home versus at a restaurant to minimize discomfort and/or embarrassment as you're learning what you can tolerate. Food logs can greatly increase awareness of which foods you can tolerate and help you keep track of how many grams protein you've been able to get into your diet (see the sample food logs in Appendix B).

> ### Cooking Tip
>
> If loose stools are a problem for you after your D/S, probiotics in active yogurt cultures may help, or "medical grade" probiotics with much higher concentrations and good quality. If not, your doctor may prescribe medication to help.

Mindful eating is essential to optimal tolerance after your D/S procedure. Diarrhea and/or loose stools, which may happen anyway after this surgery, can really be exaggerated if you're eating too fast and/or your portions are too large. Keep in close contact with your surgical center's dietitian to help ensure you're meeting your extensive nutritional needs.

The talked-about and sometimes experienced body odor post-op D/S can be alleviated or at least managed with a host of products such as Devrom, an "internal body deodorant" available online.

As with any weight loss procedure, chewing food until it's liquid and being aware of chest fullness and chest pressure while eating and stopping immediately can minimize symptoms and even help avoid or minimize loose stools, in at least some patients.

The Least You Need to Know

♦ Gastric bypass surgery is a metabolic surgery, although it does not involve significant malabsorption.

♦ Gastric banding surgery is a purely restrictive weight loss surgery, so foods that are liquid and/or easily absorbed can make weight loss success more challenging.

♦ Gastric sleeve surgery is more than just a "banana stomach" because it is also a metabolic surgery.

♦ D/S is a truly malabsorptive surgery with the best weight loss results of all the weight loss procedures.

Carbs, Fiber, Sugars, and More

In This Chapter

- Separating the good carbs from the bad
- The skinny on fiber
- The inside scoop on the glycemic index
- The lowdown on sugar substitutes

Carbohydrates … the mere mention of the word sends shivers down the spines of many people who have dieted for what seems like their whole lives—and that includes almost all weight loss surgery patients, perhaps even you.

But are carbs really bad? How much do our bodies need, and how much is too much? In this chapter, we answer these questions. We also take an honest look at fiber, the glycemic index, and sugar substitutes.

The Good, the Bad, and the Ugly—Carbs

The principal job of carbohydrates is to provide energy to all the cells in your body. But not all carbs are created equal. There are good-for-you carbs, carbs that aren't so good for you, and those that are just plain ugly, health-wise. Knowing which is which is important for weight loss as well as your overall health.

At 4 calories per gram, carbohydrates (a.k.a. carbs) are an energy bargain compared to fats, which contain 9 calories per gram, and alcohol, with 7 calories per gram. Protein, tied at 4 calories per gram, is the most comparable food source in terms of calories. But still, a calorie is not a calorie, and there are different kinds of carbohydrates, with some better for you than others.

In the following sections, we take a closer look at carbs and help you identify the good from the bad and the ugly.

The Good Carbs

The "good" carbs are the complex carbohydrates, found in plant-based foods. Complex carbohydrates are considered good because they typically carry a healthy amount of vitamins, minerals, and fiber. These are the carbs you want in your diet.

> **Food for Thought**
>
> An examination of several studies, involving a total of about 700,000 men and women, found that eating an extra 2 servings of whole grains per day decreased the risk of type 2 diabetes by 21 percent.

Foods that contain good carbs include fruits, vegetables, and whole-grain products such as 100 percent whole-wheat pita bread or English muffins, old-fashioned oatmeal and cream of wheat, and all-natural high-fiber cereals—some of which contain up to 14 grams fiber per serving.

These healthy carbs can help you feel full and lower your risk of constipation. Certain kinds of carbs can even help with diarrhea. (More on fiber a bit later in the chapter.)

The Bad and the Ugly Carbs

If the good carbs are the complex carbs, the bad carbs are the simple carbs, like sucrose (table sugar). Although some people might disagree with the "bad" sugar title, in relative terms, simple sugars (e.g., table sugar, high-fructose corn syrup) may cause increased hunger or blood sugars for some people. Also, although controversial, some scientists suggest the increased weight issues in the United States have been directly tied in with the first appearance of high-fructose corn syrup.

Why all the fuss? Because although 1 teaspoon table sugar contains only 16 calories and may not, by itself, cause danger to your health in terms of increased weight and disease risks, Americans consume far more table sugar than we should. The U.S. Department of Agriculture (USDA) has recommended that you aim for no more than 10 teaspoons table sugar a day (or 40 grams carbohydrate as simple sugars). However, the Center for Science in the Public Interest (CSPI) estimates actual consumption somewhere around 50 teaspoons sugar a day—a far cry from the USDA goal!

Measurement of simple sugars can get cloudy because natural and whole foods may contain simple sugars. For example, an 8-ounce glass of milk contains 12 grams simple sugar, while a serving of water-packed canned fruit has about 12 grams. So it gets confusing. Even those of you who read food labels may find "sugars" on a label confusing because milk and fruit in its own juice has simple sugar (as lactose and fructose, respectively), but are not simple or refined, like table sugar or high-fructose corn syrup, so they may not raise your blood sugar like table sugar. (Read more about calculating grams of sugar in Chapter 8.) However, most scientists would agree that excessive table sugar intake might increase risk for weight gain and could worsen some health issues, like diabetes.

Food for Thought

According to the Center for Science in the Public Interest, Americans consumed 158 pounds of table sugar in 1999, a 30 percent increase from 1983. Reports also cite that consumption of high-fructose corn syrup (HFCS) has increased more than 1,000 percent between 1979 and 1990, far exceeding changes in consumption of any other food or food group. New concerns regarding HFCS include its high mercury content, as highlighted in a January 2009 *Washington Post* article, where almost half of tested samples of commercial HFCS contained mercury.

Then you have the "ugly" carbohydrates, which are not only refined/simple carbs, but are then processed further, such as high-fructose corn syrup (HFCS). Although you might have seen the commercials on TV stating HFCS is natural and fine in moderation, scientific studies on this highly processed syrup have revealed that chronic intake may result in an increased risk of higher triglycerides (TG) or fat in your blood. Because TG is an independent risk factor for heart disease, HFCS could be something to avoid overall.

But it's controversial. Some scientists note that the processing tends to involve genetic modifications in fructose, so it's not the same, health-wise, as the fructose you find in fruits. The truth is that we just don't know the long-term ramifications of increased HFCS in our diets. Therefore, go very lightly on HFCS, or just try your best to avoid it in favor of whole foods with natural sugars, like fruits and vegetables.

Simple, processed carbs (like pretzels) are often well tolerated after all the weight loss surgery procedures, and most don't cause dumping with gastric bypass or diarrhea or malabsorption with the duodenal switch (D/S). However, they're easily absorbed and typically have a higher glycemic index, meaning they can increase your blood sugar more than some other foods, so they may increase your blood sugar. In addition, you may find they don't satisfy your hunger, which makes sense because they're usually low in fiber and protein. They also may cause an increased release of insulin from your pancreas with a subsequent drop in blood sugar. Ugly, indeed.

Your Carbohydrate Needs After Surgery

Carbohydrates provide your body with energy, and several months to a year or so post-op, many dietitians, including myself, recommend that around 50 percent of your calories come from carbs to help meet energy needs, although in the first few months after surgery, your diet will be mostly protein, especially since you may not have room for much more. The 50 percent carbohydrate goal may be something you may only reach about a year out. Getting adequate carbohydrates—ideally from fruits, vegetables, and whole grains—can help your body keep protein taken in the diet to heal and "feed" your muscles. Otherwise it's used to meet energy needs, which often happens in the immediate post-op period when almost all food intake is comprised of protein because of decreased appetite and intolerance of healthy carbohydrates.

Although carbohydrate needs vary by surgical procedure as well as medical issues such as diabetes or insulin resistance, 130 grams carbohydrate per day is what's often quoted in weight loss surgery scientific literature. This is in line with the U.S. Dietary Recommended Intake (DRI) for carbohydrates: 130 grams per day. This goal may seem overwhelming and most likely won't happen within the first few months after your surgery, but it's certainly something to aim for at least 6 to 9 months post-op.

See if this helps put your carbohydrate goal into perspective:

◆ 1 piece of fruit (e.g., 1 medium apple) = 15 grams carbohydrate

◆ 1 (8-ounce) glass milk = 12 grams carbohydrate

- 1 slice bread = typically 15 grams carbohydrate

- 1 serving vegetables = around 5 grams

So if you had 2 glasses of milk, 3 starches, 3 fruits, and 2 vegetables in a 24-hour period, you've met your 125 grams goal. No, this isn't likely to happen the first few months post-op, but it *is* possible. Just be sure you keep up your protein intake while you add carbohydrates to your diet to help ensure all your needs are being met.

Although it may be hard to meet your protein needs *and* get enough carbs, it's worth the effort to get them into your diet. I've seen patients several months post-op who are afraid to eat any carbs for fear of weight gain or slowed weight loss, and they typically not only have bad breath (ketosis, caused by using fats to meet the brain's sugar/glucose needs) but also report they have no energy. While there are some beneficial aspects to ketosis, such as decreased basal insulin levels, promotion of lipolysis (fat breakdown), and suppression of appetite, there are risks, particularly if ketosis becomes long term.

> **Post-Op Pitfall** _____
> Studies show ketosis is more likely to happen in diets providing less than 100 grams carbohydrate a day, which includes a vast majority of people within the first few months after weight loss surgery.

In the early stages of fasting, the use of ketones (by-products of fat breakdown) by the heart and skeletal muscles conserves blood glucose for support of the central nervous system, including the brain. However, with more prolonged starvation or when there are not enough carbohydrates in your diet to support metabolism, the brain can switch to using ketones for energy. Utilization of ketones for energy can increase the acidity of the blood and brain (decreasing the normal pH of the cells and making them more acidic) and can lead to many symptoms like possible changes in your mental status, such as feelings of confusion or "hitting the wall."

It's important to start where you are in terms of carbohydrate intake, and not sacrifice protein needs as you're adding more carbs to your meal plan. For example, if you're taking in about 30 grams carbohydrate total a day the first week or two, which is not that unusual, see if you can make short-term goals, such as an increase of 15 grams carbohydrate/day within the next week or so. Continue to work on this until you eventually get to the 130 grams carbohydrate goal, which may take you several months or even a year to reach. Working with your surgical center's registered dietitian can give you the help and support you need to maximize your nutrition after surgery.

Fiber: Make It Your Friend

Fiber is a form of carbohydrate found in fruits, vegetables, and whole grains that can provide many health benefits, including lowering your risk for developing certain kinds of cancer, among other diseases, and of course, keeping you regular by lowering your risk for constipation or diarrhea.

The American Dietetic Association recommends a daily intake of 25 to 30 grams fiber for optimal health. Don't shoot for that amount right after your weight loss surgery, though. That's a goal better suited for a few months, if not longer, post-op.

If you have issues with constipation, increasing your fiber a bit can help, but remember to increase it gradually and accompany it with plenty of water to help your body eliminate it. Otherwise, you might feel bloated and uncomfortable. (More about fluids in Chapter 5.)

Fiber contains a type of chemistry, called a beta glucan linkage for you chemists out there, your body can't absorb, so fiber can be your weight loss friend. Not only is fiber calorie free, but it can also help you feel fuller longer as it causes your stomach to empty slower.

There are two kinds of fiber, soluble and insoluble, and each has different benefits that can help you maintain a healthy body and lifestyle after your weight loss surgery. Let's examine each.

> **Food for Thought**
>
> A Harvard study of more than 40,000 male physicians revealed that high fiber intake lowered heart disease by 40 percent. A related Harvard study of female nurses revealed similar results.

If you have an apple handy, slice it and put the peel in a glass of water. The peel doesn't dissolve in the water, so that's an insoluble fiber. Insoluble fiber, including bran and the peels and skins of fruits and vegetables, goes through your gastrointestinal (GI) tract quickly and helps alleviate constipation. (If you have diarrhea, however, you'll want to hold off on the insoluble fiber because it could worsen your situation and possibly lead to low levels of potassium and other electrolytes.)

Let's get back to that apple. After you've peeled it, place the pulp in a glass of water and you'll see it eventually dissolve. This is an example of soluble fiber. This kind of fiber, which includes oatmeal, applesauce, rice, and bananas, moves through your GI tract more slowly than the insoluble kind and picks up cholesterol and bile salts and helps your body get rid of excess fat and cholesterol. It may also help bind your stools if you have diarrhea.

The Glycemic Index

Maybe you've heard or read about the glycemic index (GI), and maybe you're also aware of reports that foods like carrots and tomatoes may not be a good idea because they produce too much of a sugar response. It's important to look at the health benefits of the foods in question as well as such reports about them.

While the GI does rate blood sugar response to foods, keep in mind that most people don't eat one food at a time or foods in the amounts that were tested in these glycemic index studies. Let's take a closer look at this thing called GI, shall we?

What Is GI, and What Does It Have to Do with Me?

The glycemic index is a ranking of carbohydrates on a scale from 0 to 100 according to the extent to which they raise blood sugar levels after they're eaten. Foods (and beverages) are considered "low-GI" if they're under 55 on the glycemic index scale. Foods with a GI between 55 and 70 are "medium-GI," and foods with a GI greater than 70 are typically classified as "high-GI" foods.

Low-GI foods, by virtue of their slow digestion and absorption, produce gradual rises in blood sugar and insulin levels and have proven health benefits. Low-GI diets have been shown to improve both glucose and cholesterol levels in people with Type 1 and Type 2 diabetes. They also have weight control benefits because they help control appetite and delay hunger. Low-GI diets reduce insulin levels and insulin resistance.

Foods with a high GI are rapidly digested and absorbed and result in marked fluctuations in blood sugar levels. High-GI foods are discouraged in some diet plans because they can raise blood sugar and insulin levels significantly and may also increase hunger and sugar cravings.

In 1999, the World Health Organization (WHO) and Food and Agriculture Organization (FAO) recommended that people in industrialized countries base their diets on low-GI foods to prevent such common and devastating diseases such as heart disease, diabetes, and obesity.

> **Food for Thought**
>
> Recent studies from Harvard School of Public Health indicate that the risks for Type 2 diabetes and heart disease are strongly related to the GI of the overall diet. Research shows a 50 percent decrease in risk of diabetes found among diets rich in cereal grains and a high percentage of low-GI foods.

Low-, Medium-, and High-GI Foods

Some diets have placed a large emphasis on low-GI foods as a way of giving the green light to carbs and helping avoid carb deprivation while helping blood sugar control. Therefore, some health experts tout low-GI foods as the "right" carbohydrates to include in your diet. Recent studies and expert consensus do seem to suggest that low-GI foods have merit and can be particularly helpful not only with patients with diabetes or insulin resistance, but also anyone working on their weight because a lower blood sugar response seems to help deter sugar cravings and hunger.

Here are some examples of low-, medium-, and high-GI foods:

Low-GI foods (<55):

- *Fruits:* apples, cherries, grapefruit, grapes, kiwi, mango, peaches, pears, plums
- *Vegetables:* artichokes, asparagus, bell peppers, broccoli, brussels sprouts, cabbage, celery, mushrooms
- *Legumes:* black beans, garbanzo beans, kidney beans, navy beans
- *Grains:* barley, brown beans, cereals with barley or bulgur, pumpernickel bread, sourdough bread, stone-ground whole-wheat bread, whole-wheat spaghetti
- *Dairy:* skim or 1 percent milk; plain, nonfat, or low-fat yogurt
- *Soy:* soy milk, soybeans

Medium-GI foods (55 to 70):

- *Fruits:* apricots, bananas, papaya, pineapple, raisins
- *Vegetables:* beets, corn
- *Grains:* brown rice, couscous, deli rye bread, light popcorn, oatmeal, thin linguini pasta, white potatoes (boiled), whole-wheat bread (or whole-wheat pita bread)
- *Dairy:* ice cream (full-fat, regular ice cream)

High-GI foods (>70):

- *Fruits:* dried dates, watermelon
- *Vegetables:* carrots, parsnips
- *Legumes:* fava beans

- *Grains:* dark rye bread, graham crackers, instant white rice, plain bagels, pretzels, rice cakes, saltine-type crackers, some commercial cereals (e.g., bran flakes, corn flakes, raisin bran), vanilla wafers

- *Soy:* frozen tofu desserts

Of course, for each of the GI groups, serving size is important, so check with your dietitian for optimal serving sizes individualized for your needs and procedure.

Wrapping Up the Glycemic Index

This is not an all-encompassing look at the glycemic index, but rather a quick glimpse at what could be a good dietary tool, particularly if your doctor and dietitian have encouraged you to include foods that cause less of an increase in your blood sugar. Some foods may have different GI scores, even within the same food (e.g., an over-ripe, medium banana has a high GI of 82 while a medium banana that's not overripe has a medium GI of about 55).

Also, keep in mind that the glycemic index is only a tool and shouldn't divert you away from healthful foods, like particular fruits and vegetables, just because they might not fall into the low-GI category. We typically eat more than one food at a time, and foods with protein and fat tend to lower the total glycemic index of a meal or snack, so GI numbers are not absolute. There are many great resources available to learn more on this subject (see Appendix B).

The Skinny on Sugar Substitutes

Sugar substitutes have come a long way since they came out many years ago, but they're still not without controversy. What's the scoop on the ones available today, and are they safe?

What Are They Exactly?

Sugar substitutes, also called artificial sweeteners or non-nutritive sweeteners, are compounds that contain the sweetness of sucrose (table sugar), but have a small fraction of the calories or no calories at all. Given that the average American consumes the equivalent of 50 packets of sugar a day, with 16 calories each packet, you can see the potential difference in caloric intake by switching to noncaloric sweeteners.

Sugar substitutes also may help with diabetes or controlling your blood sugar and could potentially help you get off your diabetes medication after your weight loss surgery.

The Sugar Substitutes Available Today

Artificial sweeteners have been around in the United States since the 1950s. While popularity of these sweeteners really waned in the 1970s when cancer connections were found, they've regained their popularity in recent years. However, a good deal of controversy continues to surround these sweeteners, with some speculation that they may not be safe. Despite these fears, many scientists believe the U.S. Food and Drug Administration–approved non-nutritive sweeteners are safe. In the United States, approved artificial sweeteners typically fall under the generally recognized as safe (GRAS) list. Items found on the GRAS list have been defined by the FDA as any substance that's intentionally added to food as a food additive.

> **Cooking Tip**
>
> Sugar substitutes are 30 to 8,000 times sweeter than table sugar so they might help you keep your caloric intake and weight down because you're consuming far fewer calories versus sugar or caloric sweeteners.

These are the six FDA-approved artificial sweeteners:

- Acesulfame potassium
- Aspartame
- Neotame
- Saccharin
- Stevia
- Sucralose

Acesulfame potassium (or "ace-K") was approved as an artificial sweetener in 1988, but although it's commonly found in many foods and beverages in the United States, many Americans aren't familiar with it. Look for it on ingredient labels as acesulfame K or perhaps as ace-K, acesulfame potassium, or Sunett.

Aspartame, also known as NutraSweet and Equal, was FDA approved for limited use (e.g., in breakfast cereals, gelatins, puddings, and chewing gum) in 1981. In 1996, the FDA approved it as a "general purpose sweetener." It's now present in approximately 6,000 foods. It's 160 to 220 times sweeter than table sugar, and it does provide calories, but in very small amounts. The FDA has set the acceptable daily intake (ADI) for aspartame at 50 milligrams/kilograms (mg/kg) body weight, which is usually far more than the average adult American could reasonably consume.

Neotame was approved by the FDA in 2002 as a new take on aspartame. It's chemically related to aspartame, but it doesn't contain phenylalanine, so it's not a potential danger for people with the genetic disease phenylketonuria (PKU). Neotame is much sweeter than aspartame—7,000 to 13,000 times sweeter than table sugar. The ADI has been set at 18 mg/kg body weight. While neotame's website claims that 100 scientific studies have supported that it's safe to consume, those studies have not looked at potential long-term ramifications of its use.

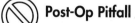 **Post-Op Pitfall** _____

People with the genetic disease phenylketonuria, who cannot metabolize phenylalanine (an amino acid/building block of protein that's a key ingredient in aspartame), should avoid aspartame.

Saccharin, probably best known in the United States as Sweet'N Low, contains zero calories and is 200 to 700 times sweeter than table sugar. Saccharin is generally believed to be the safest of the 5 approved artificial sweeteners, although if you were around in the 1970s, you might remember the research showing saccharin caused tumors in rats. Since then, more than 30 studies on humans have shown that saccharin is safe. The ADI for saccharin is 5 mg/kg of body weight, so most adults consume well under this limit.

Stevia is a new sweetener that's garnered a lot of attention in the United States lately because it's truly natural, originating from herbs and shrubs in the sunflower family native to South America and Central America. Although natives of Paraguay and Brazil have been using stevia for centuries, it's the new kid on the block in the United States, and until recently, the FDA only approved it as a dietary supplement. However, the FDA reversed its position, and this non-nutritive sweetener is now popping up on shelves everywhere, including sugar-free candies and diet beverages. Stevia was approved as a sugar substitute in December 2008, where it was classified in the GRAS category, along with the other sweeteners cited in this section.

Stevia's popularity may stem from the fact that although it's about 300 times sweeter than table sugar, it has a slower onset and longer duration, while having a negligible effect on blood sugar. This may be especially attractive to people with diabetes or anyone encouraged to watch sugar, such as people who have had weight loss surgery.

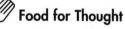 **Food for Thought** _____

The Japanese have been using stevia for more than 30 years without any reports of sensitivity or allergies.

Recently, two new stevia-based sweeteners were granted GRAS status, and because they were developed by two major food companies, expect to see stevia products everywhere in the future. The new stevia-based sweeteners are a mixture of the purified plant extract and other sweeteners, such as erythritol (a sugar alcohol), which helps reduce the sweetness and licorice-type taste in stevia some people might not like.

Sucralose, also known as Splenda, is the newest artificial sweetener to receive FDA approval. The makers of Splenda claim it's made from table sugar, and it's often touted as the most "natural" of artificial sweeteners, although it's not the same as sugar. It's about 600 times sweeter than table sugar, provides virtually no calories, and is so popular it's now found in almost 5,000 foods that are cooked or baked. The ADI is 5 mg/kg body weight.

The Nutritive Sweeteners

Nutritive sweeteners—agave, fructose, and sugar alcohols—are different from non-nutritive sweeteners or artificial sweeteners because they contain calories. However, in moderation, they may be a good alternative to artificial sweeteners, especially if you have sensitivity to artificial sweeteners or prefer more natural sweeteners.

Agave (pronounced *ah-GAH-vay*) may be known to some as the plant from which tequila is made. However, you may not know that agave has been an ingredient in foods for thousands of years. *Honey water* is the term for the nectar (also called agave syrup) that comes from the agave plant, which looks kind of like a cactus plant and originates in Mexico. Recently, some top U.S. doctors have noted agave as a preferable form of sweetener because of the fact it's more natural.

Agave syrup is most frequently made from the blue agaves found in southern Mexico among the volcanic soils. The plant has to grow for at least 7 to 10 years before the core of the plant, which looks like a pineapple, can be cut. The sap extracted from the agave is filtered and heated at a low temperature. The result is syrup that's mostly fructose.

Many people find that agave syrup tastes like honey, although not identical. Because agave syrup is concentrated, it's not low in calories—1 teaspoon provides 21 calories (versus 16 calories in 1 teaspoon table sugar). However, it has a sweet taste to it, so you might use less than table sugar. It also has a low glycemic index, so a lower blood sugar response may mean you're less hungry or less likely to crave carbs. It's just one of the alternatives, and the extra 5 grams sugars per teaspoon should be counted in your diet, particularly if you had gastric bypass and are prone to dumping.

Fructose, also known as levulose, is a monosaccharide, or simple sugar, found in many fruits and some vegetables. It is one of three monosaccharides in our diet. (The other two are glucose and galactose.) In nature, fructose is usually found in combination with glucose in the form of sucrose (a.k.a. table sugar). Fructose is also created from the digestion of sucrose and high-fructose corn syrup (HFCS).

Crystalline fructose and HFCS are typically thought of as the same thing, but they're not. HFCS results in an approximate 50/50 mixture of fructose and glucose, while crystalline fructose ends up being about 90 percent fructose. HFCS may be genetically modified, and some health experts link increased HFCS to the burgeoning problem of higher weight and obesity in the United States. Many health experts consider fructose as a sweetener (and particularly found naturally in foods) preferable over HFCS. It's important to realize both fructose and HFCS contain calories … about 16 calories per teaspoon, so it really adds up.

Sugar alcohols (or *polyols*) contain fewer calories than sugar (about 2 calories per gram [or about 8 calories per teaspoon] versus 4 calories per gram in table sugar). Despite the name, this sweetener is not an alcohol but rather a carbohydrate. Its molecule structure looks like both a sugar and an alcohol. Sugar alcohols are mainly found in low-sugar foods and items like sugar-free hard candies and gums. To identify sugar alcohols on food labels, look for words that end in -*ol*, such as *sorbitol*, *mannitol*, and *erythritol*. Sugar alcohols can be marketed as "sugar free" because they essentially take the place of full-calorie sugar sweeteners. The sweetness of sugar alcohols varies from 25 to 100 percent the sweetness of table sugar, but they don't promote tooth decay—one reason they may be in your toothpaste. Also, like agave, sugar alcohols have a low GI.

> **Food for Thought** _____
>
> Sorbitol is found naturally in fruits and vegetables. It's manufactured from corn syrup but has only 50 percent of the relative sweetness of sugar, which means twice as much must be used to deliver a similar amount of sweetness.

Unfortunately, as with almost anything, sugar alcohols come with some potential negatives. The most common side effect is abdominal bloating and diarrhea. Sugar alcohols first came on the scene in health care as *sorbitol*, used primarily as a laxative. Sugar alcohols form short chain fatty acids (SCFAs) that serve as food for the "bugs" in your colon, the end result typically being gas, bloating, and sometimes diarrhea. (So don't try sugar alcohols for the first time when you're traveling or dining out.)

The American Diabetes Association claims sugar alcohols are acceptable in a moderate amount but should be avoided in excess. Go easy on sugar alcohols overall due to possible gastrointestinal complaints, as well as the fact that your body can absorb about half of these calories—especially important to keep in mind if you have diabetes or are finding your weight inching upward.

Nutritive and non-nutritive sweeteners may have a place in a balanced and health-ful meal plan, particularly if used in moderation and in place of simple sugars. Some sweeteners, particularly non-nutritive varieties, are not without controversy and may cause sensitivities or other issues. It's important to do your research and listen to your body. If you feel ill or think a sweetener doesn't agree with you and might be causing you to gain weight, avoid it.

The Least You Need to Know

- ◆ Carbohydrates are essential for energy. Choose complex carbohydrates over processed, simple carbs for the most bang for your carb buck.

- ◆ By paying attention to a food's glycemic index, you can lower your blood sugar response to foods.

- ◆ There are two kinds of fiber, soluble and insoluble, which could help you with cholesterol and being regular, in that order.

- ◆ Nutritive and non-nutritive sweeteners are generally considered safe and could help with your weight loss efforts.

Chapter 3

Protein Power!

In This Chapter

- The importance of protein, especially after weight loss surgery
- The different kinds of protein
- Protein needs for your particular surgery
- Evaluating protein supplements

You've probably heard a lot about protein at your surgical center, and maybe you've read studies that indicate you might be at risk for protein deficiency after your procedure. Western culture has embraced protein to the point that American protein consumption is among the highest in the world. As a matter of fact, many Americans consume more than twice the amount of protein they need every day.

However, after weight loss surgery, particularly malabsorptive surgery like the D/S, you may find it difficult to get in all the protein you need. Even if you manage to get a lot of protein, you want to be sure you're getting high-quality protein your body can easily use and that your overall diet is balanced and complete. In this chapter, we show you how.

It's Not Just for Muscles!

The root origin of the word *protein* is *proteos*, which means "prime importance" or "taking the first place." And what more appropriate time for protein to take prime importance than after weight loss surgery?

Protein is a functionally active component of the human body found in the skeletal muscles, skin, blood, liver, kidneys, lungs, heart, and bones. In adults, 43 percent of the body's protein is in skeletal muscle, 15 percent in skin and blood, 10 percent in the liver and kidneys, and 32 percent in other organs.

Protein isn't stored the same way carbohydrates or fats are (see Chapter 2), but your body does maintain a reserve of it to help you sustain physiological functions—like the stress your body goes through during and soon after weight loss surgery, for example. No matter what kind of weight loss surgery you had, protein should be an important part of your daily meal plan.

Protein is linked with all forms of plant and animal life, and the molecular structure and activity of living cells depend on it. It is the major structural component of all cells in your body, making up over half of the solid content of cells. Proteins also function as enzymes (e.g., in chemical reactions), in membranes, and as transport carriers and hormones.

That's a lot of work for one component to do, so you want to be sure you're getting enough protein after your weight loss surgery so all the bases are covered.

Not All Protein Is Created Equal

Many years ago, while I was a freshman at the University of Rhode Island and studying basic nutrition, I was introduced to the concept of high and low *biological value* (*BV*) protein. I think it's important to discuss both here, especially because one kind is obviously much different from the other, and you want to be able to spot high- versus low-quality protein, especially after your weight loss surgery.

def•i•ni•tion

Biological value (BV) is a summary of the proportion of the protein your body absorbs from food. It's determined by a test that measures nitrogen, a product of protein metabolism in your body.

Back then, eggs had a BV score of 100 and were deemed perfect in protein terms. These days, however, they've been relegated to a mere 93.7 by some sources because whey protein has been discovered to have the highest-known BV around. Despite this, eggs are generally still considered a good source of

protein. However, if you have any cholesterol and/or fat restrictions, the egg white is
where you'll find the wonderful, high-
quality protein without the fat and cholesterol of the yolk. Egg whites are also low
in calories. Just be sure you cook them to
avoid the risk of salmonella and/or binding of certain vitamins. For example, if you
eat a raw egg, not only could you get food
poisoning, but biotin, a B vitamin, could
be bound by a substance called avidin, so
you might be at risk for biotin deficiency.
Bottom line: try to avoid eating raw eggs.

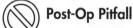 **Post-Op Pitfall**

Raw egg whites contain a
substance called avidin, which
binds to biotin, an important B
vitamin. A biotin deficiency can
lead to alopecia, or hair loss.
Hair loss is often observed after
bariatric surgery, typically related
to the stress of significant and/
or rapid weight loss, so avoid
anything that may exacerbate this
condition.

High biological value (HBV) protein is the gold standard of protein, meaning all the
amino acids or building blocks are present so your body can better utilize it—which is
especially important after surgery. Examples of HBV protein foods include eggs, whey
and casein protein (found in dairy products), meat, poultry, fish, and soy products like
soy protein and tofu. The highest score a protein can receive in this grading process is
100. The score's based not only on the presence of what are called *indispensable amino
acids* (building blocks of protein your body cannot make and must receive through the
diet) but also the amounts of each of the amino acids.

There are nine indispensable amino acids (previously called essential amino acids):
histidine, isoleucine, leucine, lysine, methionine, phenylalanine, threonine, tryptophan, and valine. Three of these—leucine, isoleucine, and valine—are called branched
chain amino acids and are considered especially important during times your body is
under physical stress because they allow your body to better utilize protein and heal
more quickly and efficiently. This certainly is important after weight loss surgery.

Think of these amino acids like actors in a play. When one is down in terms of
amount or function, the show may go on, but it might not be as well received. In a
way, this happens in your body, too. You may be taking in what you think is enough
protein, but maybe it's not the highest-quality protein because some of the important
amino acids are either missing or are in smaller amounts than necessary.

Low biological value (LBV) proteins are found in plants, legumes, seeds, nuts, and
vegetables. (The exception is the soybean, which is relatively HBV.) They're considered LBV because some of the indispensible amino acids or building blocks of protein
are either missing or too low to make the food a complete protein. However, as any
vegetarian reading this most likely knows, you can "complement" two LBV sources

to make them HBV by combining two protein sources to provide all the necessary or indispensable amino acids. For example, rice and beans alone are LBV protein sources. But together, this combination provides all the amino acids you need. It's no wonder this combination is a staple among many cultures!

Making the Grade

After the BV test, the second best method of assessing protein quality is the *protein digestibility corrected amino acid score* (PDCAAS). The PDCAAS first came on the scene in 1991 to evaluate protein quality and has been deemed a superior way to assess protein quality. It's similar to the BV in that protein quality is decreased significantly if amino acids or building blocks of protein are missing.

The PDCAAS compares the nine indispensable amino acids to the estimated average requirement (EAR), a reference value for the indispensible amino acids established by the Institute of Medicine. The EAR essentially is comparable to the least amount of each amino acid needed to make the protein complete and usable by your body. The PDCAAS score is a very helpful and accurate tool to assess protein supplement quality because it reveals the limiting amino acid and also predicts your body's capability to absorb and use that supplement to make protein. The PDCAAS for whey, milk, casein, egg whites, and soy is 100, which is a perfect score. However, not every type of protein earns this high a grade, and some downright fail, as is the case with collagen, which we discuss in a later section.

BV and PDCAAS are the two most accurate methods of assessing protein quality in your diet. With these, you now have two of the best tools for assessing protein quality and absorption in your diet and in your body. It's especially important to know about and utilize this information immediately after your weight loss surgery, when your protein needs are typically at their highest.

If you'd like to find out more about the BV and PDCAAS, a few resources include www.nal.gov, where you can enter foods high in protein and it will tell you how good the quality is. Also, the registered dietitian at your surgical center is another good source of information on this. Finally, Mary Lichford, Ph.D., R.D., wrote a book called *Protein Potions, Powders and Elixors*, available on her website, www.casesoftware. com, offers a very in-depth study of protein sources and quality protein products.

Assessing Your Protein Status

Meeting your protein needs after weight loss surgery is one of the most important goals in meeting your overall nutritional needs. The goal is to maintain a steady state of protein synthesis equal to the rate at which your protein stores break down. When your diet is low or inadequate in indispensable amino acids, the balance between rates of protein synthesis of some proteins could decrease significantly. If you find your diet sorely lacking in protein after your weight loss surgery, and you're eating low-quality protein (more about this coming up), you could be at risk for developing protein malnutrition.

 Post-Op Pitfall

Long-term protein deficiency may result in significant health issues, including lower-leg swelling due to lack of a certain kind of pressure from protein that helps move fluids around.

If your diet goes unchecked, you could even be at risk for potentially serious conditions, such as congestive heart failure from your body's inability to move fluid that could build up around your heart. In addition, the presence of infection, injury, or the physical stress of surgery could increase your protein needs further. It's critical, then, that the protein you consume be the highest quality possible.

Suggested protein goals for various weight loss procedures have been established and published as guidelines for bariatric surgery patients. (In fact, Margaret was privileged to be part of such a published committee. Find the paper in the September 2008 *SOARD* supplement, a publication of the American Society for Metabolic and Bariatric Surgery at www.asmbs.org/Newsite07/resources/bgs_final.pdf.) There's always more research to be done, but nutritional guidelines, including protein, have been suggested based on the current research and expert opinion and consensus.

But no two people are exactly alike or have the same nutritional needs, so it's important to adjust your protein needs specifically to your body. For example, a gastric bypass patient who is tall with a great deal of muscle mass and is working out with weights three times a week requires more protein than a smaller person with little muscle mass who is not doing any structured physical activity. Protein needs may vary among men and women as well, among other variables.

Methods of assessing protein in your body and whether your protein intake is appropriate include several laboratory tests, particularly for prealbumin and albumin. Albumin is a more common protein test and aside from changing status with fluid shifts (e.g., if you have a lot of fluid retention it can be falsely low and falsely high with dehydration), tells you what your protein status has been within the last 3 weeks. Albumin is a major transport protein in your body that helps move fluids from your feet and legs back up through your body and is a general marker of nutritional status.

However, if you're dehydrated, it could look like your nutrition is okay but you might be low in protein. It also tells you what your nutrition was like about 3 weeks prior to the test, so not as good a protein marker as prealbumin. Prealbumin is a protein marker which is *not* changed with dehydration, and tells you what your nutrition was like 2 or 3 days ago, so better for checking your current nutrition than albumin. At some centers, the prealbumin is more commonly checked versus the albumin for this reason, although some centers may not have access to the prealbumin lab, especially if insurance doesn't pay for prealbumin.

> **Food for Thought** _____
>
> Prealbumin has a short half life, meaning it can tell you what your protein status has been like within the past 2 or 3 days, and is not changeable with fluid shifts, unlike albumin.

If your prealbumin is low, a nutrition visit may be warranted, even if it's not within your usual post-op nutrition visit schedule. Your dietitian will most likely want to take a careful, detailed history of your diet, including protein supplements. In addition, they can help be sure the quality as well as the quantity of protein intake in your diet is optimal.

Unfortunately, both of these protein-status indicators may be unreliable if or when there's a high degree of inflammation in your body (see Chapter 4). Therefore, right after your surgery, when fighting acute infection, and when you are experiencing swelling in your extremities, values of albumin and prealbumin may not accurately reflect protein status in your body. A lab test for an inflammatory reactant called C-reactive protein may help determine the level of inflammation in your body. It's important to check C-reactive protein because if it's high, it could mean you have a higher risk for heart disease. In addition a high level could mean that your body is under a lot of stress and, therefore, may not be able to use all of the nutrition, including protein, you're taking in during the early post-op period. The prealbumin and albumin are more specific for protein markers versus C-reactive protein as a marker for general inflammation in your body.

Protein Recommendations After Surgery

Weight loss surgery experts recommend approximately 70 grams protein per day during periods of significant caloric restriction, as is often the case in the early post-op period. Due to higher protein needs after weight loss surgery, the recommended daily allowance (RDA) of 50 grams protein per day doesn't appear sufficient.

While some surgical programs assess protein needs in reference to your ideal body weight, quite a few other programs, including Margaret's, generally recommend 60 to 80 grams protein per day. Of course, everyone's an individual, so if you have a lot of muscle mass and/or are very tall or dealing with a wound infection (which happens in some patients after open gastric bypass surgery), your protein needs, at least initially, may be higher than this, perhaps approaching 100 grams per day.

Although protein malnutrition doesn't occur very frequently after gastric bypass, we certainly have seen some gastric bypass surgery patients with mild protein depletion, typically because they were taking inferior-quality protein supplements without realizing it (more on that coming up). It's imperative to keep regular appointments with your health-care team, including your dietitian, to help ensure you're taking in not only enough protein, but the highest quality possible so your body can truly use it.

How are you going to get all that protein during the early post-op period when you might not feel like eating? Try high-quality protein drinks and supplements (see the following "Protein Powders and Supplements" section) in at least three doses. Shoot for only 20 to 35 grams protein at a time, especially in the beginning, because too much protein at once, even in the form of protein drinks, can be dehydrating.

Also, don't force down a 60-gram protein drink, even if it's high-quality, to "get it over with." When the hunger hormones—or real hunger—come back after your surgery, you're more likely to overeat and get into a bad habit of eating fewer than 3 meals per day. Therefore, even if the last thing you want to do is think about protein, aim for 3 servings of 20 to 35 grams protein (typically in a high-protein drink the first several weeks post-op) no more than 5 hours apart to help meet your body's protein needs. This gets you in a 3-meals-a-day habit and can help curb hunger.

Don't neglect carbohydrates though. They're your body's chief form of energy, but they also help spare protein. If your body isn't getting enough carbohydrates, it will most likely start breaking down muscle tissue or using the protein calories for energy and not for repair and healing. *Gluconeogenesis* will most certainly be the result.

def•i•ni•tion

Gluconeogenesis means your body is making new glucose from nonglucose sources. This is not a good thing, generally, because your body won't be able to use protein you take in for your muscles and healing because it's busy making glucose for your brain. Bottom line: your protein labs (e.g., prealbumin) could be low, even if you're taking in a lot of protein, because it's not going where it's supposed to be going because your brain needs glucose.

The D/S is the only truly malabsorptive surgery of the ones discussed in this book, and estimates of protein malabsorption range from 20 to 40 percent, with the average estimated loss at about 25 percent. Therefore, it's important to aim for an even higher protein level after surgery. The average protein requirement for D/S patients is estimated at about 90 grams per day, which allows for the approximate increased need of 30 percent that results from the malabsorptive component of this procedure. Often you'll see D/S recommendations range from 80 to 120 grams protein per day, with the higher end of the range reserved for patients with larger muscle mass or perhaps increased stress after surgery. Of course, if you're several months out and doing a lot of weight or resistance training, your protein needs could be higher as well.

> **Food for Thought**
>
> Some scientific resources suggest that a total of 100 grams carbohydrate a day may lower your chance of muscle breakdown for glucose needs by as much as 40 percent, so you'll want to slowly increase your carbohydrate intake to at least 100 grams a day to help spare protein or be sure it's going to your muscles and not being used to make glucose.

It's very important to ensure your diet after D/S is balanced and includes sufficient carbohydrates (see Chapter 2) to meet your body's needs and help spare your protein. Many free online logs can do all the work of tallying your protein, as well as carbohydrates and other nutrients, so it doesn't have to be a full-time job for you (see Appendix B).

Protein Powders and Supplements

As you know, HBV protein in your diet includes eggs, meat, poultry, fish, dairy products, and tofu. However, it's very difficult for a lot of patients after weight loss surgery, even after a few months, to meet their protein needs with diet alone. That's where protein bars, powders, and drinks can fill the protein gap. Like everything else, big variations exist in quality of these products, and in the following paragraphs, we use some of the HBV information as well as the PDCAAS to help you assess the quality of these products.

The Grade-A Supplements

Whenever possible, opt for whey protein isolate over whey protein concentrate. The isolate version is a bit more expensive, but you get what you pay for. It's a higher-quality protein and doesn't contain lactose, like the concentrate does. This can be a big issue if you happen to develop lactose intolerance after surgery, especially gastric bypass surgery.

In general, all the protein powders mentioned in this section can mix well into water, diluted (50/50) juice, low-sugar drinks, and skim or 1 percent milk or soy milk, although some manufacturers strongly recommend either a blender or shaker bottle to help the protein dissolve fully. We've tried many different protein powders, and some mix well with just a spoon, while others really do need a blender or mixer. Also, protein bars are sometimes dry, but they're okay, especially if whey or protein isolate mostly, particularly if it's nothing versus a protein bar.

> **Food for Thought** _____
>
> Whey protein received the highest PDCAAS of all protein types because it contains high levels of branched chain amino acids (leucine, isoleucine, and valine), which are especially in high demand when your body is under physical stress.

If you were lactose intolerant before your surgery, definitely go with the whey protein isolate. Or you can purchase lactase enzyme pills to help your body digest lactose, or milk sugar.

Another high-quality protein is soy isolate, and this is ideal, of course, if you're vegan and/or have allergies to milk-based protein. Some great protein supplements, including some protein bars, have soy protein isolate as the first ingredient. (See Chapter 7 for more on ingredient lists and reading food labels.)

If you have both milk and soy allergies, a high-quality version of rice protein may be appropriate. However, you want to be sure it's been supplemented correctly because by nature, untreated rice protein is LBV, so it's missing some key amino acids.

Egg white protein is a good choice if you don't have egg allergies and want to avoid milk or soy products. It also mixes well and typically has no taste, although we've yet to find a protein bar with this protein. Most have milk or soy-based protein.

Supplement Failures

Collagen-based protein powders are *not* high quality, in general, unless a high-quality protein powder like whey protein isolate has been added. Collagen is missing tryptophan, an indispensible amino acid, and is also low in three other amino acids, so your body may only absorb anywhere from 16 to 50 percent of a collagen-based protein. Think of protein like a rope. If you have a thick, sturdy rope but it's weak in one area, the whole rope could break, so it's only as good as its weakest area.

We've seen post-op gastric bypass patients who were given collagen-based protein powders as a gift and used them primarily in the first few months post-op for protein.

Food for Thought

Most commercial protein supplements contain a mixture of protein sources, such as whey protein isolate and whey protein concentrate. Whey protein isolate is higher quality and has filtered-out lactose; whey protein concentrate has slightly lower quality and contains lactose.

Although the powders all had protein totals over 100 grams, which should have been more than their body needed, they all were low in protein, according to the low prealbumin levels in their blood work. This corroborates what the PDCAAS states regarding collagen—mainly that it's not absorbed or utilized well by your body due to an incomplete amino acid profile.

Stop the collagen products and switch to a high-quality protein product like whey or soy protein isolate. Whey and soy concentrates are okay, too, but keep in mind that whey concentrates contain lactose, and that may be an issue for you pre-op, as well as post-op, with surgeries like gastric bypass and D/S.

Protein, without a doubt, is absolutely essential to your long-term health and weight loss success. However, not all proteins are alike, and they can vary greatly with respect to quality and your body's ability to utilize them. Keeping the BV and PDCAAS in mind may help you better assess protein quality, both in whole foods and supplements, and allow you to make higher-quality protein choices for life-long good health. Also, more is not necessarily better, in terms of protein. For example, some gastric bypass patients say they're taking in more than 150 grams protein, or we see it in their food records. In general, most people can't use more than about 100 grams protein a day (120 grams a day for D/S), and extra protein is extra calories, and may also be dehydrating and taxing on your kidneys, particularly if you already have kidney challenges.

The Least You Need to Know

- Protein is vital for optimal healing and health after weight loss surgery.

- Your protein needs after your surgery may vary from about 60 to 120 grams per day, depending on your procedure.

- The biological value (BV) and PDCAA score are two accurate and valid ways of assessing protein quality and absorption.

- Protein supplements vary in terms of quality, but in general avoid those with collagen because your body can't use these as well.

Chapter 4

Fat Phobia

In This Chapter

- Healthful versus unhealthful fats
- The essential fats
- Fish oils and the omega family
- The post-op fat suggestions

Everyone needs some fat in his or her diet, especially after weight loss surgery. For example, your body couldn't absorb the fat-soluble vitamins A, D, E, and K without some fat in your diet. And your body couldn't sufficiently produce many hormones, including sex hormones like estrogen and testosterone, without fats. But for weight loss success, you need to have fats in the right amount and proportion. In this chapter, we introduce you to the different kinds of fats and share which ones best help you win the weight loss battle—for good.

All About Fats

It can be confusing trying to figure out which fats are the healthiest. In the next several pages, the difference between the kinds of fats you should eat, and the kinds you should avoid, will make sense. Not only that, but you'll soon find yourself differentiating between the "villain" fats and the "twisted villain" fats, as well as the "hero" fats, the good fats that help keep your heart and weight as healthy as possible.

The Villain, the Twisted Villain, and the Hero

Good fats, bad fats, villain fats—what's the difference? Plenty! Bad fats are like bad people: rigid and troublemakers! Bad fats are called saturated fats because they're saturated molecules, which makes them rigid at room temperature. This rigidity causes the molecule to have adverse health effects in your body. Another villain in the story, called trans fat, is a saturated fat with a twist—literally! This twisted villain is also blamed for wreaking havoc on the body and is implicated in conditions such as heart disease and type 2 diabetes.

The three types of fats that have influenced health the most are the saturated fats (including trans fats, which are also known as "villains" of sorts), the monounsaturated fats, and the polyunsaturated fats (the heroes).

Saturated and Trans Fats

When fats are saturated with hydrogen molecules, they're called saturated fats—these are the villain fats. Saturated fats, which are typically hard at room temperature, are created by a process called hydrogenation, which takes the fat from a liquid to a solid. Saturated fats, including trans fats, have unhealthy effects on your body. They increase total cholesterol and LDL cholesterol (low-density lipoproteins—the bad guys) and have been linked with higher risks of heart disease, among other things. The least-healthful fats around, saturated fats include animal fats, like butter or grease from cooked bacon.

Trans fats, the twisted villains, are the result of hydrogenation of liquid oils and were created to increase the shelf life of packaged foods as well as help foods withstand the stress of the food production process. Unfortunately, they've been found to stress our hearts, too. Trans fats are so bad for you—they're the fats most linked to increased heart disease risk—that it's recommended you avoid them in your diet altogether. According to a 2007 review in the *New England Journal of Medicine*, if trans fats make up even 1 or 2 percent of the fat in your diet, your risk of heart disease could be significantly increased. Examples of foods that contain trans fats include doughnuts, fried chicken, and french fries. You can fry your own foods in healthier oils, such as canola oil, but watch the high-calorie content, as all oils have the same calories—9 calories per gram, or about 45 calories per teaspoon.

Monounsaturated Fats—the True Heroes

A diet rich in monounsaturated fatty acids (MUFAs)—those fats that have one double bond between two carbons—has been shown to decrease total and LDL cholesterol but has not shown to have any adverse effects on high-density lipoproteins (HDL cholesterol), the good cholesterol. These fats may be considered "heroes" of sorts because they can help keep your body healthy. The Mediterranean diet, rich in good-for-you olive oil, has increased in popularity thanks to its positive effects on blood lipids and heart health. Studies have shown that diets rich in MUFAs were as effective as diets rich in polyunsaturated fatty acids (PUFAs) in lowering the bad guys (LDL), without significant changes in the good guys (HDL). Olive oil is a popular source of monounsaturated fat; other sources include macadamia nut oil, peanut oil, and avocados.

Monounsaturated fats are among the most heart-healthy fats and should be included in your diet as part of a balanced meal plan. Diets rich in MUFAs as well as polyunsaturated fatty acids (PUFAs; more on these coming right up) can decrease your cholesterol level and may improve *insulin sensitivity*. With improved insulin sensitivity, glucose regulation can improve, a condition called glucose homeostasis. Recent studies have shown that improvement in glucose homeostasis decreases the risk of conditions like prediabetes (also known as insulin resistance) and diabetes.

def•i•ni•tion

Insulin sensitivity is a term used to define the improved action of insulin, which allows for blood glucose (sugar) uptake into the muscle and fat cells. The cells offer less resistance to allow insulin to enter and do its job with blood sugar uptake.

Polyunsaturated Fats

Polyunsaturated fatty acids (PUFAs) are termed *poly*unsaturated because they have more than one double bond in their structure. A diet rich in PUFAs, including corn oil and sunflower oil, has been shown to decrease all types of cholesterol, including the good kind, too, unfortunately.

Let's focus on two PUFAs, the essential fatty acids: alpha-linolenic acid (ALA), an omega-3 fatty acid, and linoleic acid (LA), an omega-6 fatty acid. Your body can't make these essential fatty acids, so your diet has to supply them. Essential fatty acids are very important because they help your body make hormonelike chemicals called prostaglandins, which control a whole host of bodily functions, including the production of cholesterol and triglycerides (fats). True, production of cholesterol is bad, but your body needs a certain amount of cholesterol (a waxy, fatlike substance made in your liver) for proper cell function and to make hormones, including sex hormones. Other functions of essential fatty acids include blood clotting and blood formation. They're also key to the structural component of cell membranes.

Back to ALA and LA. These are both essential fatty acids because your body can't make them, but one is definitely healthier for you than the other. ALA is the parent of two long-chain omega-3 fatty acids, eicosapentanoic acid (EPA) and docosahexanoic acid (DHA). Although EPA and DHA can be synthesized from ALA, the conversion rate is believed to be very low, anywhere from 5 to 8 percent overall. This low conversion rate is not a good thing because you get a very small percentage of the active ingredients of omega-3s from ALA or vegetarian sources, so not very much bang for your buck compared to DHA and EPA typically found in fish oil versions of omega-3 supplements. ALA is highly concentrated in plant oils, including flaxseed oil, chia seeds, and certain nuts, especially walnuts. DHA and EPA are mainly found in fatty fish like salmon and sardines. Fish oils have the most DHA and EPA concentration.

Omega-3 fatty acids, including ALA and offspring EPA and DHA, are needed for life and for good health. They help regulate mood, sleep, reactions to stress, and hormonal actions. Several clinical trials have suggested that omega-3 fatty acids, in the form of fish oil supplements, can lower cholesterol. Although omega-3 fatty acids are an important part of your cells, and help them stay healthy, they're actually quite fragile, so it's important to take antioxidants such as vitamins E and C and minerals like selenium (more about that in Chapter 9) to help protect against cell damage of the super-healthy omega-3 fatty acids.

Omega-3s and Weight Loss

Studies have shown that a diet rich in omega-3s may increase satiety (fullness) in people who are overweight and trying to cut down on calories. This can be good news for you, especially if you're finding your weight spiraling upward before or after your weight loss surgery. More good news about omega-3s: research has shown them to have anti-obesity effects.

Food for Thought

Many studies suggest that omega-3 fish oils could help decrease the joint stiffness you might feel in the morning, thanks to their anti-inflammatory effects. They might help with hair loss as well.

Omega-3s and their anti-inflammatory properties have also been found to slow hardening of the arteries, lower blood pressure, and reduce the risk of death via heart attack. Research has also found that omega-3s may help improve a variety of psychological and neurological disorders, such as anxiety, depression, bipolar disorder, and Alzheimer's disease.

Tips for Omega-3 Beginners

The most common reason why people stop or never take fish oils is the fishy smell and aftertaste. Fish oils could make you less than popular with your family and friends because they may cause flatulence, belching, bloating, and diarrhea. Try the odorless kind. Liquid or powder fish oil preparations now exist, too, which may make it much easier to take.

The Food and Drug Administration (FDA) has determined that fish oils are "generally regarded as safe," and according to health experts, fish oils have been shown to be safe under the conditions for which they're used. That said, if your fish oil capsules didn't smell fishy when you first bought them, but progressively smell fishy as you start taking them, they might have oxidized, which would render them rancid and potentially toxic. Follow your nose to help ensure your fish oils are still okay.

A USP-Verified mark on a fish oil label means that compliance with standards set by the United States Pharmacopeia (USP) organization has been met. The FDA does not regulate dietary supplements, so a USP-Verified seal may provide assurance that the fish oil is of a higher quality.

Flaxseed is a popular ALA source for vegetarians who don't eat fish. But don't just top your cereal with some seeds. They need to be ground to convert to DHA and EPA. (A coffee grinder works well.) Also, be sure you're drinking plenty of water when consuming flaxseed to avoid bloating.

> **Post-Op Pitfall**
>
> Excessive intake of some fatty fish may increase the risk of buildup of toxic metals and chemicals, such as mercury and dioxin. Pregnant or breast-feeding women are often advised to limit high-mercury fish, such as shark and swordfish, to help decrease the risk of harm to both mom and baby.

Maximizing Your Omega-3 Benefits

The American Heart Association (AHA) recommends 1 gram (or 1,000 milligrams) EPA and DHA daily for adults with heart disease. For adults with high cholesterol levels, the AHA suggests 2 to 4 grams (or 2,000 to 4,000 milligrams) EPA and DHA daily to see the benefits of fish oils.

At this time, the exact amount of omega-3 fatty acids needed to help protect against diseases is unknown. However, amounts in the range of 200 milligrams DHA and EPA (each) and approximately 1,000 milligrams ALA are believed to be necessary in your daily diet to help make up for the omega-3 fatty acids your body loses every day through metabolism.

Certain weight loss surgeries, such as gastric bypass and the biliopancreatic diversion with duodenal switch, are believed to result in greater needs for omega-3s. Although there's no definitive answer, perhaps anywhere from 2 to 5 times the amounts of DHA and EPA than are normally recommended might be needed, especially within the first few months of surgery when weight loss is at its maximum. Research studies are needed, however, to determine optimal amounts of omega-3s, as well as whether they can be absorbed by D/S patients.

Also, we don't yet know of possible risks of excessive intake of omega-3 supplements, and what's appropriate for one person may be excessive for someone else, so check with your doctor or dietitian to find out what might be best for you. Some people on blood thinners may not be able to take omega-3s at all because of their blood-thinning action, so talk to your primary care physician or surgical center doctor to be sure it's safe for you.

Post-Op Pitfall

Because of the possibility of side effects and interactions with medications, dietary supplements such as fish oils should only be taken under the consent and supervision of your physician and should be used with caution among people who bruise easily or are taking blood-thinning medications. For this reason, they're typically avoided right before and after surgery.

The Other Essential Fatty Acid: Omega-6

Linoleic acid (LA) is the parent of the omega-6 series. Although your body can't make LA, it's capable of manufacturing long-chain (20 carbons +) omega-6 fatty acids, including arachidonic acid. Examples of omega-6 fats include corn oil, safflower oil, and sunflower oil.

Both essential fatty acids, omega-6s and omega-3s, influence cellular activity in the body, but they have opposite effects on inflammation. We're not talking about acute inflammation like what would occur if you sprained your ankle, but rather the chronic inflammation in your body that results from cell injury from reactive oxygen species (see Chapter 9) and damage to your cells. Why is this a potential problem? Because prolonged inflammation can lead to atherosclerosis (hardening of the arteries), heart disease, diabetes, and Alzheimer's disease, among others.

Consider omega-6 fats the ugly step-sister of PUFAs because they have pro-inflammatory actions in your body. Omega-3 fats, on the other hand, are considered anti-inflammatory—they're the "beauty queens" of the essential fatty acid world!

The diet of early humans—we're talking cavemen days—were estimated to be in a ratio of about 1:1 omega-6 to omega-3 fatty acids. The typical modern Western diet is more like 10:1 omega-6s to omega-3s, due to a sharp increase in the intake of vegetable oils like sunflower oil rich in LA and decreased consumption of fatty fish, a rich source of omega-3s via EPA and DHA. A ratio of 2:1 omega-6s to omega-3s is recommended to help decrease the risk of chronic inflammation and heart disease.

It seems like we're seeing a lot more issues with inflammation these days, and higher weight and obesity are kinds of inflammatory diseases, so who knows what this skewed fat ratio could be doing to our health long term. It seems like a good idea to try to keep the ratio of omega-6 to omega-3 fats around 2:1 to optimize your health by minimizing your risk for inflammation.

Fat Recommendations by Procedure

It's sometimes difficult to make general fat recommendations after weight loss surgery because each of the procedures is different and may affect the way your body handles and absorbs fat. Therefore, let's discuss each surgery separately. However, keep in mind that there are some definite gray areas when it comes to some fats, even the good ones such as the omega-3s.

Most health experts agree omega-3 fats are healthy for your heart, but the topic is still controversial. For example, some physicians are hesitant to recommend them for someone who had a malabsorptive surgery, like the duodenal switch (D/S), because it's unknown whether the patient will absorb enough of these good fats to be worthwhile.

The truth is, until there's more research, we just don't have the answers to those questions yet. However, we can tell you what level of fat intake seems to work for the different procedures, in terms of tolerance and limiting the risk for issues such as diarrhea. Of course, you do need to watch the fat levels in your diet to meet your needs while helping keep your weight down.

Gastric Banding

In the first few months after a gastric banding procedure, keep your fat content low and your protein high (like ½ cup low-fat cottage cheese or Greek yogurt as snacks) and no more than about 10 grams or so fat at a meal (2 ounces low-fat fish, such as sole or scrod) because higher fat intakes in the beginning can cause issues with heaviness, indigestion, and possibly vomiting or diarrhea.

Why is that? After your band is placed, your stomach kind of stresses out and swells at least a little bit because it doesn't know what just happened or why your surgeon placed a band at the top of your stomach. If you were to eat a high-fat meal at this time, you might have issues because fats delay the emptying of your stomach. A tighter band could leave you at higher risk for gastrointestinal issues, or at least abdominal discomfort.

What if you're about 3 or 4 months post-op band and have had a couple fills or adjustments to your band? If you're doing well with your protein and fluid intake (see Chapters 3 and 5 for more details), and you're able to eat about 3 ounces or a deck of playing cards' worth of meat, chicken, fish, or tofu without feeling chest pain or vomiting, about 30 to 40 grams fat or so a day is okay, provided you don't add gravy other than nonfat or at least low-fat varieties, and you don't eat fried foods. High-fat foods and those foods with cream sauces or regular ice cream can really slow down the emptying of your stomach from top to bottom and leave you feeling heavy or possibly increase your risk of diarrhea.

Okay, what if you're about 9 to 12 months out after your band, have had at least 3 or 4 fills/adjustments, and feel you've hit the "sweet spot," or the point where you feel you have just the right amount of restriction? Go with a general low-fat diet by avoiding fried foods, those with cream sauces, and foods with skin, like chicken.

> **Cooking Tip**
>
> As with all weight loss surgery procedures, it's important to keep foods moist because dry, grilled chicken breast or steak can get stuck in your throat or esophagus.

If you're using an online food log (see Appendix B), your fat calories shouldn't be more than $^1/_3$ of your total calories. This is not only for calorie reasons (fats have twice the calories of carbohydrates and protein), but also because a higher fat diet can increase your risk of heart disease.

Gastric Bypass

During the first month after gastric bypass, you may be on liquids or puréed foods, for at least a few weeks, and it's important to watch your fat intake, even with high-protein drinks and puréed foods. As you've learned, fats slow down the emptying of your stomach, and your pouch is just sitting there for the first 6 weeks or so after your surgery. You can keep your fat intake down by choosing fat-free yogurts that are low in sugar (see Chapters 2 and 7) and avoiding high-fat foods.

About 3 months after your gastric bypass procedure, go with low-fat meats and fish, with fat-free or low-fat sauces, gravies, etc., and be sure you're chewing until everything is absolutely liquid. Stop eating when you feel chest fullness.

About a year or so after your gastric bypass surgery, you should find you're able to eat a pretty large variety of foods, maybe more than you thought.

Gastric Sleeve

In the first month or so after a gastric sleeve procedure, aim for all foods to be either low-fat or nonfat. Stay away from high-fat foods like regular gravies and sauces, as well as fried foods because these could stress your banana stomach's smaller size if you challenge it, especially in the beginning.

About 3 months after your sleeve, you're probably able to eat at least a deck of cards' worth of meat, chicken, or fish at a time, and maybe $1/2$ cup vegetables and $1/2$ cup starch, which, if it's all lean, should keep your fat intake in check. Avoid fried foods and sauces to help with tolerance, as well as to keep the fat and calories down.

After a year or so, you should be able to eat quite a large variety of foods. Focus on variety, about 3 or 4 ounces (a deck of cards' worth) of lean and tender meat, chicken, fish, tofu, etc., with at least a few fruits and vegetables and whole grains a day, and chew until it's absolutely liquid. Fewer than $1/3$ of calories from fat is generally recommended for a heart-healthy diet, which helps keep calories down, too.

Duodenal Switch (D/S)

In the first month or so after a D/S, it's likely that most of your calories are coming from protein, specifically high-protein supplements due to your higher protein needs and possible inability to take in much food, and you want to be sure they're not high in fat. Although your stomach is larger than the pouch that gastric bypass patients have, your surgery is a true malabsorptive one, and roughly 72 percent of your fat intake isn't absorbed, which could mean you might have, at least initially, some issues with loose stools or diarrhea. Hang in there! Many things may help. Probiotics are live bacterial cultures added to foods, like some yogurts, that may help with diarrhea after weight loss surgery (see the "Probiotics Prebiotics" section in Chapter 8). Anti-gas medications and body deodorants may also alleviate or help prevent gastrointestinal issues after surgery.

If you're 3 or 4 months post-op D/S, you may be coasting along finding yourself able to eat the majority of foods you like, including tender meats, chicken, and maybe even some foods with sauce, gravy, and/or skin. However, given the D/S malabsorption rate of fat, you may want to keep the fats in your diet lower to decrease your risk of diarrhea and abdominal discomfort.

About a year or so post-op D/S, you're probably enjoying many different foods and perhaps are able to tolerate larger quantities, and higher-fat foods, than you ever thought possible. However, if you're at risk for heart disease or are finding that your weight is climbing and the rest of your diet (e.g., carbohydrate intake) is okay, you may want to reevaluate how much fat you're taking in.

Some D/S patients have lost *more* weight than is healthy, and they may need to *increase* their fat intake. No, not those dreaded trans fats or saturated fats, but healthful monounsaturated fats and omega-3 fats like almonds, walnuts, salmon, etc. Bringing your food logs to appointments with your dietitian is a good idea to evaluate your progress and your needs.

Certainly, an important way to help prevent or lower your risk for heart disease includes a healthy, balanced diet low in fat, particularly saturated fat and those ugly trans fats. Get most of your fats from monounsaturated fats (MUFAs) and to a lesser extent, polyunsaturated fats (PUFAs). Keeping your overall fat intake low will also keep calories down and improve your chances of maintaining your weight loss.

The Least You Need to Know

- Polyunsaturated fats include essential omega-3 and omega-6 fatty acids, with omega-3s decreasing inflammation and omega-6s increasing inflammation.

- Trans fat, a type of saturated fat, is the least healthy and should be limited as much as possible in your diet.

- Monounsaturated fats are generally considered the most heart-healthy fats and could help decrease your bad (LDL) cholesterol.

- Cholesterol is not a type of fat, but rather a waxy, fatlike substance made in your liver, so it only comes from animal sources.

Fluid for Life

In This Chapter

- The importance of fluids after surgery

- Signs and symptoms of dehydration

- Fluid requirements after surgery

- Reasons to stay away from carbonated beverages, caffeine, alcohol, and energy drinks post-op

Adequate fluid intake is extremely important after your weight loss surgery. Mild dehydration is the number-one issue Margaret sees post-op, across all the bariatric procedures, generally because of decreased fluid intake. Gastric banding patients, for example, might experience post-op swelling around the band and decreased ability to get in much fluid at a time. D/S patients might have additional fluid losses via loose or watery stools, particularly in the early post-op period or after eating higher-fat foods. Additional fluid losses could come from vomiting or diarrhea, sometimes seen with gastric bypass surgery patients who experience dumping.

Think of fluid's importance in your body like gas in a car—your body just can't run without it. In this chapter, we show you how to get enough of the right kinds of fluids after your surgery.

Why You Need Fluids

Your body is about $^2/_3$ water, and every day, you lose some of that water through various ways, including your breath, perspiration, urine, and bowel movements. For your body to function at its best, you must constantly replace your water supply by consuming beverages and foods that contain water.

Post-Op Pitfall

Persistent vomiting after weight loss surgery is not normal and could be a source of increased fluid loss, as well as a symptom of a serious issue. Contact your surgeon immediately.

That's sometimes easier said than done though, particularly in the first few weeks after your procedure. Inadequate fluid intake may increase the risk and severity of constipation, a common complaint after surgery. In addition, improper fluid intake may hamper your weight loss success because many of the metabolic processes that occur in the immediate post-op period require water.

When to Drink Up

When you get your fluids can be as important in combating dehydration as how much and what kind of fluids you get. For example, spend the first 30 minutes or so in the morning after you wake catching up on fluids. After all, you just went all night without drinking. And because drinking fluids with meals is discouraged, waiting 30 minutes after you finish breakfast to drink could put you at further risk of dehydration.

Your surgery center might want you to avoid liquids 30 minutes before a meal, as well as 30 minutes after. The meal itself should take about 30 minutes, particularly when you've advanced to solid foods, so skipping the morning fluid means you have to wait as long as an hour to drink again, which could set you up for dehydration. However, it's possible, particularly in the first several weeks post-op, that at least one of your meals consists of a high-protein drink, so in this case the fluid *is* your meal, so no need to wait 30 minutes before or after a liquid meal. In this case, the protein drink *is* the liquid, and you could drink water or another approved beverage right before the protein drink.

In the hospital, most bariatric surgery patients are introduced to fluid with 1-ounce medicine cups on their clear liquid tray the day after their surgery. When you're discharged from the hospital, you'll be aiming for a lot more fluid than 1 or 2 small medicine cups per hour, or otherwise you're headed for dehydration for sure.

Everyone's fluid needs may vary though, and guidelines aren't one-size-fits-all. How much fluid do you need? Let's find out.

How Much Do You Need?

Fluid needs are like gas needs for cars: there are many different situations where your fluid needs may change, such as if you're doing a cross-country journey or a leisurely Sunday drive. However, everyone agrees that you need to keep a certain amount in your tank, regardless of your destination, for your car to run properly.

Different factors could influence your individual fluid needs, including exercise, the heat and humidity of your environment, illnesses or health conditions, and medications, as well as if you're pregnant or breast-feeding. However, a general rule of thumb for bariatric surgery patients is 48 to 64 ounces fluid per day. You may, of course, need more than this, and we talk in a bit about why, when, and how much that might be, but at least this is a starting goal.

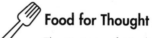

Food for Thought

The Institute of Medicine recommends that men consume about 13 (8-ounce) cups fluid a day and women about 9 (8-ounce) cups fluid a day.

Factors That May Influence Your Fluid Needs

Everyone's fluid needs are different, even if the same two people are performing the same physical activity in the same physical environment or climate. Fluid needs may also be different depending on medical conditions and ailments. Pregnancy and breast-feeding—at least 18 months after weight loss surgery—may vastly change fluid needs as well. Let's examine these factors more closely.

Physical Activity

Exercise may cause you to sweat a great deal, particularly if you're in a very warm climate or environment or participating in strenuous activity.

Sweat is comprised of more than just fluid; it contains minerals like sodium and chloride as well. Sodium, chloride, and other minerals that help maintain fluid balance in the body are called electrolytes. Electrolyte imbalances can be serious, even life-threatening, so if you lose a lot of sweat during your workouts, a replacement beverage containing electrolyte replenishment may be necessary.

It's estimated that you need an extra 2 cups or so fluid a day if you're exercising regularly. However, as you might imagine, this is highly variable and might be an underestimation, particularly if you're exercising for long bouts of time or noticing that your urine is dark despite drinking more water. Another way to estimate fluid needs with exercise is to weigh yourself right before you exercise and again right after you finish. If you find, for example, that you're 1 pound lighter after your workout, you need to replenish that lost fluid with 16 ounces fluid, preferably water. If you've

had a longer or more strenuous workout and lost, say, 2 pounds, you need to add 32 ounces fluid to your day. That's in addition to the 48 to 64 ounces fluid a day recommended after your surgery. However, avoid gulping, using straws, and drinking with meals or within 30 minutes after meals to decrease your risk of intolerance issues. Straws, especially if they're the very wide variety, might cause you to suck in too fast and increase gas, bloating, and chest pressure or pain due to taking in too much at one time.

> **⊘ Post-Op Pitfall** _____
>
> Using a straw may result in an overfill of air in your pouch if you've had gastric bypass and may cause general discomfort for patients who have had other bariatric procedures.

Ideal beverages to consume during bouts of exercise longer than an hour may include some sugar, but watch out for sugary drinks, even if they're touted as energy drinks. These can add unnecessary calories and may cause osmotic diarrhea. Whether you had gastric bypass or not, look for drinks with less than 15 grams sugars per serving to lower the risk of dumping (if you had gastric bypass) and decrease consumption of simple sugars in your diet. Even fruit juices may be dehydrating if they're used as sports-type beverages, so dilute them at least 50 percent with water. Ideally, water or beverages containing 10 calories or less per serving (not carbonated or caffeinated though—more on that later in this chapter) are your best bet. A sports-type drink may be warranted if you're exercising for an hour or longer, but even then, you might want to dilute it by 50 percent or so to decrease the concentration and caloric content.

As a general rule of thumb, drink at least 4 ounces fluid every 15 minutes into your workout, if possible, so you're well hydrated, and so you won't feel as overwhelmed when you try to make up your fluid losses after your exercise session is over.

> **✎ Food for Thought** _____
>
> The American College of Sports Medicine (ACSM) recommends consuming extra fluid several hours before you exercise to better enable fluid absorption and allow your urinary production or output to return to normal levels. ACSM also suggests that people needing to achieve rapid and complete recovery from dehydration drink about 1.5 liters, or about 6 cups, for each kilogram of body weight lost. (Note: 1 kilogram = 2.2 pounds.)

Environmental Factors

Temperature and humidity level can really make a difference in your fluid needs, particularly if you're taking your physical activity outside. Hot or humid weather could increase your sweat production as well as your fluid needs, sometimes significantly. Heated indoor air is drying and could deplete your skin of moisture during the winter. Higher altitudes could also increase your risk for dehydration.

Illnesses or Medical Conditions

Fever, vomiting, and diarrhea could result in greater fluid and electrolyte losses. In general, if you're feeling under the weather, it's a good idea to increase your fluid intake, particularly water, and possibly sports drinks (diluted by 50 percent). If you have heart failure or kidney disease, your doctor may restrict your fluid intake after your weight loss surgery.

Signs and Symptoms of Dehydration

There are some tell-tale signs of dehydration, and your urine color, or lack thereof, can be the first indicator you're not getting enough fluids. Your urine should be clear—clear enough, in fact, that you could read through it. It's important to regularly take note of the color of your urine, particularly in the early post-op period, to help combat dehydration before it progresses to a dangerous level.

Some general signs of mild to moderate dehydration include the following:

- Dry, sticky mouth
- Thirst
- Headache
- Dizziness or lightheadedness
- Darker urine
- Decreased urination

Food for Thought

The average urinary output for adults is 6.3 cups a day. You lose another 4 cups water a day through breathing, sweating, and bowel movements. Beverages consumed account for about 80 percent of your fluid intake, while foods account for the remaining 20 percent.

Your body typically decreases urinary production if you're dehydrated, so not urinating as often is another red flag for dehydration. If you don't have any significant health conditions, such as uncontrolled diabetes or a serious heart condition, you can usually treat mild to moderate dehydration by simply drinking more fluids.

If you're finding that water feels heavy after surgery, consider sugar-free popsicles and granitas or water ices. (For yummy high-protein granita recipes, check out Chapter 22.) Also, keep in mind that you may be getting more fluid than you think from the foods you're eating, especially if you're a few months post-op and able to eat a varied diet. Many fruits and vegetables, such as tomatoes and watermelon, are 90 to 100 percent water by weight and can help you meet your fluid needs in a nutritious way. Decaffeinated tea and coffee can also help, but stay away from their caffeinated versions.

On the flip side, very high protein supplements—40 grams or more per serving— can be dehydrating and provide less free water than you might have thought, which is another reason to limit protein to no more than 20 to 30 grams in a single serving of protein drink. Your kidneys have to work harder to flush out the waste products from protein breakdown, so it's important to provide your body with plenty of water before and after a higher-protein meal or supplement to ensure adequate fluid repletion.

Mild to moderate dehydration that's untreated can lead to significant dehydration, so seek medical attention if you find any of the following apply:

♦ Can't keep fluids down

♦ Are having issues with continuous vomiting

♦ Have moderate diarrhea for 3 or more days

♦ Develop severe diarrhea, with or without vomiting or fever

♦ Feel irritable or disoriented and much sleepier or less active than usual

Post-Op Pitfall

Severe dehydration is a medical emergency and may manifest as extreme thirst; lack of sweating; little or no urination; low blood pressure; rapid heartbeat; extremely dry mouth, skin, and mucous membranes; and, rarely, delirium and unconsciousness.

Go to the nearest hospital or emergency room or call 911 or your emergency medical number if you think you're severely dehydrated or have any of these symptoms.

You'll improve your chances of avoiding severe dehydration if you focus on getting continuous fluid throughout the day (bring a water bottle with you everywhere you go, for example), but of course not with meals or directly after, and possibly not right before meals. Knowing the signs of dehydration might just help you minimize it.

Fluids to Avoid After Weight Loss Surgery

Although avoiding dehydration is key, all beverages are not alike, in terms of tolerance and hydration, and you should avoid some at all costs because they may be linked with possible risks, such as gas pain and pressure, gastrointestinal issues, ulcer formation, and even possible stretching of your pouch (if you had gastric bypass surgery). Let's run through the list of common offenders.

Carbonated Beverages

Carbonated beverages are generally discouraged after weight loss surgery, particularly in the early post-op period, when they're often linked with gas, chest pain or pressure, and general abdominal bloating or discomfort. Tolerance to carbonated beverages may vary among the surgical procedures.

Gastric banding patients might find particular discomfort with carbonated beverage intake after they've had more fills as the stoma, or opening through the band, becomes more narrow and gas and bloating are more common. The tighter the band, the higher the risk for GI discomfort with carbonated beverages, so it's important to keep this in mind, especially if you're dining out.

Gastric sleeve and D/S patients have a fairly large stomach area, especially compared to gastric bypass patients, so carbonation sensitivity may not be an issue. Although surgical centers typically vary in their nutrition protocols, carbonated beverages are generally discouraged across all procedures to minimize flatulence and general abdominal bloating and discomfort.

In general, carbonated drinks are ill tolerated among gastric bypass patients, and there's at least speculation that they may stretch the anastamosis (the connection leading from your pouch), leaving you feeling hungry all the time.

Margaret worked with a few gastric bypass patients who started drinking carbonated beverages a few years out and had a common complaint of sudden hunger. These same patients shared the same bariatric surgeon, and when she did an upper endoscopy to look at their anatomy, they all had the same thing in common: the anastamoses were all wider than they should have been, possibly the result of continuous carbonation ingestion. Of course, it's impossible to say this was the absolute cause, but this knowledge might help you see the point of limiting or avoiding carbonated beverages altogether. At the very least, avoiding carbonated drinks can help minimize gas and bloating.

Alcohol

Alcohol after surgery is a sensitive and sometimes complicated issue. Maybe some patients' doctors may have recommended they drink a glass of red wine a day to help lower the risk of heart disease. Others feel life is too short not to have at least an occasional celebratory drink. For others, alcohol may be their sole means of stress reduction.

Alcohol is one of the few substances absorbed directly from your stomach. Because the surface area in your stomach is decreased for most surgeries, including banding, gastric bypass, D/S, and gastric sleeve, the smaller area becomes saturated with alcohol more quickly. In addition, alcohol is actually digested as a fat. Therefore, it adds to acetylaldehyde, a toxin in your body.

Research cites an alteration in alcohol metabolism among gastric bypass surgery patients, with an increase in reports of driving under the influence (DUI) with small amounts of alcohol. The study suggested caution in the use of alcohol even a year or greater post-op. In addition, the authors of the study suggested gastric bypass patients be informed that their blood alcohol concentrations after just one drink may be quite a bit higher than their symptoms might indicate.

Alcohol is generally discouraged for several reasons, including the fact it contains empty calories overall (other than some antioxidant benefits from some wines), and some patients may be at risk for excessive alcohol use, sometimes trading food for alcohol. Although this concept of a "new addiction" may be overblown somewhat in the media, some patients do newly discover alcohol post-op and need to seek professional help. A couple of Margaret's gastric bypass patients exhibited what has come to be termed "hollow leg syndrome," whereby they didn't feel the effects of the alcohol, even with higher amounts, and found they had to drink more and more to feel the high, thus contributing a great deal of calories and possibly putting them at risk for endangering themselves and others by driving afterward.

> **⊘ Post-Op Pitfall**
>
> A Stanford University case-control study revealed blood alcohol concentrations among gastric bypass patients peaked about 0.03 percent higher and took 40 minutes longer to normalize. Always avoid drinking and driving, but especially after your surgery.

The bottom line when it comes to alcohol and gastric bypass surgery: don't drink and drive, ever. It seems prudent to avoid alcohol altogether, if at all possible, after your surgery. Alcohol is a diuretic, so you'll lose some fluid, and it provides too many calories in general, so it may hamper your weight loss efforts long term. However, if your doctor gives you the okay to drink alcohol in moderation after your procedure, avoid carbonated alcoholic beverages and sweet drinks, which are high in calories and may cause dumping in gastric bypass patients; sip versus gulping; and don't plan to drive or operate heavy machinery.

 Food for Thought _____

Gastric bypass surgery alters all the factors involved in alcohol metabolism, including weight, liver function, and the production of the enzyme alcohol dehydro-genase.

High-Sugar Drinks and/or Energy Drinks

You've probably seen the ads for the energy drinks that are supposed to boost your energy and health, but are they truly good for you? Some of the energy drinks are not only unhealthful, but can be downright dangerous for you after your surgery, particularly if you have sensitivities to caffeine or are prone to dumping. Believe it or not, some of the so-called super-healthful drinks contain the equivalent of 14 packets of table sugar and the caffeine of 3 cups of coffee in one can!

Some of the drinks also contained mysterious ingredients, such as guarana. This is a natural stimulant originating from Brazil, and many people aren't aware that it's in many energy drinks and has an effect in your body similar to caffeine. However because it's not technically caffeine, you might not even realize it, perhaps until you get a jolt of energy after drinking it.

 Food for Thought _____

Most energy drinks contain about 80 milligrams caffeine, at least as much as found in an 8-ounce cup of coffee. A 12-ounce can of soda contains 18 to 48 milligrams caffeine.

In addition, these drinks are typically "hot-filled," meaning the liquid was pumped in a hot container, which has brought up speculation regarding the risk of aluminum absorption from the can. As you can imagine, this is a very unhealthy scenario, for several reasons, so I strongly discourage these types of drinks.

Caffeinated Beverages

In addition to limiting caffeine via energy drinks and soda, watch out for other sources of caffeine that may be sneaking into your diet, including coffee-flavored drinks and protein supplements. Some may contain legal stimulants found in energy drinks, such as guarana, so you may not be aware you're ingesting caffeine. However, especially if you're sensitive to caffeine, you may feel jittery or downright anxious. Or it could drive up your blood pressure, so being unaware of caffeine in your diet can be downright dangerous.

Caffeine is generally discouraged after weight loss surgery for several reasons, including the fact that it's a diuretic, meaning your body tends to lose more fluid than it's gaining because of fluid release from the stimulatory effects of caffeine. Caffeine also has a significant link to risk for marginal ulcers among gastric bypass patients. A marginal ulcer occurs just below your pouch and can be potentially dangerous, so it's not worth the risk. However, if you feel you can't go without your morning cup of coffee, check with your doctor to see if perhaps one cup a day would be okay. If you're given the go-ahead, still look out for any burning or pain in your pouch area, particularly around the time of your morning joe, to help lower your risk of developing a marginal ulcer.

In general, it's a good idea to keep caffeine to a minimum after your surgery because, at the very least, chronic caffeine intake, especially if it involves several cups a day, can leave you at higher risk for dehydration. In addition, caffeine may increase the release of cortisol and other stress-related hormones and leave you feeling depleted in energy and craving sugar and fat about an hour or so afterward. This could set you up for a roller-coaster ride, in terms of low blood sugars and irritability, followed by continuous cravings for more caffeine. However, if you're working on cutting down your caffeine intake and you're drinking more than a cup a day, do it slowly and gradually to minimize your risk for caffeine-withdrawal headaches.

Other Fluids to Avoid

A few other fluids you might not tolerate well after your surgery include high-fat beverages and soups, particularly after gastric bypass and D/S procedures. High-fat liquids, particularly if very hot or cold versus room temperature, tend to increase the likelihood of dumping among gastric bypass patients. D/S patients may be at increased risk for loose stools because of their high rate of fat malabsorption. Even gastric sleeve and gastric banding patients may find they're intolerant to high-fat soups or other liquids because the higher fat content results in a delay of stomach emptying. A smaller stomach overall could be more sensitive to fats and the end result could be bloating, gas, and a higher likelihood of loose stools or diarrhea.

High-fat beverages are also calorically dense, so they may hamper weight loss success, especially if there's no malabsorptive component to your surgery. Bottom line: go with the lower-fat soups and beverages.

Of all the components of the post-op nutritional regimen, none is more important than adequate fluid intake. Without proper hydration, nothing else will work in terms of weight loss and your overall health, and in the worst-case scenario, life-threatening dehydration can develop. If you're confused, or concerned that your fluid intake is suboptimal in terms of quantity and/or quality of fluids chosen, it's a good idea to check in with your surgical center's doctor and dietitian.

The Least You Need to Know

- Adequate fluid intake is absolutely essential after weight loss surgery.

- A minimum of 48 to 64 ounces fluid a day is recommended after bariatric surgery.

- Dehydration is one of the most common issues after surgery, and may be potentially life-threatening if untreated.

- Caffeine, alcohol, energy drinks, and carbonated beverages are generally discouraged after weight loss surgery.

Chapter 6

Vital Vitamins and Minerals

In This Chapter

- ◆ Pre-op vitamin and mineral deficiencies
- ◆ Managing vitamins and minerals after surgery
- ◆ Finding the best vitamin and mineral supplements

Vitamin and mineral deficiencies after weight loss surgery are not uncommon, particularly among D/S patients, and also occur among a fair amount of gastric bypass patients. Deficiencies in vitamins and minerals, also known as micronutrients, may develop slowly after surgery and also affect patients with purely restrictive surgeries, such as gastric banding and gastric sleeve, although they're more likely to be an issue with gastric bypass and the D/S procedure. Therefore, it's imperative that all bariatric patients, regardless of procedure, adhere to the suggested nutritional regimen, laboratory assessments, and surgical team appointments to minimize the risk of deficiencies.

When it comes to vitamin and mineral deficiencies, it's important to realize that there have been reports of sudden or acute vitamin deficiencies, some of them potentially life-threatening, even amongst purely restrictive procedures such as gastric banding. Let's find out more about which vitamin and mineral deficiencies you may be at risk for, and how you may be able to prevent or minimize them.

Common Vitamin and Mineral Deficiencies Pre-Op

You're probably aware that you could be at risk for certain vitamin or mineral deficiencies after your surgery, especially with the procedures with malabsorptive components, such as the D/S and, to a lesser extent, gastric bypass surgery. However, you might also be deficient in certain vitamins and minerals *before* your surgery—and you might not even realize it. It's possible all the recommended tests were done and might have come back normal.

However, research is revealing that some of the standard lab tests might miss many deficiencies because of measurement at too superficial a level, which is the case with many mineral deficiencies that are unable to be measured by a standard lab test. You might be low in a certain vitamin or mineral but your blood tests won't show it in some cases because either the test was too general or you're in the early stages of deficiency and it can't be detected yet.

Whether you've had your surgery already or not, it's important to know what, if any, vitamin or mineral deficiencies you have.

Vitamin D

Vitamin D is a complex vitamin that also functions as a hormone and exists in several forms. However, for the sake of our discussion, it's a fat-soluble vitamin that's very likely to be low if you're overweight. Many people are vitamin D–deficient and aren't aware of it because the vast majority of patients seeking weight loss surgery had never checked their vitamin D levels previously.

Although there are at least a few theories on why this is the case, one possibility is that vitamin D wants to "hide out" in your fat cells and becomes unavailable to your body. Another possibility is that weight loss surgery patients may, in general, not get enough sun—a major way your body can absorb vitamin D—because sunscreens block your body's ability to make vitamin D. However, this theory may be flawed because it's been well documented that bariatric patients living in warm, sunny climates are just as likely to be vitamin D–deficient as any other patient, even prior to surgery.

> **Food for Thought**
>
> Research reveals the higher your body mass index (BMI), the lower your vitamin D level is likely to be. Statistics cite up to 80 percent of pre-op bariatric patients are low in vitamin D.

People of particular ethnic or cultural backgrounds may be at particular risk for low vitamin D levels pre-op. One research study cites vitamin D deficiency is less common among Hispanics (56.4 percent) than Caucasians (78.8 percent) and African Americans (70.4 percent).

Your doctor most likely has checked your 25(OH) vitamin D level (that's the chemical form of vitamin D with OH, hydroxyl, or an "OH" group on the vitamin D molecule), which experts consider the most accurate measure of true vitamin D available in your body. Your doctor might measure other kinds of vitamin D in your blood, like 1,25 dihydroxy vitamin D, but by the time this level is low, you're *really* low in vitamin D. Bottom line: 25(OH) vitamin D test is better at measuring early vitamin D deficiency. Although the optimal blood level of vitamin D is debatable and somewhat controversial, it's generally agreed that ideal levels are increasing, from 20 ng/mL to 32 ng/mL, and some surgical centers are aiming for levels upward of 50 to 80 nanograms per deciliter (ng/mL) for optimal health.

If your vitamin D level is low, your doctor may write a prescription for high levels (e.g., 50,000 *IUs*) of vitamin D as ergocalciferol (vitamin D_2) once a week for 6 to 8 weeks. Vitamin D_3 (cholecalciferol) is believed to be better used in your body than D_2 but isn't available in the United States by prescription as D_2 is, although some people buy it online, including in some bariatric vitamin companies. Some centers use D_2 and still have good results, even if not using D_3, although some evidence certainly suggests D_3 is better absorbed and more effective over time than D_2.

def•i•ni•tion

IUs are International Units, the unit of measure used for vitamin D supplements.

If your vitamin D level was only slightly low—which is very relative these days, given changing optimal levels varying—your doctor may recommend you start an over-the-counter vitamin D supplement, such as 1,000 or 2,000 IUs per day, in conjunction with a calcium supplement for optimal absorption and repletion. Other health-care providers may aim for at least 5,000 IUs vitamin D per day to help keep levels normal, but check with your surgical team about *your* recommendations.

Calcium

Vitamin D deficiency is often accompanied by a calcium deficiency because they work in conjunction with one another. Adequate calcium intake and supplementation before your surgery is vital, since research shows your bones could show signs of calcium loss post-op, even if you had the gastric banding procedure. Banding patients may not get in proper nutrition, including calcium, which could place bones at risk for weakening and even fractures. Significant weight loss, among other factors, could put your bones at risk for depletion or calcium losses, and ultimately place you in danger of bone depletion of minerals or weakening of your bones and possible risk of breaking your bones.

However, there is good news in all this, and it involves knowing your calcium and vitamin D status before surgery, or at least as soon as possible, so you can take action and nip potential issues in the bud.

Calcium supplementation *before* your surgery is ideal, especially if you're low pre-op. However, not all calcium supplements are alike. Calcium carbonate supplements are now generally discouraged, regardless of surgical procedure, because they require a high degree of acidity for absorption, and antacids and other medications, as well as getting older, can decrease your stomach's acidity. Studies in women who never had bariatric surgery reveal calcium carbonate was absorbed at a rate of 27 percent below that of calcium citrate. Calcium citrate does not require acid for absorption—a handy thing, considering you have very little acid in your pouch if you're a gastric bypass patient. The gastric sleeve, D/S, and, to a certain extent, gastric banding procedure, also limit acid availability, so calcium citrate is the way to go.

Just keep in mind that your body can only absorb about 500 to 600 milligrams calcium at a time, so it's likely you'll need at least 3 doses a day to meet the general recommendation of 1,500 milligrams per day pre-op. Your post-op calcium needs may be higher than this, particularly with the D/S. You also want to be sure your calcium supplement has other "bone-friendly" minerals, such as magnesium.

Cooking Tip _____

Ninety-nine percent of calcium in your body is in your bones, so a serum (blood) calcium test is not an accurate calcium measurement. Parathyroid hormone (PTH) is a much better reflection of calcium status in your body. A high PTH level suggests your calcium is too low and is commonly seen with vitamin D deficiency.

Post-Op Pitfall _____

Calcium citrate supplements are not recommended among patients with kidney disease because it results in a higher risk for aluminum toxicity. Calcium acetate doesn't require acid, like calcium citrate, and is the preferred type of calcium if your kidney function is compromised.

Iron

Iron deficiency is not uncommon pre-op, particularly among pre-menopausal women. One study revealed up to 50 percent of pre-op gastric bypass patients were low in iron, which can hamper energy and place you at risk for shortness of breath, fainting, and anemia.

Because iron absorption is significantly dependent on an acidic environment, levels of this vital mineral will most likely go down after surgery, even among the restrictive surgeries, because tolerance to high-iron foods, such as meats and chicken, may be significantly compromised. In addition, surgeries with a malabsorptive component may further exacerbate iron deficiency issues. Iron supplementation as soon as deficiency is discovered is key, both pre- and post-op.

B Vitamins

Research reveals several of the B-complex vitamins, including thiamin, vitamin B_{12}, and folic acid, may be low before surgery. B vitamins serve many functions, including participation in important energy reactions in your body and carbohydrate metabolism, so it's important to identify deficiencies as soon as possible. Also, because B vitamins typically work together, being low in one B vitamin could mean other B vitamins are low, so your surgical center might recommend a B_{50} complex, with many B vitamins in it, to lower your risk for deficiency.

This takes on even greater significance when you realize that B vitamin deficiencies, particularly vitamin B_{12} and thiamin, may be low after surgery, even with restrictive procedures. B vitamins, like thiamin and vitamin B_{12}, could result in irreversible nerve damage if you have a long-term deficiency in either one that goes untreated, so it's really important to take these and your other vitamins as recommended by your center.

Miscellaneous Pre-Op Deficiencies

One study found vitamin A levels low among some pre-op patients. The greatest source of this vitamin is fruits and vegetables, so it's possible this was reflective of suboptimal variety and perhaps low intake of fruits and vegetables. There have also been published reports of low pre-op levels of minerals, specifically potassium and magnesium. These minerals are vital for proper heart function, as well as normal muscle contraction and various energy reactions in your body, so many weight loss surgery professionals recommend supplementation with a high-quality, easily absorbed vitamin and mineral supplement *before* surgery.

Failure to treat pre-op deficiencies could have serious consequences, particularly with higher risks for vitamin and mineral deficiencies post-op, so take your vitamins!

Possible Vitamin and Mineral Deficiencies Post-Op

Vitamin and mineral deficiencies are, not surprisingly, most common among patients who've had malabsorptive procedures, such as the D/S, and to a somewhat lesser extent, gastric bypass surgery. Although your risk for vitamin and mineral deficiencies is lower if you had a restrictive procedure such as gastric banding or gastric sleeve, it's still a possibility, especially with vomiting or inability to take in much in your diet in the first several weeks after surgery. Adherence to your prescribed vitamin and mineral regimen is imperative.

Thiamin

Thiamin is a water-soluble B vitamin that has garnered a lot of attention due to its rapid half life, or turnover, and, therefore, potential for deficiency in a very short amount of time. Although rare, post-op bariatric surgery patients who rapidly developed thiamin deficiency resulting in significant, irreversible health issues have been reported.

Thiamin deficiency, or beriberi, has also been called bariatric beriberi in light of the increasing frequency among weight loss surgery patients, particularly those with sudden, uncontrollable vomiting who are not quickly treated. Another presentation of thiamin deficiency is Wernicke encephalopathy, a serious neurological disorder typically associated with alcoholism in the past, but now also seen among some bariatric patients, including post-op gastric banding patients, although more common among the malabsorptive procedures.

🚫 **Post-Op Pitfall**

Uncontrollable vomiting may cause acute thiamin deficiency, which, if untreated, could result in irreversible nerve damage and, although rare, even death. Alert your doctor if you're vomiting, and take your vitamins as prescribed.

Vitamin D and Calcium

Several research studies have documented *metabolic bone disease* (MBD) among D/S and gastric bypass patients, and there has been a suggestion of increased MBD risk among gastric banding patients, as seen by special markers measured in the blood predicting future bone loss. Because the gastric sleeve is a newer procedure, reliable studies are not available as of this writing. Despite the gastric sleeve's purely restrictive nature, significant weight loss already being seen with this procedure typically results in the loss of calcium and vitamin D from your bones, so you could be at risk for MBD.

def•i•ni•tion

> **Metabolic bone disease** (MBD) is an umbrella term encompassing many disorders involving weakened bones or an imbalance in vitamin D or other minerals important for bone health. After bariatric surgery, MBD may occur due to the decreased bioavailability or absorption of vitamin D, calcium, and phosphorus, particularly among D/S and gastric bypass patients.

It's important to recognize and treat both calcium and vitamin D deficiencies because it's not just your bones at risk. Studies show low levels can increase your risk of certain cancers as well as chronic inflammatory and autoimmune diseases, such as diabetes, inflammatory bowel disease, multiple sclerosis, and rheumatoid arthritis.

The preferred site of calcium and vitamin D absorption, the duodenum (first part of your small intestine), is bypassed with gastric bypass surgery, so it's no surprise you're at increased risk for deficiencies post-op. The malabsorptive nature of the D/S places you at high risk, of course, and the absorption of vitamin D, a fat-soluble vitamin, may be severely diminished post-op, with some patients taking very high levels (e.g., 50,000 IUs) on a weekly and sometimes daily basis to keep or achieve normalization. Calcium goals are also increased after surgery, particularly with D/S patients, with estimated needs as high as 2,400 milligrams calcium daily. Calcium citrate, once again, is the preferred source for most patients (other than those with kidney disease) and should not be taken in doses greater than 600 milligrams at a time to maximize absorption. Many foods highly regarded for their calcium content, including spinach; carrots; chards; collards; and other thick, leafy greens, really aren't absorbed due to natural binders in vegetables called calcium oxalates.

Vitamin B$_{12}$

Although vitamin B$_{12}$ absorption is complex, the first problem after gastric bypass involves the inability of vitamin B$_{12}$ to be unbound from the protein in foods because of lack of acid in the pouch. This is believed to be more of a factor in B$_{12}$ absorption

def•i•ni•tion

Intrinsic factor (IF) is a type of protein made in your stomach that's absorbed in the ileum, the last part of your small intestine. Impairment in production or function of IF may lead to vitamin B_{12} deficiency and result in pernicious anemia.

than the decreased availability of *intrinsic factor* (IF). Therefore, despite the fact that your surgical center most likely had you on a regimen of two complete vitamin and mineral doses a day, research suggests additional vitamin B_{12} supplementation, such as sublingual (under your tongue), a monthly shot, or nasal sprays, is absolutely essential to help prevent post-op deficiency.

Although vitamin B_{12} (also known as cobalamin) is known to be stored in your body for up to 5 years, certain medications, a vegan diet, and of course bariatric surgeries, including gastric bypass, D/S, and even restrictive surgeries, could put you at risk for deficiency. Be sure to keep up with your recommended labs and supplements, as directed by your doctor or dietitian.

Vitamin B_{12} deficiency has been seen in other bariatric surgeries, but gastric bypass patients are particularly at risk due to the combination of both decreased stomach acid in the pouch and decreased available IF, so be extra diligent about checking your B_{12} levels if you had this procedure. The methylmalonic acid (MMA) test can detect up to 50 percent of vitamin B_{12} deficiencies not found with a standard B_{12} test, so your surgical center doctor may check your MMA if your B_{12} is on the low end of normal and/or your blood work suggests you might have pernicious anemia.

The Folic Acid Connection

Your doctor may also order tests to check your folic acid (a.k.a. folate, a B vitamin) because folate and vitamin B_{12} are both needed for the maturation of red blood cells. Therefore, if you're low in one, you're often low in the other. You might also be low in other B vitamins because they tend to work in tandem. A homocysteine test can detect folate deficiency sooner and better than a blood folic acid level, which is more indicative of whether you're taking your vitamins.

Talk to your doctor if you experience possible signs and symptoms of vitamin deficiency, such as numbness and tingling in your fingers and toes (also seen with thiamin deficiency), sudden memory issues, confusion, or sudden-onset lethargy.

Remember that failure to treat a deficiency of one of these B vitamins may put you at risk for irreversible nerve damage, especially if long periods of time have elapsed without supplementation.

Iron

Iron deficiency is the most common deficiency seen after gastric bypass surgery, with studies showing gastric bypass patients have a 50 percent chance of being low in iron within 20 years of their procedure. It's particularly common among post-op women who are pre-menopausal; one study identified up to 52 percent of patients in this category to have iron deficiency. The cause is varied, but the combination of low acid in the pouch after gastric bypass surgery as well as lower intake of red meat due to tolerance issues are certainly major factors.

Both gastric bypass and D/S procedures reroute the stream of vitamins and minerals from your small intestine, so lifetime iron deficiency may be an issue. In addition, studies reveal gastric bypass patients who have had longer-limb procedures for greater weight loss are at higher risk for iron deficiency. The D/S, unlike gastric bypass, keeps the duodenum, or first part of your small intestine, intact, but bypasses all your jejunum, the second part of your small intestine and absorption site for a majority of your vitamins and minerals, including iron.

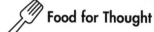

Food for Thought

There have been recent reports of pica (the consumption of ice, dirt, clay, or other items not in the typical diet and seemingly in response to a mineral deficiency) after gastric bypass surgery related to iron deficiency.

While some studies have reported a much higher rate of iron deficiency among D/S patients versus gastric bypass, the drop-out rates and subsequent sample sizes were too small to really extrapolate. However, it seems reasonable to assume D/S, as well as gastric bypass, implies a higher risk for iron deficiency long term, even with supplementation. However, all is not lost because early detection and supplementation can go a long way toward minimizing and even preventing some cases of deficiency.

About 50 to 60 milligrams elemental iron twice a day for at least 3 months is recommended to replenish iron-deficiency anemia. Elemental iron is the actual iron portion of your iron supplement compound and is usually found in the equivalent of 300 milligrams iron sulfate, for example. In some cases where oral iron supplementation still hasn't arrested deficiency, high-quality

Cooking Tip

Some oral iron preparations may cause constipation, so be sure to drink plenty of fluid. In addition, many people find that fiber supplements, even with a balanced, high-fiber diet, may be needed to override iron's binding effects.

and low-risk intravenous iron infusions are available if your doctor feels they're appropriate and necessary.

Vitamin A

Vitamin A is a fat-soluble vitamin that may be low after surgery, particularly with the D/S procedure, because the jejunum is totally bypassed. One researcher found a 52 percent incidence of vitamin A deficiency after malabsorptive surgery at only 1 year out, and the risk increased to 69 percent by 4 years post-op. Low vitamin A levels have also been found among gastric bypass patients, with one study citing more than 52 percent prevalence.

Surprisingly, gastric banding patients had a greater than 25 percent rate of vitamin A deficiency, despite the purely restrictive nature of this procedure. This may be related, perhaps, to decreased intake of high–vitamin A foods, such as fruits and vegetables, particularly after several fills and subsequent diminished ability to consume these high-fiber foods.

Some people who have gastric bypass surgery have a longer Roux limb, which is the part of your small intestine connected to your new pouch/small stomach. The length of your Roux limb may vary due to your starting weight or your surgeon's recommendation or preference. While a longer limb may enhance your weight loss success, it's important to keep in mind you'll need to be extra diligent with monitoring your vitamins and minerals. One study, however, revealed that 10,000 IUs vitamin A, in addition to other vitamins and minerals in a standard D/S post-op regimen, was enough to prevent deficiency. However, it's a good idea to know the possible signs of vitamin A deficiency and to report them to your doctor immediately if you notice them. Night blindness is the first sign of vitamin A deficiency. Additional signs and symptoms include dry eyes, corneal and/or eye inflammation, and rough or dry skin.

As of this writing, vitamin A levels have not yet been researched in gastric sleeve patients, perhaps due to the fact this is a newer bariatric procedure. However, it seems prudent to adhere to the vitamin and mineral supplementation guidelines recommended by your surgical center to help decrease the risk for vitamin A deficiency, among other vitamins and minerals.

Copper

Despite the fact that copper is absorbed in your stomach and proximal (beginning) area of your small intestine, this important mineral is infrequently measured after gastric bypass and D/S procedures. If your copper is low, it could result in anemia and even nerve issues sometimes seen with vitamin B_{12} deficiency. To date, two case reports of copper deficiency have been cited, both involving gastric bypass patients who experienced neurological issues, such as ataxia, a disorder relating to poor coordination of your muscles. Especially if you have symptoms like these, your doctor or health-care provider might want to check the copper in your blood, usually measured as a test called ceruloplasmin.

Bariatric patients with signs of neuropathy or neurological issues such as ataxia should alert their physicians immediately. In addition, if your vitamin B_{12} level is normal. The most accurate test for vitamin B_{12} deficiency is methyl malonic acid (MMA), an intermediate of B_{12}, with urinary MMA being more accurate (and cheaper to obtain) than blood MMA levels. If you're still having neurological symptoms, it may be a copper deficiency that has yet to be diagnosed. It's also important to rule out vitamin A deficiency because these vitamins and minerals appear to be interrelated when it comes to prevention and formation of certain types of anemia.

Zinc

Zinc, like copper, is an important mineral you may be at risk of not having enough of after weight loss surgery, particularly gastric bypass and D/S procedures. One researcher found greater than 50 percent of malabsorptive surgery patients had low zinc levels at 1 year post-op and the same amount remained low at 4 years out. Among gastric bypass patients, zinc levels were found to be low among 36 percent of post-op patients 1 year out. Another researcher corroborated this, and mentioned that standard blood tests for zinc were not as sensitive to diagnosing zinc deficiency as were the erythrocyte (red blood cell) and urinary zinc tests. Therefore, it's important to utilize the more accurate zinc tests available, especially if you strongly suspect deficiency.

Bariatric surgery patients may be at risk for zinc deficiency for several reasons, including decreased absorption (for gastric bypass and D/S) and frequent intolerance to high-zinc food sources, such as red meat. Patients who have had restrictive surgeries, such as gastric banding and the gastric sleeve, are not immune to zinc deficiency because red meat is poorly tolerated, in general, across the bariatric procedures. Additional factors, such as a vegan diet, may also place you at higher risk for deficiency.

Post-Op Pitfall

Zinc supplements exceeding 50 milligrams elemental zinc (e.g., found in 220 milligrams zinc sulfate) should not be used because they may result in copper depletion if used long term.

Zinc deficiency has many possible signs and symptoms, including hair loss, metallic taste, impaired immune function, and diarrhea. Your doctor may want to check your zinc levels and perhaps add 50 milligrams elemental zinc to your supplementation regimen to help prevent deficiency.

Vitamin and Mineral Quality and Absorption

Although every surgical center may have a slightly different philosophy on what constitutes a high-quality vitamin and mineral supplement, increasing data suggests that solid or hard vitamin and mineral pills are absorbed at a low rate, especially among patients who have had gastric bypass surgery and D/S. In fact, a pharmacist friend of Margaret's has noted research studies citing that gastric bypass patients are incapable of absorbing the type of salts used in the formulation of a popular multivitamin supplement on the market in the United States. Therefore, hard multivitamin pills should be avoided after these bariatric procedures.

This is a controversial area, but the newer, bariatric-specific vitamin and mineral supplements appear to emphasize chewable or liquid formulations, which seem to have evidence of better absorption or utilization in your body, especially after gastric bypass and D/S. I also recommend these formulations for gastric banding and sleeve patients because these procedures result in a decrease in gastric (stomach) acidity that may result in poor absorption of the solid supplements.

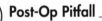 **Post-Op Pitfall** _____

Iron and calcium supplements should not be taken simultaneously because they compete for the same receptor sites in your body. Your vitamin and mineral supplement should also be taken separately from calcium for maximum absorption.

Websites and organizations such as Consumer Labs provide independent testing results of various vitamin and mineral supplements, so you may want to see if your desired supplement is on the list. Ultimately, it's between you and your surgical center's doctor and dietitian to decide which vitamin and mineral supplements are best and most feasible for you.

Wrapping Up Vitamins and Minerals

It's evident that vitamin and mineral deficiencies are potential post-op risks, especially among patients who have had a procedure with a malabsorptive component. However, people who have had purely restrictive procedures, such as gastric banding and sleeve, are not immune to deficiencies and should be just as diligent about adhering to the suggested post-op vitamin and mineral supplementation.

Hair loss is a common concern among both pre- and post-op bariatric patients. A deficiency in biotin, a B vitamin, has also been linked to hair loss, particularly after weight loss surgery, and is sometimes added to the post-op bariatric vitamin regimen. While biotin is not believed to be toxic, and may be helpful, many times post-op hair loss is more related to the stress related to significant weight loss than to a biotin or zinc deficiency. The good news is that hair loss, which typically occurs about 3 to 6 months post-op, typically goes away in another 3 to 9 months. Additional possible factors in hair loss include dehydration, prolonged inadequate protein intake, mineral deficiency (e.g., zinc and iron), and thyroid issues.

Never has taking your vitamins and minerals been more important than after weight loss surgery. Adherence needs to be for a lifetime to help ensure optimal health and weight loss success. In addition to striving for a healthful, balanced diet and a healthful lifestyle overall, it's vital that you keep regular appointments with your surgical team, including your dietitian. In addition, keeping to their suggested lab test regimen, and following up with your doctor if deficiencies are found, is absolutely imperative.

The Least You Need to Know

- ◆ Vitamin and mineral deficiencies may exist even before weight loss surgery.

- ◆ Certain bariatric surgery procedures are linked with higher risks for vitamin and mineral deficiencies.

- ◆ It's important to select a high-quality vitamin and mineral supplement that your body can absorb well.

- ◆ Adherence with your vitamin and mineral supplement regimen is key for long-term health and weight loss, as is following up with your surgical center's recommended labs, prescriptions, and appointments.

Part  2

Demystifying Food Labels and Nutrition Buzzwords

In Part 2, we share what you need to know to successfully read and understand food labels so you can negotiate the grocery aisles more easily, knowing where to find true nutritional bargains. This knowledge could really enhance your weight loss efforts and ensure your continued success down the road.

Next, we take a look at the new buzzwords and technologies in nutrition that could potentially put you a notch ahead in the weight loss and health game. Join us as we talk organic foods, antioxidants, and gut hormones. We've got some great stuff in store for you in the following pages that could turn you into an honorary nutritionist!

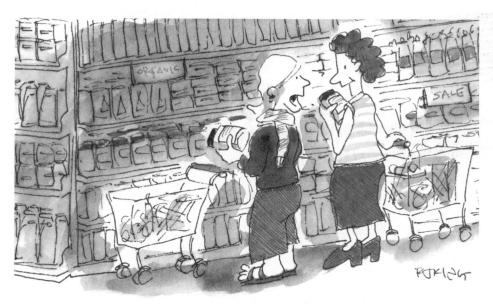

"Couldn't these labels just say 'good for you' or 'naughty'?"

Chapter 7

Deciphering Food Labels

In This Chapter

- Identifying carbs, proteins, and fats
- Determining a food's cholesterol
- Sodium and potassium uncovered
- The low-down on additives and preservatives

When it comes to reading food labels, you probably know the basics. But by the end of this chapter, you'll know how to read a food label like a pro. In this chapter, we take a close look at food labels and delve into some of the more complicated or hidden aspects of food labeling you may not be familiar with.

So keep reading. Soon you'll feel confident about deciphering just about any food label you encounter.

Food Label Basics

You've probably seen countless food labels in your lifetime. But do you really know what you're looking at? Maybe you know to look at the calories and fat content, but there's so much more to food labels. Let's have a look.

Sample label for macaroni and cheese.

(Courtesy of the FDA; www. cfsan.fda.gov/~dms/foodlab. html#twoparts)

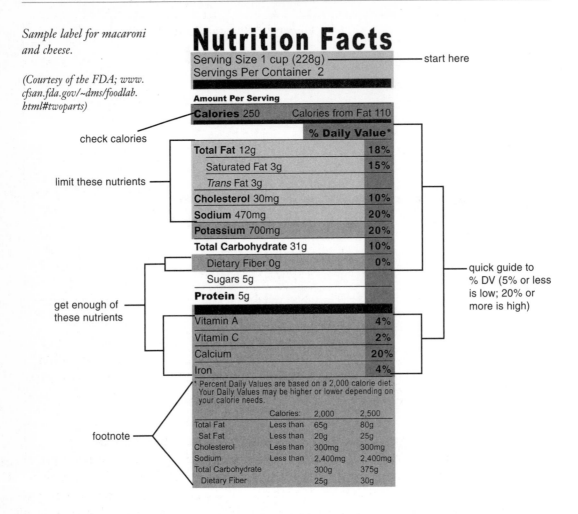

Nutrition Facts

Serving Size 1 cup (228g) —————— start here
Servings Per Container 2

Amount Per Serving

Calories 250   Calories from Fat 110

check calories

% Daily Value*

Total Fat 12g	**18%**
Saturated Fat 3g	**15%**
Trans Fat 3g	
Cholesterol 30mg	**10%**
Sodium 470mg	**20%**
Potassium 700mg	**20%**
Total Carbohydrate 31g	**10%**
Dietary Fiber 0g	**0%**
Sugars 5g	
Protein 5g	

limit these nutrients

get enough of these nutrients

Vitamin A	**4%**
Vitamin C	**2%**
Calcium	**20%**
Iron	**4%**

quick guide to % DV (5% or less is low; 20% or more is high)

* Percent Daily Values are based on a 2,000 calorie diet. Your Daily Values may be higher or lower depending on your calorie needs.

		Calories:	2,000	2,500
Total Fat	Less than		65g	80g
Sat Fat	Less than		20g	25g
Cholesterol	Less than		300mg	300mg
Sodium	Less than		2,400mg	2,400mg
Total Carbohydrate			300g	375g
Dietary Fiber			25g	30g

footnote

When looking at a food label, first and foremost, it's important to look at the serving size. Many times a seemingly small container or package contains more than one serving size, sometimes even three or four. Also, food manufacturers often cite larger serving sizes than what's generally recommended because they want you to buy more of their product. For example, a standard serving size of cooked pasta, per the Food Guide Pyramid (www.mypyramid.gov), is 1/2 cup cooked. However, many pasta manufacturers cite 1 cup cooked as a serving. Over time, this difference could add up to a lot of calories, so it's important to keep standard servings, shown in the following table, in mind.

Food	Generally Recommended Serving Size
Meat, chicken, fish, or tofu	3 ounces cooked (about the size of a deck of cards) at lunch and dinner
	1 ounce (about the size of an egg) at breakfast
Pasta, rice, or the equivalent	$^1/_2$ cup cooked
Vegetables	$^1/_2$ cup cooked veggies or 1 cup raw (broccoli, lettuce, etc.)
Fruit	1 medium piece fruit (exceptions include $^1/_2$ grapefruit) or 1 cup raw fruit (for example, melon, cantaloupe, strawberries, or blueberries)
Dairy	8 ounces skim or 1 percent milk, $^1/_2$ cup low-fat cottage cheese, or 1 ounce low-fat cheese (like part–skim milk mozzarella)

Looking at the calories and the number of servings per container is also key, especially if you're finding, several months or even years after surgery, you're eating more and more at one sitting, including snacks, and the calories and pounds are adding up. If you haven't looked at the serving size, calories, and number of servings per container, you could find your weight loss stopping or even notice weight regain when you thought your caloric intake was lower than it actually was.

The Percent Daily Value (%DV) is another important part of a standard food label, although your %DV may be very different after your surgery, especially if you had the D/S procedure. However, in general, 5 percent or less of the %DV on a label means a food or beverage is low in that nutrient. You want a low DV when it comes to things like cholesterol, trans or saturated fats, and sodium. (On the sample food label shown earlier, 12 grams fat is high, 3 grams trans fats is too high—you want to avoid this altogether—and 3 grams saturated fat is not ideal.)

If the %DV is 10 to 19 percent, it's a good source of that nutrient. You'd want 10 to 19 percent for fiber, vitamins, and minerals in general. And 20 percent or more of the DV in a food or beverage means it's high in that nutrient. If fresh fruits and vegetables all had food labels, they'd almost all have 20 percent or greater %DV for vitamins A and C and fiber. You'll find very few canned or processed food labels that could say that. (On the sample mac and cheese label earlier, calcium is 20 percent of DV, which is good, but it's low in vitamins A and C and in iron, so overall this is not a healthy food to include in your diet, certainly not on a regular basis.)

Food labels also cite calories, fat, cholesterol, sodium, and carbohydrate goals for Americans based on 2,000- and 2,500-calorie diets, with the lower level typically aimed for women and the higher calorie amount for men. However, after your weight loss surgery, it's highly likely neither of these caloric levels will be appropriate for you … at least not for several months post-op, even if you're tall and muscular and getting a lot of physical activity.

> **Food for Thought**
>
> In 1990, Congress passed the Nutrition Labeling and Education Act. This authorized some health claims for foods and standardized the food ingredient panel, including serving sizes and terms such as *low fat* and *light*.

Calories for the day: if you need to know how many calories you should be taking in after your surgery, check in with your center's dietitian. He or she may give you some pointers on the amount of food you're eating and the quality of your diet, which is just as important, if not more so, than the calories in your diet.

If you'd like to know how many calories your body is burning at rest, you can look into a place in your community that tests your resting energy expenditure (REE) via a metabolic cart (indirect calorimetry). Less accurate but sometimes helpful is a smaller device that can check your calories burned in a day; your dietitian may be able to recommend one. An appropriate activity factor will need to be added to know how many calories you really need in a day to maintain your current weight.

If you're working on weight loss, your dietitian can tell you how much you would need to reduce a day to lose about 1 pound per week. However, you'll want to avoid the dieting mentality or over-restricting of calories, which could possibly lead to rebound eating or overeating in the future if you feel chronically deprived.

Finally, a food label lists the ingredients in the food. The ingredient list goes from highest to lowest in order of weight, so the first 3 or 4 ingredients are the ones most represented in that food or beverage. Also, beware of certain terms in the ingredient list that may not be clear on the food label, such as *partially hydrogenated oils*, which are often a sign of trans fats that might not be listed on the label.

Carbohydrates

Carbohydrates, as you might remember from Chapter 2, come in many shapes and sizes. Some, like the simple carbs and processed carbs—high-fructose corn syrup (HFCS), for example—are probably best to avoid as much as possible. But can you spot the bad carbs on a food label among the good ones?

You'll see "Total Carbohydrate" on a food label, but as you know, that's not the whole story ... not by a long shot. Carbohydrates are further broken down into generally two parts: Dietary Fiber and Sugars. Dietary Fiber is sometimes broken down again to soluble and insoluble fiber (as we discussed in Chapter 2). Total Carbohydrate and Dietary Fiber can be helpful information if you have diabetes or blood sugar issues, particularly if you're on insulin therapy, when it's important to have the right ratio of carbs to insulin for proper blood sugar control and health.

"Sugars" refers to the simple versus complex carbohydrates, namely sucrose (table sugar), fructose (fruit sugar), lactose (milk sugar), galactose (milk sugar), maltose (grain sugar), and dextrose or glucose. Sugar alcohols such as sorbitol and maltitol are also found on a food label's ingredient list but may or may not be under the Total Carbohydrate heading. You typically want to limit sugars and sugar alcohols, especially after weight loss surgery. However, as you know, all sugars are not alike, so let's dig a little deeper.

> **Cooking Tip**
>
> When looking at carbohydrates on food labels, choose whole grains and at least 3 grams fiber per serving. Try to avoid breads and other foods that have simple sugars (e.g., HFCS, dextrose, sucrose) in the first three places on the ingredient list.

Carbs Versus Sugars Versus Sugar Alcohols

Take a look at the two yogurt labels on the following page. The plain yogurt has 10 grams sugars while the fruit yogurt has 44 grams. Now look at the ingredient list. Notice anything different between the two yogurts? The first one has natural sugar only from milk so the package can say "no added sugars." The fruit yogurt, however, has high-fructose corn syrup, which is not a naturally occurring sugar and most likely represents a great deal of the 44 grams sugars.

No daily reference value has been established for Sugars because no recommendations have been made for the total amount you should eat in a day. The Sugars listed on the Nutrition Facts label include the naturally occurring fruit (fructose) and milk (lactose) sugars, as well as simple table sugar that might be added, so it's important to check the ingredient list to understand the kinds of sugars in a food or beverage.

Nutrition Facts
Plain Yogurt

Serving Size 1 cup (226g)
Servings Per Container 1

Amount Per Serving

Calories 110   Calories from Fat 0

          % Daily Value*

Total Fat 0g	0%
Saturated Fat 0g	0%
Trans Fat 0g	
Cholesterol Less than 5mg	1%
Sodium 160mg	7%
Total Carbohydrate 15g	5%
Dietary Fiber 0g	0%
Sugars 10g	
Protein 13g	
Vitamin A	0%
Vitamin C	4%
Calcium	45%
Iron	0%

* Percent Daily Values based on a 2,000 calorie diet.
Your Daily Values may be higher or lower depending on
your calorie needs.

	Calories	2,000	2,500
Total Fat	Less than	65g	80g
Sat Fat	Less than	20g	25g
Cholesterol	Less than	300mg	300mg
Sodium	Less than	2,400mg	2,400mg
Total Carbohydrate		300g	375g
Dietary Fiber		25g	30g

Ingredients: Cultured pasteurized grade A
nonfat milk, whey protein concentrate,
pectin, carrageenan.

Nutrition Facts
Fruit Yogurt

Serving Size 1 cup (227g)
Servings Per Container 1

Amount Per Serving

Calories 240   Calories from Fat 25

          % Daily Value*

Total Fat 3g	4%
Saturated Fat 1.5g	9%
Trans Fat 0g	
Cholesterol 15mg	5%
Sodium 140mg	6%
Total Carbohydrate 46g	15%
Dietary Fiber 1g	3%
Sugars 44g	
Protein 9g	
Vitamin A	2%
Vitamin C	4%
Calcium	35%
Iron	0%

* Percent Daily Values based on a 2,000 calorie diet.
Your Daily Values may be higher or lower depending on
your calorie needs.

	Calories	2,000	2,500
Total Fat	Less than	65g	80g
Sat Fat	Less than	20g	25g
Cholesterol	Less than	300mg	300mg
Sodium	Less than	2,400mg	2,400mg
Total Carbohydrate		300g	375g
Dietary Fiber		25g	30g

Ingredients: Cultured grade A reduced
fat milk, apples, high fructose corn syrup,
cinnamon, nutmeg, natural flavors, and
pectin. Contains active yogurt and I,
acidophilus cultures.

Nutrition Facts labels for two kinds of yogurt, plain (left) and fruit (right).

Some healthy carbs may *look* like they're unhealthy because the label lists Sugars
in higher amounts than you might think the food would have. For example, an
8-ounce glass of skim milk is healthful, of course, but lists about 12 grams "sugars" on
the label, due to the lactose, or milk sugar. Lactose is a simple sugar, so it shows up as
table sugar would. This happens with fruit, too. If you're buying canned fruit in water,
you might be surprised to see about 12 grams sugars in a small can. Has the manufacturer lied and added table sugar? No, but remember that fruit contains a simple sugar
called fructose.

Sugars on a label often point out simple sugars, such as table sugar. However, they may also include natural sugars found in milk (lactose) and fruit (fructose), so they're not necessarily all bad, and this makes it hard to recommend foods with 0 sugars. After gastric bypass surgery, try to eat food with around 15 grams or less sugars at a sitting to lower the risk of dumping syndrome. However, even patients who don't dump or those of you who've had other bariatric procedures probably don't need extra simple sugars, so still keep it around 15 grams. This doesn't mean, of course, that something that has 16 or even 20 grams sugars is going to make you ill or gain all your weight back. These are certainly just guidelines and may help you with your weight as well as possibly blood sugar control and hunger.

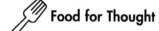

Food for Thought

Every 4 grams sugars on a label represents 16 calories and the equivalent of a packet of table sugar.

As you learned in Chapter 2, sugar alcohols aren't the kind of alcohol you drink from a bottle, or ethanol, but since they have a sugar backbone and OH added to it, or hydroxyl group in chemistry terms, they're in the alcohol family. Sugar alcohols ferment in your colon to short chain fatty acids (SCFAs) and may cause gas, bloating, and diarrhea, so you may want to look closely for them on a food label. They'll have their own section under Total Carbohydrates called "Sugar Alcohols," and they typically end in *-ol*, as in *sorbitol*, *mannitol*, and *erythritol*. If you see sugar alcohols on a label, be extra careful, especially if a label lists more than 10 grams per serving of sugar alcohols because you may get diarrhea or feel pretty uncomfortable after consuming that food. (So don't try that food while you're away on a hiking trip, for example.)

"Net Carbs" and Fiber

Net carbs has become a popular term these days, but what does it really mean, and is it valid? Net carbs is more of a marketing term aimed at appealing to the low-carb-diet consumer. It essentially involves subtracting grams of carbohydrate cited as fiber and sugar alcohols due to the notion that your body cannot absorb those calories or non-caloric sweeteners, so it's okay to subtract these carb grams from the label and call the resulting amount of carbs "net" carbs. In this way, it appears the consumer is taking in fewer calories and better adhering to a low-carb meal plan. However, this is not really the case.

Although humans don't possess the enzyme to digest fiber for calories, the same isn't true with sugar alcohols. It's estimated that your body can absorb about half of the calories from sugar alcohols, so people with diabetes and those watching their carb intakes should take this into account.

How Much Is Right for Me?

If you have diabetes or blood sugar issues, counting your carbs may be something your doctor and dietitian have asked you to do. Although weight loss surgery may have improved and maybe (hopefully) put your diabetes in remission, it's still probably a good idea to watch your simple carbs and keep your overall carbs down to minimize caloric intake.

It's impossible to arbitrarily suggest carb goals per meal or snack, but keep in mind that your brain needs a minimum of about 125 grams carbs a day to ensure its glucose needs. If you divide that among 3 meals and perhaps a couple snacks, then you're looking at a minimum of 25 grams carbohydrates at every meal and 25 grams at snacks. This might sound like a lot, but 1 large banana contains about 30 grams carbohydrates.

Protein

Protein is one of the most important components in your diet, not only for healing post-op but to help with hunger as well. Luckily, it's also pretty straightforward on the food label (unlike carbs and sugars!).

Depending on your procedure, your protein needs may vary from 60 to 120 grams per day, so you'll most likely want to aim for at least 20 grams each at lunch and dinner (about the size of a deck of playing cards' worth of meat, chicken, fish, or tofu) and ideally a minimum of 10 grams at breakfast, with at least 10 to 15 grams at each snack. Of course, if you had the D/S, these goals may need to be adjusted or high-protein drinks continued indefinitely after surgery to help you meet your protein goals.

Reading Into It

As discussed in Chapter 3, certain kinds of protein are higher in quality than others, and some are downright failures. Collagen is among the failures, so you'll want to know key words in the ingredient list that could tip you off to the issue, such as *collagen*, of course, but also *hydrolyzed animal protein*, *predigested protein*, etc.

When you're reading protein labels for a supplement, look for high-quality whey protein isolate or soy protein isolate, which have excellent protein scores. Whey protein concentrate is also generally high quality, but not quite as high as whey protein isolate. Important to note is that the concentrate form has lactose, so if you have gas, bloating, or diarrhea after your gastric bypass or D/S procedure, and you chose a whey concentrate versus isolate, a lactase pill to digest lactose could be just what the doctor ordered.

 Post-Op Pitfall _____

Collagen-based supplements are made up of animal connective tissue and are poor quality because they're missing tryptophan, an important amino acid or building block of protein. Avoid these supplements, as their absorption rate is estimated at only 16 to 50 percent of the protein listed on the label.

How Much Is Too Much?

Maybe you've heard that your body can't absorb more than 30 grams protein at a time. That's a myth, although there is some debate about how much protein you can absorb with certain procedures, such as the D/S. Studies seem to confirm that at least several months out, you should be able to absorb more than 30 grams protein at a time. However, Margaret generally doesn't recommend this, for several reasons.

The first involves a "get it over with" scenario in the honeymoon stage. Having just one meal a day is setting yourself up for hunger and overeating or eating too fast, especially when the hunger hormones come back. Instead, your body will appreciate it more if you plan on 20 to 35 grams protein at least every 5 hours or so, even if you're not hungry, to get in the habit of 3 meals a day.

Another reason to avoid supplements with 50 to 60 grams protein each, even if they're high quality, is the potential for dehydration. Your kidneys need a lot more water to flush out the waste products and toxins from a very high-protein supplement. You might notice this if your urine is very foamy. Also, darker urine may be confirmation that you're dehydrated (see Chapter 5).

 Cooking Tip _____

Aim for at least 3 servings of 20 to 35 grams protein a day when you're starting out on post-op supplements, no more than 5 hours apart. It will not only be less dehydrating than 50+-gram protein shakes, but also more weight friendly.

The Skinny on What You Need

We touched on estimating protein needs after weight loss surgery in Chapter 3, with the goal around 60 to 80 grams a day for gastric banding, sleeve, and gastric bypass, and 80 to 120 grams a day for D/S—with exceptions, of course, based on physical activity, weight training, and overall muscle mass. If you're taking in the recommended amounts, however, and your lab work (your prealbumin and albumin) reveals your protein status might be low, check with your dietitian to evaluate your diet.

If you're eating high-quality protein like meat, chicken, eggs, or tofu and avoiding low-quality supplements like collagen, you might not be getting enough carbohydrates to spare protein, or to allow the protein in your diet to be used for your muscles, etc., instead of for energy needs. This can happen with very-low-carb diets, and you get that less-than-lovely breath from ketosis to prove it.

Working with your dietitian to add healthy carbs in the right amounts your body needs and wants is important. Your ultimate goal should be around 130 grams carbohydrates per day, say by the time you're about 6 months post-op, although it may take several months to get there. Protein is something you really want to work on to get at least 60 grams protein in as soon as possible after your surgery, with your goal possibly as high as 120 grams protein per day if you had the D/S procedure or have other reasons for needing more protein. If you're already doing this and still low in your protein labs, it may be that the total amount of grams protein or the quality of the protein in your diet may need to be increased, despite the goals set for you at your center.

Fats

When it comes to meat, chicken, and fish, certain cuts or parts of the various animals are leaner and may help you keep down your overall fat and calories. They can also help decrease the risk of dumping from increased fat content because fats slow the emptying of your stomach and may cause diarrhea, especially if eaten too fast. High fat intakes could increase your risk of dumping and diarrhea because they may be too much for your body to handle, especially early after your surgery when you're getting used to your new anatomy. At the very least, high-fat foods could feel very heavy and cause you to feel lethargic or sluggish. In addition, they're high in calories, so they may slow down your weight loss, especially if you didn't have the D/S where malabsorption of fat is expected.

If you're buying a frozen meal, for example, that lists the amount of fat as 20 percent of the Daily Value (DV) or higher, you'll probably want to select another one that's lower, unless the fat is coming from healthy fat, like salmon. Having some meatless meals and opting instead for tofu or beans and rice (ideally brown) can help decrease fat and calories as well as cholesterol.

Your entrées should generally contain less than 30 percent of calories from fat to keep down not only the calories, but also your risk of heart disease, although D/S patients may need higher amounts of fat.

> **Cooking Tip**
>
> When shopping for meats, look for loin or round cuts, which are leaner. And when cooking, cut away fat and remove the skin from the meat, chicken, or poultry to reduce a lot of the fat and calories.

Mono, Poly, Sat, and Trans Uncovered

Monounsaturated fats, you'll recall, are the hero fats in your diet, as are, to a lesser extent, the polyunsaturated fats, although the latter should be consumed in smaller percentages to decrease the risk for inflammation. When you're looking at a food label, fats will first be listed as a total number, followed by saturated fats, trans fats, polyunsaturated fats, and monounsaturated fats.

As we saw in Chapter 4, trans fats are the twisted villains and should be limited as much as possible in your diet. As of January 1, 2006, the Food and Drug Administration (FDA) mandated that all foods be labeled as containing trans fats if they contained 0.5 grams or more per serving. A food with 0.49 grams per serving would not, technically, need to list it. This is currently being debated because it's believed that even small amounts of trans fats can be harmful to your health, so you may see this law get stricter with regard to the amount of trans fats per serving that must be identified on the food label. If trans fat isn't declared on a label and you're curious, contact the manufacturer and ask for this information.

You *Can* Eat Too Little

The recommended daily allowance (RDA) is nonexistent for fats. However, there is an acceptable macronutrient distribution range (AMDR) set at 20 to 35 grams fat per day. The AMDR is the range of intake for fat that's linked with reduced risk of chronic disease, such as heart disease. Although everyone's individual needs are different, especially after weight loss surgery, someone consuming less than 20 grams fat per day several months after surgery may be at risk for inadequate fat intake. This can be a problem because your body can't make all the fat it needs. You must get two essential fatty acids—linoleic (omega-6) and alpha-linolenic (omega-3)—from your diet.

In addition, your body needs at least 10 grams fat or so to best absorb vitamins A, D, E, and K, the fat-soluble vitamins. D/S patients need much more than the AMDR because an estimated 73 percent fat malabsorption occurs after this procedure. Finally, your body needs a certain amount to properly manufacture hormones, including estrogen, testosterone, and cholesterol (more about cholesterol later in this chapter).

Possible Perils of Too Much

As there are possible dangers to eating too little fat, there are also perils to consuming too much fat, including dumping or diarrhea for gastric bypass patients and risk for chronic loose stools if you had the D/S procedure.

Even if you don't have these issues, particularly if you had the gastric banding or gastric sleeve, keep in mind that fats have more than twice the calories of carbohydrates and proteins, so they may cause the scale to tip in an unfavorable way if you continually increase your fat intake, especially if you're not a D/S patient.

 Food for Thought

When reading a food label, keep in mind that every 5 grams fat is the equivalent to the fat in a pat of butter, or about 45 calories.

De-"Livering" the Facts About Cholesterol

When you look at a food label, Cholesterol has a section of its own, below the fats section, but not part of it. You may be surprised to learn that cholesterol is not a fat at all but a waxylike substance that's made in your liver. Your body only needs about 1 gram a day, but some people's livers make too much cholesterol.

Because your body makes it, you may not need to get cholesterol from your diet. However, I've certainly seen post-op patients with low cholesterol levels (less than 150 milligrams per deciliter or mg/dL) that could be due to malnutrition. Your doctor will want to assess your cholesterol level because sometimes staying on cholesterol-lowering medications after surgery when they're no longer needed can cause a too-low cholesterol level. A truly low cholesterol level should be evaluated for possible malnutrition, as this can be a red flag for health issues.

Why It's Not All About Cholesterol

Many people feel that cholesterol is one of the most important things to watch in your diet if your doctor has told you that your cholesterol level is high. Although it's not a bad idea to watch your cholesterol as part of a low-fat, heart-healthy diet, studies show trans fats, saturated fats, and total fat have a larger influence on cholesterol production in your body.

Which foods have cholesterol? Well, cholesterol is made in the liver of animals and humans alike, and that's the only place where it's made. Therefore, as Margaret has said for years in classes she's taught, "if it doesn't have a mother, it doesn't have cholesterol." This doesn't mean it's healthy if it doesn't have cholesterol because trans and saturated fats can have more of a negative effect on your cholesterol than cholesterol in foods, and your genetics could affect this a great deal, in terms of how much cholesterol your liver naturally makes.

However, saturated fats and trans fats are building blocks of cholesterol synthesis in your body. In a sense, the more saturated and trans fats that you eat, the more cholesterol your body will make.

Food Label Cues to Help Lower Your Cholesterol

As you know, trans and saturated fats can increase your cholesterol level higher and faster than cholesterol in your diet. Therefore, try to keep them as low as possible, avoiding trans fats altogether, and keeping saturated fats to less than 10 percent of your fat calories, if not lower, because your body can make these fats if necessary, and most people have too much on board.

Soluble fiber is important to help lower your cholesterol level because it appears to bind fatty acids and bile and helps your body get rid of them. Therefore, your daily bowl of old-fashioned oatmeal, as part of a low-fat balanced meal plan, might just help your cholesterol level stay or get healthy. In terms of low-cholesterol guidelines, less than 300 milligrams a day is recommended, or about the equivalent of 1½ eggs.

If your doctor wants you to limit cholesterol and fat from your diet and you love eggs, keep the egg white and discard the yolk. That's where all the fat and cholesterol lies. About 3 days a week, you could keep one of the yolks and discard the others, so your 2- or 3-egg omelet tastes richer but only has the fat and cholesterol of 1 egg. Or you could have a 2-egg omelet (with 2 egg yolks) one day and 1-egg omelet (1 egg yolk) another day. In other words, aiming for a total of 3 eggs yolks per week (e.g., egg white only omelet most days, but allowing yourself 3 egg yolks a week total), could help you stay within the American Heart Association's guidelines for lower cholesterol intake.

Sodium

On the food label, Sodium is listed below Cholesterol and above Total Carbohydrate. This is important to know because studies show most Americans consume far more sodium than their bodies need, especially if they eat fast foods and convenience foods. Your body usually doesn't need more than 2 grams per day—unless you're running marathons or triathlons, work in construction, live in a very hot climate, or otherwise are sweating a great deal every day.

Food for Thought

One teaspoon salt contains approximately 2,000 milligrams sodium. The average American is estimated to consume more than 3,500 milligrams sodium per day.

How much do *you* need? According to the Institute of Medicine, adults 50 and older and those with high blood pressure should aim for about 1,500 milligrams sodium a day. Younger adults who are healthy should aim for a maximum of approximately 2,300 milligrams per day. Food labels list, toward the bottom, guidelines for sodium suggesting less than 2,400 milligrams sodium per day. A good rule of thumb is usually no more than 600 milligrams sodium per meal.

It's important to read ingredient labels carefully and avoid foods that have sodium in the first three ingredients. For example, watch out for soups and other canned and frozen foods because they commonly have added sodium for preservation as well as taste. But sodium can wear many masks. Let's find out what some of the common forms of sodium are and how you can recognize them.

Nitrites, MSG, and More

Nitrites are a food additive, often added to cured meats such as bacon to help lengthen the shelf life. Unfortunately, they also add quite a bit of sodium. What's more, when used together with salt, nitrites become a food preservative as well as flavor enhancer. These nitrite salts react with amines in foods, and the result is the production of substances called nitrosamines, which are believed to cause cancer. For this reason, keep foods containing nitrites to a bare minimum, if avoiding them altogether isn't possible.

Monosodium glutamate (MSG), the salt of *glutamate*, is used as a flavor enhancer in foods. MSG is made commercially via a fermentation process that's actually natural and utilizes sugar and starch. It's been estimated that MSG is included in a large number of foods but is disguised on the ingredient labels. If you see *hydrolyzed protein* on an ingredient label, know that it often contains MSG, so avoid it if you have MSG sensitivities.

def•i•ni•tion

Glutamate, an amino acid or building block of protein, is found naturally in protein-containing foods such as cheese, milk, meat, mushrooms, fish, and even vegetables.

Although there have been reports of MSG-triggered asthma and headaches, MSG has been deemed a safe food additive at normal consumption levels by several respected organizations, including the American Medical Association, the United Nations, the National Academy of Sciences, and the World Health Organization.

What Level Might Be Best for You

It's estimated that at least 30 percent of people who have high blood pressure are salt-sensitive, meaning it can increase their blood pressure. According to the American Heart Association, a third of American adults have high blood pressure, and many don't know it. Although your blood pressure may be in good control, especially after weight loss surgery, it makes sense to keep to the Institute of Medicine's guidelines of around 2,300 milligrams sodium per day if you're healthy and about 1,500 milligrams a day if you have heart or blood pressure issues.

Potassium Is A-OK!

Potassium, known chemically as K+, is an important mineral for your heart. Studies have shown that you're at higher risk for high blood pressure if your diet is low in potassium, especially if it's low in calcium as well. Potassium may not be something you're used to seeing on food labels, however, because the greatest source of this precious mineral is fruits and vegetables. Therefore, unless you're eating canned fruits, you won't see potassium on labels on a regular basis.

Food for Thought

Research has concluded that a high-potassium diet may help lower blood pressure and your risk for heart disease.

However, this is an important mineral that could be depleted after surgery, particularly if you're having diarrhea or loose stool issues, because a great amount of potassium is lost in stools. Of course, if you have kidney disease your doctor may ask you to limit your potassium.

If your kidneys are healthy and there's no other reason to limit potassium, aim for an eventual goal of at least 2,000 milligrams per day, which you could get from at least 5 or 6 fruits and vegetables per day. These are the greatest sources of this mineral, especially the brightly colored fruits and vegetables.

Don't worry if you can't meet this goal the first few months after surgery; hopefully by 6 to 9 months post-op you'll be able to meet it easily.

Additives and Preservatives

The FDA defines *additive* as "any substance, the intended use of which results or may reasonably be expected to result, directly or indirectly, in its becoming a component or otherwise affecting the characteristics of any food." In other words, an additive is any substance that's added to food to enhance or preserve flavor or improve the appearance.

Direct additives are those intentionally added for a specific purpose. Indirect additives are those the food is exposed to during processing, packaging, or storing. Preservatives are additives that inhibit the growth of bacteria, yeasts, or molds in foods.

The safety and overall benefits of many artificial food additives have been hotly debated of late, with some people citing food dyes and colorings as a prime contributor in the seemingly sharp rise in food allergies and sensitivities among American children. Some people also link the apparent increase in attention deficit hyperactivity disorder (ADHD) to the rise of food colors and dyes in the food supply. Still other reports suggest chronic inflammation from food additives that may possibly contribute, over the course of many years, to a higher risk for diseases such as diabetes and heart disease. Of course, this area is not without controversy, and more research is needed.

Food additives and preservatives play a very important role, ensuring the food supply stays safe and abundant. The FDA is charged with regulating the use and approval of thousands of approved food

Food for Thought

As a result of the 1958 Food Additives Amendment to the Federal Food, Drug, and Cosmetic Act of 1938, the FDA must approve the use of all additives. It's the manufacturer's responsibility to ensure the additive is safe for its intended use.

additives, as well as evaluating their safety. Scientific evidence is lacking when it comes to consumers' concerns and complaints of food additives and preservatives, despite the media's portrayal of their health risks.

The FDA constantly monitors the safety of all food additives and takes into account any new scientific evidence called to its attention. However, it's faced with a difficult and daunting task, especially amid the vast numbers of existing preservatives and additives. While use of known dangerous substances such as FD & C No. 3 in cosmetics and certain externally applied drugs are banned due to findings of tumors in rats, complaints regarding other substances such as mild itching or hives in a small percent of the population may be less harmful. Therefore, the FDA must weigh what is generally recognized as safe (GRAS) in the final analysis.

The Least You Need to Know

- Carbohydrates, proteins, and fats can be easily deciphered on food labels if you know the basics.

- Limiting trans and saturated fats is a better way to lower your cholesterol level than limiting cholesterol.

- Most people take in more sodium than their body needs.

- Potassium is an important mineral that may help control blood pressure.

- Additives and preservatives are not without controversy but are generally regarded as safe.

Chapter 8

Food as Medicine

In This Chapter

- ◆ Nutraceuticals and other healing foods
- ◆ The skinny on antioxidants
- ◆ Probiotics and how they can help you
- ◆ Gut hormones made simple

This chapter gives you a glimpse into some of the new supplements and technology available to help you maximize your health and possibly enhance your weight loss. Some sections may be a little on the technical side, but we've tried to give you an overview of possibly new tools to help you make the most of your surgery and health.

Some of the buzz words mentioned in the following pages could help you better understand some of the exciting new products and supplements out in the market, and the highlights we give you are designed to provide just the right amount of information so you can make good choices in terms of whether they might be right for you. However, it's always recommended that you check with your surgical team and primary-care doctor before starting on any supplements that haven't been approved already.

Foods That Can Help Cure

This chapter is chock full of exciting new developments in the field of nutrition and information on how you can capitalize on these developments to maximize not only your weight loss success, but also your quality of life and longevity. Let's take a look into the latest and greatest happenings in nutrition and how they pertain to you.

The New Nutrition Buzzword: *Nutraceuticals*

Stephen DeFelic, M.D., an endocrinologist and founder of the Foundation for Innovation in Medicine (FIM), coined the term *nutraceutical* back in 1989 by combining the words *nutrition* and *pharmaceutical*. That was 20 years ago, but most Americans still aren't very familiar with it. Maybe it's the first time you're even hearing it. You can bet you'll be hearing more and more about nutraceuticals in the years to come.

Nutraceutical is mostly a marketing term, but people using the word are generally referring to food or ingredient(s) that somehow provide health or medical benefits to either prevent or treat disease. Nutraceuticals range from vitamins and minerals, dietary supplements, and specific diets to genetically engineered designer foods, herbal and botanical products, and even processed beverages, soups, and cereals.

For example, it's believed that a large proportion of the U.S. population is deficient in vitamin D. Nutraceuticals may include vitamin D at high levels—50,000 international units (IUs) once a week—so it works at a pharmacological dose or drug level to help normalize your vitamin D if it's low, which is not uncommon before and after weight loss surgery. Therefore, use of vitamin D in this way could be viewed as a nutraceutical. In contrast, the amount of vitamin D found in a glass of skim milk would not qualify as a neutraceutical because the vitamin D is not found in pharmacological doses.

Another example of nutraceuticals includes omega-3 fatty acids (see Chapter 4). Eating fatty fish like salmon a few times a week to help lower your risk of heart disease is one thing, but taking omega-3 capsules daily at the level the American Heart Association recommends for people with high triglyceride levels (2,000 to 4,000 milligrams DHA and EPA combined) is a whole new ballgame. However, if your doctor approves this for you and it helps bring down your triglyceride and cholesterol without the side effects of meds, it might be worth it to you. Check with your doctor and surgical team at your center, including your dietitian, to see if nutraceuticals may be right for you. It's highly possible that you're already on one (e.g., vitamin D at high levels) and didn't realize it.

Other examples of nutraceuticals include usage of herbs in place of traditional medicine, such as kava or lavender for anxiety (see Appendix B). Talk to your doctor before trying one of these remedies. Despite the fact they're natural, they might interfere with a medication you're taking or possibly cause a dangerous situation. For example, taking pharmacological or very high doses of garlic or St. John's wort could potentially make your blood too thin. However, if you're looking for a more holistic way to treat common ailments, such as a headache or minor ache or pain, you may want to talk with your doctor about alternative treatments that may include nutraceuticals. Nutraceuticals fit under the umbrella of natural foods products, which fit under the Dietary Supplement Health and Education Act (DSHEA) of 1994 and, therefore, are not regulated by the FDA.

These days, the supplement industry, including nutraceuticals, is a multibillion-dollar business, and it gets a little tricky to define a nutraceutical from a run-of-the-mill vitamin or protein drink. However, the main idea behind nutraceuticals is that selected organic extracts may have beneficial effects on both the body and mind and have far fewer side effects, if any, compared to the well-published risks of standard drugs on the market today.

Nutraceuticals, along with *functional foods*, appear to be taking their place comfortably between drugs and traditional foods, and more and more Americans are gladly making room on their shelves. Nutraceuticals and functional foods hold promise in clinical therapy because they have the potential to significantly reduce the risks or side effects linked with traditional drugs and may help reduce global health-care costs.

def•i•ni•tion

Foods that provide nutraceutical-type benefits have come to be known as **functional foods**. For example, eggs fortified with omega-3 fatty acids to help fight or prevent heart disease are a functional food.

Organic Foods ... Worth the Money?

In Margaret's 20 or so years working as a dietitian, she's been asked many times if organic foods are really worth the apparent hype surrounding them. She used to say "no" and cite their higher cost and little or no difference in quality. However, after researching organic foods fully, her answer has certainly changed.

Organic foods need to be "certified organic" to truly meet the high standards they are known for. This certification involves many rules and years of work for farmers to ensure the soil is free of synthetic chemicals and pesticides—typically at least 3 years before even being considered for a site inspection. Also, in most countries, including the United States, producers must obtain organic certification to market their food as organic. Certified organic means the food was grown without pesticides, additives, and genetically modified (GM) crops. Organic farming also helps protect wildlife and the environment, including fighting global warming.

If you're aware of the possible benefits of organic foods but are wary of the higher prices, we hear you loud and clear. Fortunately, some fruits and vegetables are less prone to contamination by pesticides and other harmful chemicals. The foods that may be safe to buy nonorganic are as follows:

◆ Asparagus	◆ Cabbage	◆ Papayas
◆ Avocados	◆ Kiwi	◆ Pineapple
◆ Bananas	◆ Mangoes	
◆ Broccoli	◆ Onions	

Other fruits and vegetables are at a much higher risk for contamination from pesticides or harmful chemicals. Go organic with the following if you can afford it:

◆ Apples	◆ Peaches	◆ Spinach
◆ Cantaloupe	◆ Pears	◆ Strawberries
◆ Grapes	◆ Potatoes	◆ Tomatoes
◆ Green beans	◆ Raspberries	◆ Winter squash

Although organic foods are more expensive than traditional farming produce, farmers' markets are usually more wallet friendly, so if you can spring for it, try to go organic with the high-risk produce.

Food for Thought

Fewer pesticides are used on yellow and green apples than on red apples.

In addition to lowering your risks for contamination, organic fruits and vegetables have been found to contain more minerals such as chromium, selenium, and calcium and lower amounts of potentially toxic minerals like aluminum, lead, and mercury. (To learn more about organic foods, check out Appendix B.)

Amazing Antioxidants

Antioxidants are phytochemicals, vitamins, and other nutrients that protect cells from damage as a result of *free radicals*, and in doing so are believed to help lower the risk of diseases such as cancer and heart disease. Ironically, antioxidants have the ability to neutralize free radicals by actually becoming free radicals themselves. However, antioxidants change afterward to become inactive, rather than becoming another free radical. Bottom line: antioxidants are constantly in battle, for your sake, to help your body get rid of bad/unhealthy free radicals by accepting some of their energy, in essence, but then getting rid of it and helping your body stay in healthy balance. If your body is short on antioxidants or free radicals go unchecked, they could not only increase the aging process, but also raise your risk of developing cancers and possibly increasing your risk of diseases, such as heart disease.

def•i•ni•tion

Free radicals are "radical" molecules, created in your body as part of your natural metabolism, that are unstable and react with the essential molecules, including DNA, fat, and proteins. Free radicals try to either steal or give electrons to other molecules, and in so doing, change their chemical structure. Environmental factors such as smoking, pollution, pesticides, and radiation can cause free radicals on a regular basis. Some health experts recommend daily antioxidant therapy to help combat free radicals.

Antioxidants are found in foods as vitamins like C and E, minerals such as selenium, carotenoids like beta-carotene or provitamin A, polyphenols, and other compounds found in plants. Antioxidants are most abundant in fruits and vegetables, as well as medicinal herbs and some culinary herbs. Many are often identified by their bright colors, such as the deep orange of carrots, the deep reds of tomatoes and cherries, and the blue-purple of blueberries and blackberries.

What the Studies Say

Research done in 2006 revealed that increasing the variety of fruits and vegetables in your diet may increase the positive effects of antioxidants in your body and lower your risk of cancer and heart disease. It's believed to be better to consume a small amount of many different antioxidants than a large amount of only a few phytochemicals or antioxidants. The American Heart Association and the American Cancer Society recommend healthy adults consume 5 or more servings of fruits and vegetables a day, and the National Cancer Institute ran a "5-A-Day for Better Health" campaign based on antioxidants.

Antioxidant research is ongoing and continues to confirm that antioxidants from fruits and vegetables, as well as whole grains, may reduce disease risk. While our bodies have defenses against oxidative stress, recent studies have revealed that people with higher weight or obesity have significantly higher levels of oxidative stress than lower-weight individuals. Therefore, antioxidant therapy may help counteract some of the negative health associations with higher weight and potentially help reduce the risk of associated diseases such as diabetes and cancer.

The Hot Antioxidants

What's old is new again, and that's the case with many of the hot antioxidants today, although some new ones, such as resveratrol in grapes, are being highly regarded as well. Let's look at some of the most popular antioxidants.

Vitamin E is a fat-soluble vitamin that's part of a family of eight antioxidants, the most famous being alpha-tocopherol. The main function of alpha-tocopherol in humans is as an antioxidant. Vitamin E intercepts the free radicals formed during normal metabolism and upon exposure to cigarette smoke or other environmental pollutants and then prevents a chain reaction of fat destruction. Alpha-tocopherol also protects cell membranes throughout your body, as well as fats in low-density lipoproteins (LDL, the bad cholesterol) from oxidizing. Therefore, this helpful vitamin and antioxidant may possibly help lower your risk of heart disease. Sources of vitamin E in your diet are limited though, so vitamin and mineral supplementation is the best way to go to get what your body needs.

Food for Thought

While warding off free radicals, alpha-tocopherol is altered in such a way that its antioxidant powers are lost. Fortunately, other antioxidants, such as vitamin C, are able to regenerate alpha-tocopherol's antioxidant abilities. Therefore, it's generally a good idea to take a supplement with more than one antioxidant like both vitamin C and vitamin E.

Vitamin C is a well-known antioxidant perhaps made famous by studies suggesting it could cure the common cold. Although this remains under debate, vitamin C is certainly known for its role in the growth and repair of tissues in all parts of your body. Vitamin C is critical for the formation of collagen, a vital protein needed to make skin, tendons, ligaments, and blood vessels. It's essential for healing of wounds and repair and maintenance of bones, teeth, and cartilage. As an antioxidant, vitamin C helps block damage from free radicals.

Like other vitamins, such as vitamins E and A, your body doesn't make vitamin C, so you need to get it from your diet. All fruits and vegetables contain at least some vitamin C, but the highest sources are found in green peppers, citrus fruits, strawberries, tomatoes, broccoli, and leafy green vegetables.

Vitamin C toxicity is rare, because your body can't store it, but amounts greater than 2,000 milligrams a day may lead to stomach upset and diarrhea. These higher doses, if stopped abruptly, may lead to "rebound scurvy" or signs of vitamin C deficiency, including dry, splitting hair; bleeding gums; rough, dry, scaly skin; easy bruising; nosebleeds; anemia; swollen and painful joints; weakened tooth enamel; and possible weight gain due to slowed metabolism. Generally speaking, up to about 1,000 milligrams (same as 1 gram) vitamin C per day is usually considered safe and won't increase your risk for rebound scurvy or stomach upset.

Vitamin A is an antioxidant that plays an important role in many vital bodily functions, including bone growth, vision, cell division, and reproduction. It also helps manage your immune system by making white blood cells that kill harmful bacteria and viruses, helping your body fight off infections. However, there are two forms of vitamin A, and one is certainly a higher-quality antioxidant than the other.

The vitamin A found in foods that come from animals, which is called *preformed vitamin A*, is actually absorbed in your body as retinol, one of the most active, and usable, forms of vitamin A. Retinol can be found in foods that come from animals, such as whole eggs, milk, and liver. In the United States, most skim milk and dried nonfat milk solids sold are fortified with vitamin A to replace the amount lost when the fat was removed. In addition, foods such as fortified cereals typically also have additional vitamin A, usually in the retinol form, like retinol palmitate commonly seen in cereals.

The vitamin A found in colorful fruits and vegetables is called *provitamin A carotenoid*. This form can be turned into retinol in your body. Beta-carotene is one of three common provitamin A carotenoids found in foods that come from plants and is easily made into retinol, the kind of vitamin A absorbed from animal sources. Provitamin A carotenoids, a part of the vitamin A family, are found in greatest amounts in darkly colored fruits and vegetables, such as carrots, cantaloupe, spinach, and sweet potatoes. In the United States, about 26 percent of vitamin A consumed by men and 34 percent of vitamin A consumed by women is in this form of provitamin A carotenoids. This

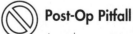 **Post-Op Pitfall**

Avoid excessive amounts of vitamin A as retinol because it has the potential for toxicity, unlike the provitamin A carotenoids.

type of vitamin A is not considered dangerous, in terms of toxicity, because whatever your body needs will be excreted. Therefore, you could ingest up to 100,000 international units (IUs) vitamin A as beta-carotene but not store it, although the palms of your hands and soles of your feet might turn orange from the beta-carotene pigment.

In contrast, your body *does* store the retinol form of vitamin A, so doses of about 25,000 IUs for anywhere from 8 to 12 months could increase your risk for toxicity, with possible signs and symptoms including blurred vision. Night blindness, in contrast, could suggest vitamin A deficiency versus toxicity, so your center should do blood tests to further investigate if you're having any visual changes.

Believe it or not, there are 563 known carotenoids, but fewer than 10 percent can be made into vitamin A in our bodies. Lycopene, lutein, zeaxanthin, and beta-cryptoxanthine don't have vitamin A activity, but do have other health benefits. Lycopene sources include tomatoes, watermelon, and grapefruit, with tomatoes having the greatest source of lycopene. As a natural antioxidant, lycopene has been linked with prevention of diseases such as heart disease, prostate cancer, and gastrointestinal cancer.

High intakes of retinyl esters (traditional vitamin A) can enhance the bioavailability (a.k.a absorption rate) of selenium, an essential constituent of several glutathione-dependent peroxidases or potent antioxidants, so it's important to be sure you're getting enough vitamin A, but not excessive amounts in the storage form or retinol versus the nonstorage form of beta-carotene.

Glutathione (GSH) is an antioxidant and detoxifying agent made in your liver, kidneys, and other tissues, including your gastrointestinal (GI) tract. GSH's availability is affected by the aging process, as well as disease, because these two conditions result in decreased tissue and blood levels. GSH in your liver is crucial for detoxification, and the higher amount you have, the better your body can ward off harmful chemicals, such as free radicals and toxins found in alcohol and other substances. Glutathione is dependent on other vitamins and minerals for optimal functioning, namely vitamin B_6, riboflavin, and selenium.

Recommended sources of dietary GSH include raw fruits and vegetables such as asparagus, avocados, squash, okra, cauliflower, broccoli, potatoes, spinach, walnuts, garlic, and raw tomatoes, with asparagus containing more glutathione than all other fruits and vegetables researched to date. Cooking greatly decreases GSH, as does processing such as the canning of vegetables.

Curcumin is an antioxidant found in the popular Indian spice turmeric. It belongs to a family called curcuminoids, which are polyphenols that have a yellow hue. Curcumin's bright yellow color is sometimes used as a food coloring. You can find curcumin at many places because it's found in mustard.

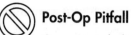 **Post-Op Pitfall**

Curcumin is believed to have anti-inflammatory and anticancer properties and may enhance the function of glutathione as an antioxidant.

Alpha lipoic acid (ALA) is an antioxidant made in your body and is found in every cell, where it assists your body in turning glucose into energy. ALA has also been found to increase glutathione levels, further increasing its antioxidant potency. Unlike other antioxidants, like vitamin C, that work only in water or like vitamin E, which works in fatty tissues, ALA is both water- and fat-soluble, so it can work throughout your body, even regenerating antioxidants that have already fought off free radicals. Research studies suggest ALA may help with diabetes and/or the nerve damage sometimes seen with this disease, so ask your doctor if you suffer from these ailments and are interested in trying an ALA supplement. In your diet, ALA is found in red meat, liver and other organ meats, and Brewer's yeast.

Selenium is a trace mineral vital for good health, although your body only needs small amounts. Selenium plays a key role as an antioxidant and is incorporated into proteins to make compounds called *selenoproteins*. These compounds help prevent damage to your cells imposed by free radicals. Selenium can be found in some meats and seafood, but by far the highest amount is found in Brazil nuts. Selenium is thought to be extremely important due to its involvement with glutathione and the formation of *glutathione peroxidase*, another potent antioxidant.

Zinc and *copper* are two important minerals in your body and are key in terms of their role in the other powerful antioxidant, *super oxide dismutase* (SOD), a potent antioxidant found naturally in your body that can help fight off diseases such as cancer and heart disease. If zinc and copper, among other antioxidants, are lacking, SOD may not be able to function at its highest level, perhaps leaving you more vulnerable to diseases.

Wrapping Up Antioxidants

Today it's virtually impossible to walk into a grocery store or convenience store without seeing antioxidant-labeled foods, some hot ones including acai berries from Brazil, and mangosteen from Southeast Asia. While these fruits are known to have a high antioxidant content (measured in ORAC value, or oxygen radical absorbance capacity), the quality may vary greatly among manufacturers, and sometimes all you're getting is high-priced juice, so buyers beware.

Your surgical center's regimen will surely include a high-quality vitamin and mineral supplement (more than one a day, typically, for gastric bypass and D/S), and this should contain a large variety of antioxidants, including vitamins A, C, and E, and possibly some of the newer antioxidants. Antioxidants shouldn't be used to excess, so always check with your center and stick with its recommendations.

Probiotics and Prebiotics

Although genetics, environment, and lifestyle can certainly all play a significant role in higher weight and obesity, emerging evidence supports that bacteria in your gut may affect nutritional metabolism as it relates to energy storage. Also, our bodies are composed of about 100 trillion bacteria—more than we have human cells—and recent reports suggest that probiotic supplements may help us have or get more good bacteria in our gastrointestinal tract, particularly in our small intestines, which might help decrease the risk of certain diseases, such as diabetes and possibly obesity.

Probiotics refers to foods or dietary supplements that contain healthful bacteria similar to those found in your body. Although many people don't need probiotics like they need vitamins, these microorganisms may provide many health benefits similar to the good bacteria in your body, including helping protect against harmful bacteria and aiding digestion, which certainly may be a problem, especially after D/S. At this writing, Margaret presented on probiotics, prebiotics, gut bacteria, and obesity at an international weight loss surgery conference. At the conclusion of this presentation, some physicians and other health-care providers told Margaret they're using probiotics in their clinics with excellent results, with one center, in India, reporting greater weight loss with probiotics.

> **Food for Thought**
>
> Probiotics may help treat diarrhea, especially with certain antibiotics. They also may help with irritable bowel syndrome (IBS), as well as vaginal yeast and urinary tract infections.

Some D/S patients find probiotics very helpful in preventing loose stools. Examples of probiotics include yogurts that cite increased live bacterial cultures and help with gastrointestinal (GI) distress.

Prebiotics are the nondigestible complex carbohydrates or oligosaccharides found in foods such as bananas, onions, leeks, Jerusalem artichokes, chicory, and honey. Human breast milk also contains prebiotics. These carbohydrates are thought to stimulate the growth and activity of beneficial bacteria in the gut. Other oligosaccharides, termed fructo-oligosaccharides (FOS) and *inulin*, a fiber and carbohydrate belonging to a class of compounds called *fructans*, which are resistant to digestion in the upper GI tract, are being seen more and more commonly in nutritional supplements touting enhanced gastrointestinal health. Other fibers like guar gum (not a prebiotic) can calm the gut and decrease your risk of diarrhea.

It's a Gut Thing

The human gut contains upward of 100 trillion microbial organisms, known as the *microbiota*. The microbiota may contain about 500 to 1,000 species and almost 100 times the number of genes in the human genome. Studying the bacteria in our gastrointestinal tract is important for many reasons, including the suggestion that having certain kinds of weight-friendly bacteria in our GI tract could help with weight loss and long-term weight management.

What the Studies Say

The development of obesity has been suggested to be influenced by the relative proportions of two major phyla of bacteria, bacteroidetes and firmicutes, both present in your colon.

Recent research suggests that the gut microbiota (or the bacteria in our GI tract) and manipulation via probiotics may provide novel therapeutic treatments for a variety of diseases, including obesity. Studies in mice suggest that probiotics may modify fatty acid metabolism and increase the recycling of fats, as well as stimulating glucose and protein metabolism. Through nutrigenomic-type research, it's possible that certain techniques and bacterial "neighborhoods" may be found to contribute to obesity or lack thereof, and that probiotics may help alleviate the signs and symptoms and therefore help with weight maintenance overall.

Several studies have highlighted the finding that the gut microbiota of people with obesity changed in accordance with body weight loss after low-calorie diets. Interestingly, the bacterial changes seen in the gut with weight loss were constant 1 year later. Study conclusions seem to suggest that obesity includes a mechanism that increases the intestinal absorption of glucose and energy (a.k.a. calories) absorbed from fats, and results in higher production of insulin, all of which could play significant roles in obesity. People who are of normal weight may have far less intestinal absorption of glucose, which may help, at least in part, explain why some people who are overweight may actually be eating less than some people of normal weight.

Everyone is different and carries a unique "community" of microorganisms in their gut, so future treatments for obesity may involve the attempt to modify the intestinal microbiota through the use of probiotics and/or prebiotics. Other conclusions from researchers in probiotics include the role of the gut microbiota in controlling plasma levels of lipopolysaccharides (LPS), a potent cause of inflammatory responses believed to be linked to diseases such as diabetes and obesity.

Weight loss surgery, particularly the gastric bypass and D/S procedures, may induce weight loss by many mechanisms, including the rerouting of the gut microbiota, which may allow for decreased glucose and fatty acid absorption in the gut and, therefore, help to keep obesity at bay, hopefully for a lifetime. Research with weight loss surgery patients would help illuminate possible mechanisms of probiotics as they relate to gut microbiota and weight regulation and may help contribute to significant advances in treatment of obesity.

At this writing, Margaret had presented on a study finding that after gastric bypass surgery a whole new strain of bacteria in the GI tract was found, and that the bacteria in the post-op gastric bypass patients was more similar to subjects in the study that were normal weight and less like the bacteria of overweight subjects. More research is needed, of course, but could weight and/or obesity be influenced by our bacteria?

Gut Hormones After Metabolic Surgery

While we're on the topic of your gut, let's take a brief look at some of the key changes after weight loss surgery, particularly gastric bypass and D/S procedures.

The Real Players

Metabolic surgeries like gastric bypass and D/S involve alterations in the connections from your gut to your brain, which ultimately help you lose weight and keep a good percentage of it off for good. In plain terms, certain pathways between your brain and gut help protect your body to not resist weight loss, and changes in hormones help you stop feeling hungry, at least for several months after surgery. After you eat food post-op, sensory information travels to your central nervous system and your GI tract and your brain gets the message that you're full. Let's start with the players that help you feel full and those that may be weight friendly. We've highlighted some of the important "players" in your weight loss that may help you to better see the overall picture, in terms of the metabolic effects of some of the surgeries.

Glucagon-like peptide 1 (GLP-1) is a peptide (a.k.a. protein) made in the cells of your ileum (the last segment of your small intestine) and also in your colon. GLP-1 is stimulated by the release of carbohydrates and fats. It stimulates insulin secretion and slows the emptying of your stomach. GLP-1 acts as a fullness hormone by decreasing your appetite at the brain level during a meal. It's also a factor in the *incretin effect* seen in people with diabetes after metabolic surgery. In other words, it helps your pancreas make insulin and enhances weight loss overall.

def•i•ni•tion

The **incretin effect** is a greater insulin response of the pancreas to oral versus intravenous glucose and is thought to be related to gut hormones, including GLP-1. The improvement in blood sugar control occurs during the first week after gastric bypass surgery, so weight loss may not be the driving mechanism.

Peptide YY (PYY) is a long protein found throughout the small intestine, but the highest levels are in the large intestine and rectum. It delays emptying of your stomach and contributes to satiety or fullness by inhibiting activity of the early part of your small intestine. The increase of PYY after gastric bypass, D/S, and also possibly the sleeve gastrectomy, may help, at least in part, explain weight loss and improvement in diseases such as diabetes.

Now let's turn to a hormone that may *not* be weight friendly. *Ghrelin* is a key player in hunger. It's a well-studied hunger hormone that goes up before a meal and down afterward, and it's vastly diminished after gastric bypass and D/S, and many times the gastric sleeve as well, for about 3 to 6 months post-op, and sometimes much longer. Because 80 to 90 percent of ghrelin is produced in your stomach, primarily the top part, it's no wonder that these surgeries, which reduce your stomach capacity (particularly gastric bypass), result in at least temporary decreases in ghrelin and subsequent decrease in hunger, although other factors are also involved in the lack of appetite typically seen initially.

What the Studies Say

Clinical trials with GLP-1 have reported a decrease in food intake in humans. The drug Exenatide actually stimulates GLP-1 production and has been approved by the FDA for treatment of type 2 diabetes but not obesity.

PYY has been studied in humans, and IV infusion of PYY was found to decrease hunger, as well as resulting in a 30 percent decrease in buffet-meal intake, without causing nausea or affecting food palatability or fluid intake. Although exciting advances have been made in weight loss surgery and important, groundbreaking research conducted, there is still much to learn about the mechanisms of weight loss and weight regulation long term. With the advent of tools for long-term weight loss such as bariatric surgery, particularly the metabolic surgeries, there are certain to be many additional breakthroughs to help get diabetes, and even obesity, into remission once and for all.

The Least You Need to Know

- Nutraceuticals are nutrients or supplements that have benefits and actions similar to some drugs.

- Antioxidants may help fight free radicals and, therefore, diseases such as cancer.

- Probiotics and prebiotics may help with weight management as well as post-op loose stools.

- Gut hormones and changes after metabolic procedures may provide the key to long-lasting weight loss success.

Part 3

Ensuring Your Continued Success

In Part 3, we've included some chapters dealing with strategies for long-term weight loss success, so you won't want to miss them! We delve into mindful eating, setting SMART goals, advice for multitasking in the kitchen, and tips for grocery shopping and dining out.

Next, we tackle the topic of how to stay successful, including how to get the support you need. We also discuss stress management and alternative medicine and how they can help you with your weight loss efforts.

Finally, you'll read about red flags, in terms of weight regain and/or unhealthy lifestyle habits, and how you can get back on track if you find it's happening to you.

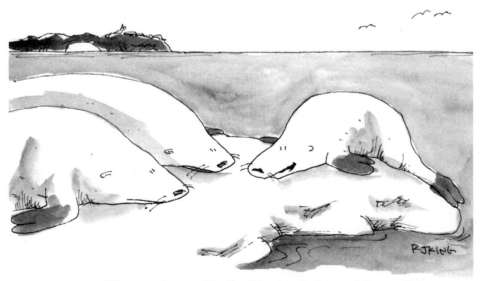

"Keeping the weight off will be the challenge, fellas.
Can I count on you to be my support system?"

Strategies for Winning at Weight Loss

In This Chapter

◆ An exercise in mindful eating

◆ The importance of setting SMART goals

◆ Setting up your kitchen

◆ At the grocery and dining out

Weight loss surgery is a fantastic tool to help you lose weight and keep it off for good. But sometimes life gets in the way while you're carrying through on the best-laid plans, so in this chapter, we give you some of our favorite tools to help you meet your life-long weight and health goals.

We start by talking about ways to set goals that will knock the ball out of the park, so to speak, and keep you focused on your goals. We incorporate some mindfulness training and continue that into the next two chapters, so get ready for winning ways your whole family can use. Joe, an award-winning chef, gives you some kitchen tricks of the trade to make your time spent there more enjoyable. And he makes it seem easy as he gives you the low-down on kitchen multitasking.

Weight-Friendly Strategies

You've had your surgery, and thanks to Part 1, you're well versed in carbs, proteins, fats, fluids, and vitamins and minerals. You know how to decipher food labels and are, perhaps, intrigued by some of the foods as medicines from Chapter 8. You have all this information at hand, but now where do you go? How do you start a post-op eating plan without feeling deprived or, worse, backsliding to your old eating habits? That's what this section is all about: tools and techniques to help you get off on the right foot and stay on track for life.

The Importance of Mindful Eating

Thanks to our fast-paced society, many of us eat while we're doing one or many other things—driving, handling work or family demands, and even walking. Approximately 66 percent of Americans eat in front of the TV, which makes it hard, if not impossible, to really focus on what you're eating and whether you're feeling full or not. Studies cite the average American watches about 3 hours of TV a day, yet spends just 72 minutes a day—*total*—on eating.

In short, the art of dining and taking your time is often a luxury perhaps reserved for weekends and days off. When you factor in that it takes your brain about 20 minutes to get the signal that you're full, you can see that if you're eating too fast, you may get this signal too late, causing you to eat too much.

That's where mindful eating can help. Mindfulness practices, including mindful eating, stem from thousands of years ago and have regained popularity in the United States over the past 25 years. Mindless eating, or eating without awareness, can impact your health in a negative way.

Research also reveals that even the way you eat a protein bar can influence your feeling of satisfaction and fullness. Subjects who ate their protein bar on the run, from the package, felt much less satisfied and much hungrier than those who sat down at a table with a plate and nothing to distract them. They cut their protein bar in small pieces and ate it mindfully and had much less hunger and much greater feeling of satisfaction and fullness, as well as better weight loss overall.

Mindful eating has been shown to have a positive impact on weight management, including binge eating disorders, and the benefits of this practice extend to emotional and physical health as well. While the feeling of fullness may vary depending on your surgical procedure and how far out you are from your surgery, some common fullness signals, such as chest fullness and pressure, that indicate you should stop eating or you'll feel chest pain and possibly run the risk of vomiting.

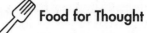 **Food for Thought** _____

Scientific studies reveal that "tuning out" during mealtime may affect your digestive process, making them 30 to 40 percent less effective. This can increase your risk of gastrointestinal distress, including gas, bloating, and constipation or diarrhea, and may decrease your feeling of satisfaction.

Eating mindfully incorporates all your senses and awareness, as this mindful eating exercise you and your family and friends can do at home illustrates:

1. Distribute one raisin (or craisin or dried cranberry) to everyone doing this exercise.

2. Have everyone, including yourself, pick up their raisin and take a true, solid look at it, examining every angle.

3. Start massaging the raisin gently with your fingers and note what it feels like and what it might be similar to.

4. Smell the raisin; really take in its aroma and see if you can describe it in as many terms as possible.

5. Place the raisin in your mouth. Don't chew or swallow it, but let it sit on your tongue and note how it feels. Close your eyes and sense the raisin fully in your mouth. If thoughts other than the raisin pop into your mind, let them go and go back to focusing fully on the raisin.

6. Start gently moving the raisin around in your mouth, and gently take a few bites of it, noting how it tastes and what it might be similar to. Notice every minute movement of your jaw, and let any distracting thoughts that might come to mind float away, and refocus on the raisin in your mouth.

7. Chew the raisin completely now, and note the full flavor and texture of it. Notice the raisin moving toward the back of your tongue and into your throat. Swallow the raisin, and trace it down your throat until you can't feel the sensation any longer.

8. Discuss with your family and friends how the raisin felt and tasted and smelled and how it might be different from how you perceived raisins in the past. Was it hard to focus entirely on the raisin and this experience the entire time? Were you bored? Did the raisin taste entirely different from what you remembered? Did it taste better?

Cooking Tip

To enhance mindful eating, try eating with chopsticks, with your nondominant hand, or with no distractions at all, like TV or work. Aim for dime-size bites, and see how many times you can chew without swallowing. Eating the portions recommended by your surgical center, see if your meal can last 30 minutes.

Chances are, this was a new experience to you, and perhaps it brought a new awareness to eating a raisin that you might want to carry over into other foods and eating in general. It might just help you enjoy food more and possibly eat more slowly and lose more weight or help you maintain your weight loss more easily. You might discover something about your usual eating habits or those of your family and friends that can be helpful for you in your healthy lifestyle. Some people try doing a shorter version of this exercise with the first bite of every meal and snack as part of a mindful eating practice, so you might want to try it, too!

By implementing mindful eating techniques in your everyday life, you'll be able to make better food and meal choices based on awareness of hunger and how your body is feeling. You'll also be better equipped to handle personal triggers for mindless eating and emotions or situations that may put you at risk for overeating or mindless eating. Also, by appreciating and savoring every bite of food, you and your family might thoroughly enjoy eating more, which could help you win the battle at weight loss for good. (We've included some great mindful eating resources in Appendix B.)

Setting SMART Goals

So many people plan so many things, including vacations and work projects, but sometimes our life goals may fall by the wayside. It's true that those who fail to plan, plan to fail, so let's go over some *SMART* goals.

def•i•ni•tion

SMART is an acronym that stands for specific, measurable, attainable, realistic, and timely goals.

Chances are, you may be doing this already, and if so, great! Even so, maybe you could tweak your goals a bit using this goal-setting technique. If you've never done anything like this, that's great, too, because it could be a fantastic new tool for you to get to the bottom of your true health, fitness, and life goals. Let's look at what makes up SMART goals:

Specific: adding as much detail as possible to your goal will really help you achieve it. Answering a lot of "W" questions can really help, such as: *What do I want to accomplish? Who might I involve? Where will I do it? When? Which things or situations (like bad weather) might call for plan B? Why do I want to do this?* You might think the statement, "I want to join a gym and get in shape," might be specific. But a SMART goal might sound more like, "Every Monday, Wednesday, and Friday from 6 to 6:30 A.M., I'm going to walk 20 minutes with my neighbor Mary."

Measurable means you're establishing some sort of way to evaluate if you're making progress toward your goal. Measuring your progress helps you stay on course and reach your target dates and goals. It also helps add a sense of accomplishment. Continuing with the exercise example, you can measure your progress by asking yourself some questions beginning with "H" such as: *How much walking am I doing compared to my set goal of 20 minutes at a time? How many days this week have I walked with Mary?*

Attainable goals are important and involve taking a long look at yourself, your life, and what's really possible or realistic for you in this moment in time, even if it may change in the future, especially with continued weight loss if you've recently had your surgery. When you list your goals, you get that much closer to achieving them. However, be sure to break them down into many steps. In our example, perhaps walking 20 minutes 3 times a week is a little overwhelming at first, so breaking it up into 10 minutes a day might make it more attainable, and building up endurance over several weeks or months could result in walking 30 minutes or longer a day.

The journey of a thousand miles begins with a single step. When you pinpoint the goals that mean the most to you, you help develop your abilities and skills and may find that you can attain just about any goal you want to achieve!

Realistic goals involve those you're both willing and able to reach for, so it should be something near and dear to your heart to have the best chance for success. For example, if you're not a skier and you don't like the cold weather, if you set your goals based on skiing, you'd be setting yourself up for failure for many reasons.

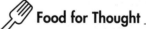 **Food for Thought**

It's estimated that only about 5 percent of the population actually takes the time to write down their goals. Write them down! It helps!

This happens also when people have treadmills or other equipment in their houses they absolutely detest using, but feel they have to include them in their goals.

Consider selling that treadmill and perhaps buying another piece of cardio equipment that doesn't hurt your joints and that you truly find more enjoyable. Or if you're much more motivated exercising with other people, consider walking with your neighbor or a walking club, or perhaps join a gym you feel comfortable going to and that's not too far out of the way from your home or work.

Timely goals involve a specific time frame. Without that, there just isn't any accountability, as in the vague statement, "I want to work out more." Instead, our earlier example noted a specific time: walking 20 minutes 3 times a week, and that could be expanded to walking 30 minutes 3 times a week after a month of reaching the first goal, increasing to 30 minutes 4 times a week the next month. The following month's goal might include increasing time to 40 minutes and continuing 4 times a week. Alternatively, if 30 minutes is your max before you feel tired, try increasing to 5 days a week while continuing at 30 minutes at a time. Also, have a plan B such as walking on your treadmill or in the mall if the weather is bad.

SMART goals, like anything else, can truly be tangible if you break them down into tiny steps, so go for it!

Visualizing Success

In addition to using SMART goals, increasing evidence shows that you have a much better chance of attaining your goals if you truly can picture yourself achieving them. There have been several accounts of extremely successful athletes who have pictured the ball going in the basket or over the tennis net over and over again and their lifting up the trophy. Studies show that visualization can truly make or break your success overall, including on the playing field of life. It's been said, "if you can see it, you can achieve it," and that's a much better way to look at things than the "I'll believe it when I see it" perspective so common today. Many extremely successful people have cited visualization of their dreams and goals as playing a major part in achieving them. But where do you start?

Act as if you've already achieved your goals. This might sound a little crazy, but if you want more vitality in your life, think of some positive affirmations, such as, "Every day, I'm feeling healthier and more energetic in every way." Of course, you don't have to say these affirmations out loud, especially if you're outside around a lot of people. (But if you have an iPod or a cell phone earpiece, they might think you're singing or talking to someone else!)

Make your goal as detailed as possible. Sift through some magazines to find some pictures of what you want in your life, like maybe a picture of someone who truly looks happy and healthy or maybe a peaceful place you'd like to vacation with your family. Put these pictures on a bulletin board, and share it with special people in your life you trust and who can help make your deepest dreams a reality. This is called a vision board and is something a few highly successful people have mentioned as a wonderful tool for motivating success. Look at your vision board often, perhaps more than once a day, and truly picture yourself and your life as you've designed it.

Review your goals often, and reassess to see if they're still what you really want in your life. You might get so good at visualizing and achieving your goals that you need to reach higher!

Kitchen Essentials

Eating well involves preparing good, healthful, fresh food, and you won't want to do that if you're not comfortable in the kitchen or have a kitchen setup you're not happy with. So let's fix that. In this section we help you set up your kitchen so you can work efficiently—and enjoy yourself.

Must-Have Kitchen Tools

First things first, it's very important to have a good set of sharp knives. These knives don't have to be expensive, just comfortable for you to work with. A number of different brands of knives are available, so you should be able to find something you prefer.

Be sure you have a good set of spoons and spatulas as well. Go for wooden as well as metal spoons, and for the spatulas, have both rubber and metal. Each of these has its own purpose in the kitchen and will come in handy when you least expect it.

A set of measuring spoons and measuring cups, both liquid and dry, are essential in the kitchen, *especially* when it comes to cooking by the book, especially if you're not the most experienced chef in the world. Your new eating plan, particularly right after your surgery, might be fairly limited, so measuring your ingredients is very important to ensure you're getting the proper nutrition.

> **Post-Op Pitfall** _____
>
> Stay away from the knife sets where the chef knife, paring knife, well ... every knife is serrated. These knives are hard to use because you basically have to saw through everything, and the final product is rarely attractive.

If you can swing it, I would even invest in a small scale. This can be very helpful when it comes to preparing your 3-ounce protein choice. Visually, that's about the size of a deck of cards, but it's often faster and easier to just weigh 3 ounces as opposed to battling with yourself about whether that piece of meat is the size of a deck of cards or not.

Cutting boards and mixing bowls are very important for a well-functioning kitchen. You need something to chop your food on, something to put it in after you've prepped it, and a nice place for mixing.

A good set of nonstick pots and pans are also very important. Why nonstick? Because you don't have to use as much oil to cook in nonstick pans because the food shouldn't stick to the pan.

A fine mesh strainer and colander are also good to have on hand. If you can only have one, pick a fine mesh strainer, but get a large one. It can do the same job as a colander.

Now, let's move on to some of the more exciting kitchen necessities, such as a blender and a food processor. A blender is useful for preparing smoothies and purée-ing soups and sauces. A food processor is good for chopping, and if you get a good one, grating, slicing, etc. For the most part, a blender is used for liquids and a food processor is used for solid foods, although you can use a food processor for some liquid applications. A blender, however, needs liquids for the blending to work.

A Microplane grater is another great tool to have in your kitchen. These are a little more expensive, but they're worth it. However, a box grater will do, too. They're good to have around to zest citrus fruits, grate fresh spices, and shred cheese.

An electric mixer is also good to have in your kitchen. In a perfect world, we would all have stand mixers, but in reality, they're no better than hand mixers, just slightly more convenient. If you have the cash, treat yourself to a nice stand mixer; if not, a hand mixer will do just fine.

Stocking Up on Staples

A cupboard filled with your favorite seasonings and spices is invaluable when cooking at home. Be sure you have salt (unless your doctor or your dietitian say you should avoid it), a pepper mill filled with whole peppercorns, ground cinnamon, ground nutmeg, and so on.

When it comes to meats, it doesn't matter what kind of meat you have, as long as it's lean. Keep some lean chicken breast, ground turkey, and fish on hand at all times, whether in the refrigerator or freezer. After your surgery, it's extremely important that you get the protein you need, and having a variety on hand will make your life easier.

Having tons of vegetables available increases the likelihood that you'll eat them. Get fresh when you can, and frozen when you can't … and even when you can. Joe gets fresh vegetables usually on a whim or when he's cooking for friends or family, but when he's cooking for himself, he usually just grabs a bag of steam-in-the-bag vegetables from the freezer and tosses them in the microwave. Frozen vegetables are quick, easy, and just as healthful as fresh—and more convenient. (But stay away from frozen cauliflower. It doesn't always handle the freezing and thawing well.)

Fresh and frozen fruits are delicious and good for you. Keep fresh fruits to snack on and frozen fruits for smoothies and shakes. After your surgery, you'll become very much acquainted with protein shakes, and over time, they might become a little boring. It's easy to liven them up by tossing in some frozen berries.

Tofu is a great source of protein and can take on a ton of different flavors. Tofu is also very versatile; it can be puréed, grilled, baked, sautéed, and so much more. Try silken tofu, which is good for soups and smoothies as well as firm and extra firm tofu, which are better for sautéing and baking. To get the best flavor, freeze your tofu and then thaw it before you marinate it. This enables the tofu to absorb more flavor from the marinade.

Beans are a great source of protein and fiber. Keep a few cans of a few different kinds of beans in your pantry. Beans are so versatile, and you never know when you're going to be able to sneak them into a recipe. Worried about the gas that comes with eating a lot of beans? Take heart because the more you eat beans, the better your body gets at breaking down the *oligosaccharides* that cause the gas and the fewer problems you'll have with it.

Yogurt is good for your body and is a terrific source of protein, especially Greek yogurt. Greek yogurt is used in many of the recipes in this book because of its high protein and low sugar content.

def•i•ni•tion

Oligosaccharides are carbohydrates containing 3 to 10 simple sugars joined together and are an example of prebiotics (see Chapter 8). Examples include onions, leeks, garlic, legumes, wheat, asparagus, and other plant foods. Americans eat about 1 to 3 grams a day; Europeans, 3 to 10 grams a day.

Finally, whole grains are a must-have. Whole grains are healthier for your body than the bleached enriched wheat products and have a low glycemic index (GI) response. Cook with whole grains whenever possible.

Too Busy to Cook?

Yes, you're busy, but you have to make time for yourself. Setting aside some time in your busy schedule for some home cooking can be beneficial for you, your health, and your success in your weight loss goals. Plus, foods prepared in the home can be much healthier for you than food you pick up on the go.

With the following tips and tricks, you'll look forward to the time you spend in the kitchen—and your body and weight will thank you.

Kitchen Multitasking Made Simple

Multitasking is the easiest way to make meals at home—and do it efficiently. The best way to do this is to prepare foods with like ingredients at the same time. If you're working on making a turkey meatloaf, why not make some turkey burgers, too? If you're making hummus with some garbanzo beans, why not open a couple cans of different beans and make a mixed-bean salad? This might seem difficult, but the easiest way to do this is to think ahead. While you're grocery shopping, plan what you're going to make and think about what other things you could make with the same ingredients.

> **Cooking Tip**
>
> Carry a small notebook or other note-taking device (try the notes feature on your cell phone) with you to jot down any ideas or recipes that might interest you. You can also keep a food diary and journal here. This can help you succeed in your weight loss goals and also give you a reference to look back on later.

Slow cooker recipes are great for multitasking. Throw all the ingredients for a slow cooker recipe into the cooker and set it. While this is cooking, make another recipe. Then you'll have two recipes going at once, and it will feel like you're doing one.

As you become more and more acquainted with the ingredients and cooking, you'll become more efficient in your multitasking.

Freeze Me, Please!

One of the greatest things about multitasking in the kitchen is the ability to store multiple meals for the week. Make one, two, even three recipes at a time, and in bulk, and freeze them in individual servings so you can grab them on your way to work, play, etc.

If you take one day of your week (preferably after you go grocery shopping) and prep as much as you can, you can get all the cooking out of the way for the week, and then just have to heat things up later. If you portion out vegetables, sandwich meats and breads, soups, salads, etc., and put them in their respective homes in the refrigerator or freezer, you'll have a healthful meal already prepared and waiting for you every day of the week.

Negotiating the Grocery and Restaurants

The grocery store can be intimidating, especially if you're really hungry when you go. Studies show that grocery shopping and dining out when you're very hungry or have gone several hours without eating leaves you more likely to overeat or make less-than-healthful choices—neither of which are good for you. Even if you're in the honeymoon phase after your surgery, going several hours (i.e., 6 or more) without eating could increase your risk for eating too quickly, which could be a recipe for disaster, in terms of chest pain, pressure, and even higher risk for vomiting and diarrhea. Some simple tips to keep in mind while grocery shopping and dining out can help prevent this.

Acing the Grocery Aisle

You've probably always heard you should shop the perimeter or outside of the grocery store, and this is generally true, although you don't want to necessarily avoid some of the healthy items in the middle aisles.

For example, in moderation, you can enjoy nuts such as natural almonds and walnuts, although you'll want to keep an eye on the servings, particularly if you didn't have the D/S procedure or you find your weight creeping upward after your surgery. Cereals are in the middle aisles as well, but there are, of course, certain healthful cereals to look for such as the high-fiber varieties with lower sugar (like any of the Kashi brands, Fiber One, All-Bran, etc.).

Of course, you'll need to go to the perimeter of the store to get your milk to go with the cereal. We recommend skim, 1 percent milk, or lower-sugar soy milk. If you're lactose and/or soy intolerant, you might want to try almond or rice milk. However, keep in mind it won't provide quite as much protein. If you like and tolerate soy milk, remember that some are higher in sugar, such as a few brands of chocolate soy milk. Sugar-free soy milk brands could help you keep down the calories and keep up the protein, as long as you're not sensitive to the artificial sweetener used.

If negotiating the grocery store is overwhelming, call your local market to see if it offers tours. Many of them are guided by registered dietitians who can point out where to shop and what to look for—and avoid.

Decoding Restaurant Menus

Dining out can be a challenge and a source of anxiety right after your surgery, and you may think it's impossible to dine out for several months, if ever again. However, it *is* possible to dine out without getting off track from your new eating regimen.

If you're in the first few weeks after surgery, such as 2 or 3 weeks post-op, and your center suggests you stay on puréed foods until 4 weeks out, look for fat-free cream soups or broth-based soups that are low in fat. Puréed-type appetizers, especially low-fat and healthful appetizers such as hummus, provide protein, carbohydrate, and fiber with a small amount of healthful (monounsaturated) fat. And the smaller appetizer portions may be perfect for you, because 2 tablespoons may be all you might feel like at 3 weeks out.

If you're 4 to 6 weeks post-op and/or your center's guidelines suggest you're ready for soft foods, look for vegetarian or turkey burgers—without the lettuce, tomato, and bread. Other possible selections include shrimp cocktail with plenty of lime and lemon and perhaps a little cocktail sauce, although not everyone is ready for spicy items this early. Keep in mind that each shrimp might suggest 4 or 5 bites, and be sure to chew completely until it's liquid before swallowing.

Another possible dining out choice at this time might be a very lean hamburger with mustard or ketchup. Some gastric bypass patients dump on ketchup, so be sure you can tolerate it or bring sugar-free ketchup with you if the regular kind doesn't agree with you.

Finally, a soft baked or broiled fish such as tilapia, scrod, or haddock might be a good bet, if it's moistened with lemon or lime and not covered with butter or oil.

Salmon and other fatty fishes may be okay, but remember that higher-fat foods, even healthful ones, take longer to empty from your stomach. Try these at home first, and remember to chew thoroughly before swallowing to maximize tolerance to foods, regardless of which surgery you had.

Cooking Tip

Looking at a menu in advance, either online or from a take-out menu, can help you plan ahead so you know exactly what you'll order that's in line with your surgical center's recommended regimen. If you can, try whatever food(s) you're thinking about ordering at the restaurant at home beforehand so you'll know if you can tolerate the food and avoid a potentially painful or awkward situation at the restaurant if you suddenly realize that food didn't sit well with you.

At 6 to 8 weeks post-op, you may be able to eat a larger variety of foods, such as salads or fresh fruits and vegetables. Just keep in mind that eating at least a few bites of protein-based foods like fish, tofu, soft meats, chicken, etc., versus fruits, vegetables, or starches will help you meet your protein needs. Otherwise, you'll fill up on salad and miss out on protein, which you don't want to do, especially with the higher protein needs of D/S patients. If you had the D/S, you'll want to try to get some (healthful) fats in your diet to help you absorb your fat-soluble vitamins, especially given the approximate 73 percent fat malabsorption with this procedure.

If you're several weeks post-op, your options should be fairly broad, but your procedure may somewhat limit the ideal selections, such as sugars for gastric bypass patients, although it's generally a good idea to limit simple sugars due to their low nutrient content and empty calories. Most restaurants have at least a few healthier entrées on their menus. And more and more restaurants have their own websites where you can read how the entrées are prepared and how to lower the calories and fat content.

The Least You Need to Know

- Mindful eating is important, regardless of which weight loss surgery procedure you had.

- Setting SMART goals can help enhance your chances for long-term weight loss success.

◆ Knowing how to stock your kitchen for healthy eating can help you stick with your new eating regimen.

◆ Grocery shopping and dining out can be made easy if you plan ahead and know what to buy or order beforehand.

Chapter 10

Setting Yourself Up for Success

In This Chapter

- Getting the support you need
- Setting up your A team
- Invaluable stress-management techniques
- Help from alternative medicine

If you watch interviews of very successful people, you'll notice that they often mention all the people who helped them get there. Invariably, they'll talk about their team, perhaps in more ways than one, and how they couldn't have achieved what they did without them.

In a similar way, weight loss success, which includes the all-important weight maintenance, will most likely involve a team of people who help you get to where you're going. Even more importantly, they'll help you stay on the right path.

The Importance of Support

People who've had surgery and attend post-op groups on a regular basis tend to be more successful than people who don't. Even the best-laid plans can go sour if you're busy or life just gets in the way. One day you're doing great and feeling on top of the world after your procedure, and then one day, you notice your clothes getting tighter and your eating and exercise regimen going astray. Post-op support groups help you remember why you had the surgery and give you practical tips and perhaps professional advice for getting back on track.

Many people find the first several months after weight loss surgery to be the honeymoon period, with typical drops in hunger, particularly for the metabolic procedures such as gastric bypass and D/S, and the weight, for many people, seems to drop off fairly easily during this time. However, as the months go by and the hunger hormones start waking up, life could get more and more challenging. Your weight might go in the wrong direction, or just plateau. This is when you need support the most, and it can make a big difference in people who are truly successful versus those who flounder a bit with their weight loss and then have to work to get back on track. (Read more about red flags in Chapter 11.)

Weight loss and hunger vary among the bariatric procedures, and some studies reveal that gastric banding patients have higher levels of ghrelin, the hunger hormone. This could be especially challenging. You may find you're hungry, especially prior to your first fill, which is typically 4 to 6 weeks post-op. This is the time when you might wonder what's wrong and why you're hungry. It's the ghrelin, and it's temporary. This is when support is absolutely necessary to stay the course and not panic if the hunger and weight loss are not what you expected. Keeping in touch with your surgical team, including your dietitian, could make a huge difference in how you feel and your confidence level in the band as a weight loss tool.

If you had the gastric sleeve, gastric bypass, or D/S procedure, it's possible you've had a honeymoon or a total lack of appetite the first 3 to 6 months or so post-op. Shortly after this time, you might have noticed your appetite starting to wake up suddenly. Perhaps your weight loss has tapered off a bit or even stalled. This is when support groups are absolutely crucial—you can hear from patients further out from you and how they were able to get past the challenging times. Even if you find you're not hungry or experiencing weight loss plateaus several months out from your surgery, it's really key to *stay* feeling positive and supported.

Your Best Support Group: You

Studies reveal that ongoing support after weight loss surgery can significantly increase your chances for success. That's why most surgical centers not only recommend support groups, but have at least monthly groups.

Not only are support groups an avenue for you to address any issues or concerns you may be having, but they're also a way to develop connections and relationships with your peers and perhaps help them or serve as a mentor at some point after your procedure. Although receiving support is key, studies also show helping others can actually cause endorphins or "feel-good" hormones to be produced in your body. Your helping others may serve as reinforcement to you of how important it is to stay on track and continue to serve as a role model.

Support groups can help you set realistic weight loss and maintenance goals, as well as create and maintain a healthy perspective about change and your future. They also can assist you in nipping food issues in the bud and staying on a healthful meal plan. They may even help you successfully manage relationships in your life, and develop or maintain skills for coping with life's changes, including dealing with people jealous of your weight loss or those who aren't supportive of your new lifestyle.

By regularly attending weight loss surgery support groups, you'll be able to get and stay connected with various members of your surgical team, including mental health providers who can help you deal with possible issues that arise or continue to be issues post-op. Some great online support groups are available as well. However, it's important not to compare yourself to anyone, especially when some people cite tremendous weight loss and you might not be experiencing the same results.

> **Cooking Tip**
>
> It's absolutely essential that you remember that everyone is different, and absolute pounds lost is not the ultimate measure of your success, but rather a healthy lifestyle and outlook on life and your goals.

Supporting yourself via regular visits with your center's dietitian is key because what you should or shouldn't be eating can get truly confusing, even if you had great counseling pre-op. Your dietitian can help you make sense out of all the information and take a good look at your diet and vitamin and mineral regimen to be sure you're meeting your nutritional goals. It truly can make or break your success if you know how to optimize your nutrition and your dietitian can pick up on areas that might need to be tweaked, such as fluid, protein, fat, or carbohydrate intake.

Skipping meals is not uncommon in the first few months post-op, but it could really sabotage your long-term weight loss, so check in with your nutritionist to be sure your diet, including your fluid intake and vitamin and mineral regimen, is in top shape.

Sometimes, no matter how hard you try, you might be feeling like a weight loss surgery failure, and it's hard to know if or when you might need professional behavioral help, so be sure to check out Chapter 11 on red flags. Regardless of which procedure you had, weight loss surgery encompasses every area of your life, from your daily eating regimen to your activity program to your relationships with your significant other and other family members, so receiving and keeping support is priceless.

Setting Up Your "A Team" to Maximize Success

Building your "A team" for success after your surgery is not unlike building a successful team in any other area of your life, be it business or family life. You need to start with good players on your team, and it's important to work together. And it's important to have goals—and good ones—in place to help you get to the finish line and stay successful for life.

If you think about this in your personal and family life, your significant other might be great at supporting you in your personal weight and wellness goals, but maybe another family member or friend is better able to help you with your career goals. Although these two goals may seem separate from each other, succeeding in your career goals may have an enormous impact on your eating and lifestyle.

Your team may include your significant other and family members, but also close friends who truly want the best for you and keep you to task. Your A team might also include a clergy member, behavioral therapist, and dietitian, as well as your primary care physician. It's important to think outside the box when it comes to support because there may be some people you never thought of who can not only provide support, but truly help you strive for and achieve your goals, and stick around to help you maintain your success. These are the people you may want to share your SMART goals with (see Chapter 9) and who truly help you strive for dreams and goals maybe you never believed you could achieve.

> **Cooking Tip**
>
> Your A team should include people who genuinely care about you and want to support you for life, not those who are secretly trying to sabotage your success.

Even if you have the best A team possible, however, it's important to keep yourself motivated and supported for ultimate success. Sometimes stress can get in the way of motivation and success, so let's talk about ways to manage stress.

Stress Management Help

Just about everyone on the planet has experienced stress to some extent, and it's no coincidence that the majority of heart attacks occur on Monday mornings, when many people are about to face what they feel is a stressful job. However, what is stress exactly, and can it affect your weight in a negative way?

Stress is in the eye of the beholder, meaning it's not a negative situation if you have the time, experience, or resources to manage the situation or challenge. However, if you don't have any of these, suddenly the situation could become a stressful situation because it's overwhelmed you or caused you to feel helpless. Stress may have negative effects on your health and your weight, especially if you have chronic stress that isn't managed well. Stress can have a negative impact on just about every part of your body and can affect your mental and emotional health as well.

Researchers have discovered that your body produces unhealthy chemicals and hormones, including cortisol, when you're under stress, which may lead to insulin resistance and weight gain. Cortisol, in turn, is believed to cause a surge of glucose into your bloodstream, resulting in increased insulin levels. High blood levels of insulin, called hyperinsulinemia, can cause many adverse health effects, including insulin resistance. Insulin can also promote fat production and storage, working against your weight loss efforts. In addition, cortisol release typically results in cravings for sugars and fats, and not healthful ones.

> **Food for Thought**
>
> Research reveals that about 10 to 25 percent of Americans have insulin resistance, which may be induced by or worsened by stress.

Stress and subsequent increases in cortisol are linked with weight gain, specifically weight gain right around your belly area, which is particularly dangerous because it's associated with a higher risk for diabetes, heart disease, and fatty liver. Cortisol triggers the well-known fight or flight response leading to the release of other chemicals, such as adrenaline (also called epinephrine). This response was okay in the caveman days when it helped men and women flee danger and survive. However, these days, stress is often emotional or psychological, and we may be sitting at our desk at work trying to meet a deadline rather than physically running away, which doesn't help matters in terms of your weight.

The stress response typically increases cravings for carbs like chocolates and typically not fruit. This craving is caused by the fact that carbs are used as a fuel for the fight or flight response. When you eat more carbs, more tryptophan, an aromatic amino acid, can cross your blood-brain-barrier and stimulate the production of a brain chemical called serotonin. The increased serotonin from carbs helps your brain feel calmer, but unmanaged stress causes a vicious cycle of carb (and fat) cravings and possible emotional eating. This unhealthy cycle may ultimately lead to weight gain or weight loss failure, at least to some extent, if not controlled.

In addition, stress is often believed to worsen blood sugars in people who have diabetes. Of course, after your weight loss surgery, particularly if you had gastric bypass or the D/S, you may be enjoying remission of your diabetes. However, not only weight regain but unmanaged stress could put you at risk for returning blood sugar issues or failure to keep diabetes in remission.

It's crystal clear that chronic, uncontrolled stress can wreak havoc on your emotional and physical health and hamper your weight loss success. But there are strategies and tools that can help you continue your success as stress-free as possible.

Physical Activity

You know that exercise has many benefits, including better management of blood sugars, blood pressure, cholesterol, and, of course, your weight. But some forms of physical activity may also induce stress. Not all physical activity relieves stress, but as many runners have attested to, it can certainly induce calm and a meditative state for some people, and a significant number of research studies cite regular exercise is key for long-term weight management.

Exercise burns calories, but it also has other benefits. For example, certain weight friendly hormones and chemicals are produced, some of which mimic those produced after gastric bypass and D/S procedures. In addition, physical activity, especially if it's something you love to do, can really help you escape from the world, mostly because of your connection to your breath and the shutting down of the busy thoughts you have throughout the day. Walking is physical activity that's more accessible than running and may be meditative as well, especially if you're connecting with your breath and thinking calming thoughts.

It's key to continue connecting with your breath and adjusting your intensity as needed to avoid overexertion. In addition, especially if you haven't exercised in a long time, seek the expert guidance of an exercise physiologist or a well-educated physical or personal trainer to help ensure proper form and avoid overexertion and injuries.

Resistance training or weight training helps increase muscle, increase your metabolic rate, and strengthen your bones. For certain people who love weight training, it can also be a form of stress reduction as you connect with your breath, especially as you challenge yourself to heavier weights and need to breathe deeply to complete the exercises properly. Once again, a personal trainer or exercise specialist may be very helpful to ensure you have proper form and that you're challenging yourself regularly. Otherwise, your muscles may not respond as well after some time using the same weights and not adding other work.

> **Food for Thought**
>
> The American College of Sports Medicine (ACSM) suggests a minimum of 2½ hours of moderate-intensity exercise a week for anyone with weight issues, leading to an energy expenditure of 300 to 500 calories per day.

Physical activity is certainly a component of a healthy lifestyle, and in this chapter, we touched on a couple ways exercise can help with stress. If you can, go for a walk when you're feeling stressed out. Feel-good hormones called endorphins may just be the ticket to get you and your body to release the pent-up tension. If you're an emotional eater, you may find that going for a walk helps you avoid reaching for a sugary or fatty food you thought you wanted when your body really needed to release physical stress through activity.

Sometimes, if you're feeling anxious or stressed, you might find that physical activity doesn't help you calm down. Please don't stop exercising, but as a complement to it, consider a traditional form of stress management like deep breathing, meditation, or yoga.

Deep Breathing: It's All in Your Belly

Deep breathing is a very simple yet highly effective technique for relaxation. An important component is deep belly breathing rather than the shallow chest breathing so common in today's harried lifestyle. Margaret sometimes sees patients who appear stressed and when she asks them if they'd like to do breathing exercises for a minute or so, they report feeling better after 5 breaths.

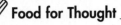

Food for Thought

Herbert Benson, M.D., conducted a series of experiments on popular meditation techniques and found they had a real effect on reducing stress and controlling the fight or flight response by slowing heartbeat and breathing and reducing oxygen consumption. This is commonly termed the relaxation response.

Belly breathing is easy. All you do is inhale deeply, with your belly puffing out as much as possible, and then exhale deeply, with your belly going back in as much as possible. Practicing at least 5 minutes of deep breathing a day helps your body get into the relaxation response. Deep breathing can help with stress, which might also result in help with long-term weight loss success.

Many good books and CDs are available on deep breathing and the relaxation response, and we've included some of them in Appendix B, so be sure to check them out!

Relaxing Meditation

Meditation slows down your heart rate and breathing, lowers your blood pressure, helps your body use oxygen more efficiently, and calms your adrenal glands, which helps minimize cortisol production and the fight or flight response to stress. People who meditate often have been found to deal with stress more effectively, and some studies show a regular meditation practice helps slow down the effects of aging. In addition, regular meditation practitioners are less likely to struggle with stress or emotional eating.

Some people think of meditation as sitting quietly on a cushion for hours on end—boring!—and this has probably kept some people from trying it. Meditation comes in many forms, including walking meditation, so it's not one-size-fits-all by any means.

No matter which form of meditation you choose, you'll find your thoughts may be your biggest challenge. It's estimated the average human adult has about 50,000 thoughts every day, and many times they're the same few thoughts over and over again. (Hopefully, they're positive thoughts, or life could be extra-challenging, for sure.) As you work on your meditation practice, try to let go of those thoughts and try to be completely free of thoughts.

This can be very difficult, especially if you're thinking about all of life's responsibilities and obligations, but continue with it and you just might find meditation to be your biggest refuge from the day-to-day stresses of life. A regular meditation practice may also help you with your weight by decreasing emotional eating or mindless eating due to stress. We've included some wonderful meditation references, including some CDs, in Appendix B.

Yoga: It's Not All About Headstands

Yoga is an ancient relaxation technique that originated in India more than 5,000 years ago. Margaret, who is a registered yoga teacher, still considers herself a work in progress after 9 years. But as some yoga teachers claim, "yoga is a practice, not a perfect."

When you say the word *yoga*, many people, especially if they're overweight, think it's not for them because of all the headstands and other seemingly impossible twisting poses involved. Poses are involved, but yoga, which means "union," is more about the connection between your body, your mind, and your breath. Yoga can help you connect with your breath, and in doing so, evoke the relaxation response.

While yoga, especially more vigorous forms such as power yoga, ashtanga, Bikram yoga, or vinyasa styles, have been shown to burn a lot of calories and help with weight loss, more gentle forms of yoga have also been found to be helpful. A large study in Boston a couple years ago looked at a few thousand senior citizens who practiced gentle yoga a few times a week. They weren't asked to follow a rigid diet, but only advised to practice yoga about 30 minutes a few times a week. At the end of a year, most subjects lost at least 5 pounds. Not only did they report lower stress and better blood pressure, etc., but they also ate more mindfully due to the stress-relieving benefits of yoga. Some forms of yoga may also help with particular ailments, such as back pain, which is often an issue if your weight is high.

> **Food for Thought**
>
> *Asana,* which literally means "seat" in Sanskrit, describes the physical poses many Westerners associate with yoga. However, asanas were created essentially to calm the body enough to meditate, with corpse pose (*savasana*) being the most important for meditation.

We've included some high-quality yoga CDs and books in Appendix B, as well as some websites you can log on to practice one yoga pose at a time, which might be the right pace for you and your busy life. However, if possible, I highly recommend instruction from a qualified yoga teacher (check out www.yogaalliance.org to find one). You want to interview the teacher to be sure you connect with him or her and that their energy and philosophy gels with yours.

Just remember that yoga is not competitive, so start where you are, keep connecting with your breath, and enjoy the physical benefits of yoga, which could very well include weight loss and management as well as stress reduction.

Alternative Medicine—Is It for You?

Complementary and alternative medicine (CAM) includes nontraditional forms of healing or those not taught in most Western medical schools, including homeopathy and acupuncture. Recently, CAM has become more widely accepted in the United States as people gravitate toward nonpharmaceutical treatments to escape the side effects and perhaps gain peace of mind.

In this section, we highlight a couple forms of alternative medicine, acupuncture and massage therapy, that appear to show clinical benefits in research studies.

Acupuncture

During an acupuncture treatment, very thin needles are inserted into your skin in various parts of your body, depending on the particular issue(s) you're suffering from. Acupuncture is a great stress reliever as well as amazing treatment for a variety of ailments.

Acupuncture has been found to have the potential to treat or manage some medical ailments, including stress-related health issues. Some pressure points (like acupressure) and other tools (such as certain herbs and pressure points in certain areas, such as the back of the ear) may be helpful with hunger and weight management as well, although there may not yet be research to corroborate their effectiveness. Some people use acupuncture as an adjunct to Western medical treatments for symptomatic relief for ailments like back pain, headaches, fibromyalgia, and osteoarthritis.

> **Food for Thought**
>
> When performed properly, acupuncture is a safe practice that can complement other treatment methods and help control certain kinds of pain unresponsive to pain medications.

Acupuncture may even be covered by your insurance, so talk with your doctor if you feel you'd like to explore the possible benefits. Your physician may be able to direct you to a qualified practitioner in your area who accepts your health insurance plan. If acupuncture is something you end up exploring, you might just find it helps with relaxation and stress reduction to a great extent, and that it may help with your weight loss maintenance as well.

Massage Therapy

Massage therapy is one of the oldest healing arts, dating to more than 3,000 years ago. The ancient Hindus, Persians, and Egyptians utilized different forms of massage for a variety of ailments. Even Hippocrates apparently wrote papers recommending a form of massage to help heal joint and circulatory problems.

These days, massage therapy is being accepted by many health insurance plans because studies have shown it can help many chronic ailments, such as low back pain, arthritis, depression, diabetes, and high blood pressure. Massage therapy can also help boost your immune system, and studies are showing that the mere physical touch involved can be healing in many ways, including stress reduction. It may also help you with your weight if your eating is stress related.

Finding the Right Fit for You

In addition to your weight loss surgery procedure, many other tools are available to help you stay on your successful weight loss journey. Ultimately, it's up to you to determine which stress reduction method(s) might be right for you and how to best support yourself in your new journey.

Support is key, both in the form of traditional support groups and your personal A team. Be true to yourself, and your goals and dreams will help you determine how to best take care of yourself and your new body. Taking care of yourself emotionally is also key to long-term weight loss success, and we hope you've found this chapter helpful. Cheers to your continued success!

The Least You Need to Know

- Support is extremely important to your long-term weight loss success.
- Stress-management techniques, including deep breathing, meditation, and yoga, may also help with weight loss.
- Yoga is not about doing handstands or perfect poses but rather connecting with your breath.
- Alternative medicine techniques, such as acupuncture and massage therapy, can have far-reaching benefits.

Chapter 11

Weight Regain and Other Red Flags

In This Chapter

- ◆ Weight regain after weight loss surgery
- ◆ Common red flags to watch for
- ◆ How to get back on track if you slip
- ◆ Detoxifying your environment

In this chapter, we discuss issues that may be on your mind, including weight regain after bariatric surgery and what's normal and what's not. We also talk about tools and techniques to get you back on track if you're experiencing weight regain that's perhaps greater than average. Many wonderful resources are available to help you.

Let's start by finding out what kind of regain is normal and what you can do if you find yourself off the charts, in the wrong direction, with respect to gaining back weight, or failing to lose the average amount.

Weight Loss and Regain: How Much Is Expected?

The most common fear or anxiety mentioned during pre-op nutrition visits is often weight regain. Some patients have read horror stories online or seen celebrities talking about their significant weight regain after gastric bypass surgery, and they're convinced the same thing will happen to them.

The statistics are on your side, for the most part, although expected weight loss and regain certainly can vary by procedure. Let's find out what "normal" weight loss is first, and then look at what studies reveal is the average weight regain.

What's Normal Anyway?

A note before we go any further: the numbers discussed in this section are by no means engraved in stone, and many studies have been done on weight regain and what's "normal," and some have refuted others. The average weight loss discussed in this section is what Margaret sees at her center. Of course, every center is different, and some of the surgeons Margaret works with may have slightly different numbers, but the average weight loss numbers presented here are certainly at least the average and most common statistics quoted to patients pre-op, based upon the latest research findings. Gastric sleeve is a newer procedure, so the numbers quoted are generated from the limited research and experience so far. Your center's statistics may differ from what you read here. Regardless, you're not necessarily a "weight loss failure" if you're years out and haven't achieved this weight loss.

Currently, for gastric banding patients, the expected weight loss typically quoted is about 30 to 50 percent of excess body weight, with 50 percent of patients possibly failing to lose this much weight. These numbers have come from various research studies, although you're not destined to fail or lose only the maximum quoted amount.

Let's put this quoted weight loss into perspective. If you weigh 250 pounds and your "healthy weight," as quoted by your surgeon or dietitian, is 150 pounds, you have 100 pounds of excess weight. So if you lost between 30 and 50 pounds by about 2 years out after the band, you would be in the average weight loss range. Failed weight loss might constitute the inability to lose at least 25 pounds, if you had 100 pounds

> **Food for Thought**
>
> Many people are stunned by these numbers, but these are strictly averages in the United States. If you look at Australian studies and even some other studies within the United States and Europe, you may find "better" numbers. Of course, some band patients have lost all their excess weight, but that seems to be the exception rather than the norm.

to lose, say by 1 year out, or losing 40 pounds out of 100 to lose and gaining back 20 pounds, for a net weight loss of 25 percent of "excess weight."

Gastric sleeve is a newer procedure, but so far, the research allows a rough estimate of 40 to 50 percent excess body weight loss. In other words, losing about 40 to 50 pounds if you were told you're 100 pounds overweight. Gastric bypass expectations fall in the 60 to 75 percent excess weight loss range (60 to 75 pounds lost for every 100 pounds overweight). Duodenal switch (D/S) patients have, on average, 70 to 85 percent excess body weight loss (70 to 85 pounds lost for every 100 pounds you're overweight), based on the latest research.

BMI Basics

One way to figure out your excess body weight is by comparing your pre-op weight to a body mass index (BMI) of 25. BMI calculators are available online to help you calculate BMI of 25 based on your height and weight, but if, for example, you're 5'6" and 155 pounds, your BMI is 25.

The BMI calculation is not the end-all and be-all and may be skewed if you're very muscular and/or have a large frame size or heavier bones from being heavy many years. It also may not adjust for differences between men and women. However, BMI offers a way to measure your progress over time.

In the preceding example, someone who is 5'6" and weighs 255 pounds has 100 pounds excess weight. Therefore, if he or she lost 50 pounds 2 years after the band, that would be 50 percent excess weight loss (50 pounds lost ÷ 100 pounds excess body weight), or the upper end of expected weight loss, which many centers consider quite good. However, losing 25 pounds in this case might be considered a weight loss failure of sorts (25 ÷ 100 pounds excess weight = 25 percent excess body weight lost).

There are many factors to consider, including medications such as insulin and certain antidepressants that could increase weight, as well as the effects of stress and other factors. Hang in there if you're not in the expected weight loss range just yet.

What the Studies Say

Now let's look at what the research reveals about average weight regain. Based on mice, rat, and human studies on gastric bypass surgery, the average weight regain may fall into a range of 5 to 15 percent of excess body weight loss.

To put this into perspective, let's take the 5'6" person who weighed 255 pounds pre-op (100 pounds excess body weight), and imagine they've lost 65 pounds (65 percent excess body weight) and gained back 10 pounds from years 2 to 5 post-op. Although this may seem excessive, this is actually 15 percent weight regain (10 ÷ 65 pounds lost = 15 percent), which is still within the expected regain after gastric bypass.

You may be able to keep off more weight, perhaps, if you're eating a very healthy diet, include a lot of physical activity daily, and have a great stress-management program. As mentioned in Chapter 1, keep in mind that your body will most likely want to gain back some weight from your lowest weight as a form of "famine insurance" even if you're doing everything right.

A red flag though: if you gain back 30 pounds of the 65 pounds lost (30 ÷ 65 = 46 percent regain), that's not within the expected weight gain and could mean you're having some struggles, possibly with one of the issues discussed later in this chapter.

Gastric banding studies looking at weight loss and regain are conflicting, with a few citing similar weight loss to gastric bypass several years out and others refuting this. However, the average band patient loses about 30 to 50 percent excess body weight. Using the 5'6" example and a 255-pound starting weight, if you lost 40 pounds with the band (your lowest weight) and at 5 years out have kept off 35 pounds of this, many clinicians would say you've been successful because you had 40 percent excess weight loss (right in between the 30 to 50 percent expected excess body weight loss [EBWL]) and regained 12.5 percent, which is within the max 15 percent weight regain mark.

> ✍ **Food for Thought** _____
>
> In general, weight regain of 5 to 15 percent is expected from year 2 to year 5 post-op. Consult with your surgical team if your weight regain is higher than this.

Gastric sleeve is a newer procedure, but if 40 to 60 percent weight loss is average EBWL, then a 5'6" person who weighed 255 pounds pre-op and lost 55 pounds would be considered good weight loss. If he or she gained back 8 pounds 5 years out, it would be 14.5 percent weight regain, which is still within the acceptable range.

D/S patients enjoy the largest EBWL of 70 to 85 percent, so a 5'6" person at 255 pounds pre-op who lost 85 pounds would be considered a success initially. If he or she gained back 10 pounds or 11.7 percent EBWL, they'd still be doing well.

Now that you know what "normal" post-op weight loss and weight regain look like, perhaps you'll be able to better assess where your weight loss and weight regain stands. If you're in the expected range or better, fantastic! Congratulations! However, if you find you're failing the grade, so to speak, you can turn it around. Even if you're not having any issues presently and are enjoying excellent weight loss, you may want to read about some possible red flags to help ensure they don't stop you.

Common Red Flags and Getting Back on Track

Red flags are something to always be on the lookout for after surgery. Sometimes they're subtle, such as the slight weight regain that might seem normal but could be due to the return of a binge-eating disorder that maybe the patient isn't ready to divulge or may not be aware is recurring.

It's important to take a long, hard, honest look at your eating habits and the possibility that old, unhealthy habits might be returning. This can be especially true if you've had a lot of life changes, even good ones, and you find you're not getting enough sleep suddenly or don't have as much time to exercise. In the following sections, we cover the most common red flags and some possible ways to turn them around to win at weight loss for good.

Grazing: When a Snack Isn't Just a Snack

While we don't like the term *grazing* because it could bring to mind an image of a cow, we use it here simply to describe the eating style sometimes associated with higher weight regain, particularly for purely restrictive procedures such as gastric banding. This is a controversial area, but in Margaret's clinical experience, she's seen a higher percentage of both weight loss failures and higher weight regain among band patients, for example, who grazed throughout the day, even if they weren't hungry.

def•i•ni•tion
Grazing is eating snacks all day long or eating small amounts of different foods all day.

This is a time when a look at food logs might help identify problem areas. For example, someone who is waiting for their second fill after their band and feeling very hungry should have 4 to 6 mini-meals of high-protein foods, such as low-fat, low-sugar yogurt, cottage cheese, or ricotta cheese to help curb hunger and provide protein and calcium. However, someone who has had 4 or 5 fills and is deemed to be at the sweet spot of ultimate restriction who is eating 100-calorie snack packs, pretzels, chips, and drinking high-calorie drinks is displaying grazing behavior, which could put them at much higher risk for weight loss failure and higher-than-normal weight regain.

If you find your weight loss or weight gain isn't normal, and feel you might be grazing, contact your dietitian and schedule a consultation to review some possible strategies to get back on track. In the meantime, try making one change at a time like cutting out snack packs or pretzels and substitute with a low-fat, low-sugar yogurt or low-fat cheese stick. See if you can increase your activity, too.

If stress or emotional eating could be contributing to your grazing, read on to find out how to change that.

Emotional Eating, or What's Eating You?

Emotional eating may be something you struggled with before your surgery and, therefore, it may be an issue sometime after surgery as well, particularly if you find you have sudden issues or stress in your life you didn't expect—and that can include wonderful new opportunities, which are often stressful. Studies suggest emotional eating may be fairly common if your BMI is 35 or higher, so rest assured you're not alone if this is an issue for you or has been in the past.

When Margaret meets with patients pre- and post-op, she looks at their food logs, if available, to see if there's a pattern between how they're feeling and what and how they're eating. For example, if they're eating faster and larger amounts of food while they're studying for an exam or under deadline pressures at work, it's a pretty big red flag that either emotions or stress are factors in their eating and/or overeating. If this sounds like you, continue doing food and mood logs, and note any changes in your eating when you tune out all distractions while you're eating, such as TV and the computer.

In addition, get some physical activity or some form of stress reduction—which, as you know from Chapter 10, could be one and the same thing. If you see a therapist or counselor on a regular basis, be sure to share your food and mood logs with them as well, and enlist the help of your family and friends if you feel you're falling into emotional eating.

Eating a minimum of 3 meals a day, no more than 5 hours apart, and including protein, fiber, and some healthy carbs and fat into your diet are key to helping your body stay on an even keel physically as well as emotionally. Take your vitamins and minerals exactly as prescribed because missing your vitamins can actually increase your risk of emotional eating and the blues (more on this coming up).

Substituting Alcohol for Food

Alcohol abuse after bariatric surgery does happen, and you might have heard about some celebrities who became alcoholics after gastric bypass, for example, when they never touched alcohol before their procedure. Although the actual percentage of bariatric patients who struggle with new addictions like this may be lower than you think, the fact remains that some people do have new issues with alcohol and other food replacements, such as recreational drugs and gambling.

As discussed in Chapter 5, studies on gastric bypass patients and alcohol have revealed blood alcohol levels in the intoxicated range with small amounts of alcohol ingestion, so you never want to drink and drive, with any procedure, especially gastric bypass surgery. Alcohol contains a lot of calories and may increase your appetite, so it could spell disaster in terms of your weight loss or weight regain, as well as put your health at risk in other ways, such as increasing your risk of fatty liver.

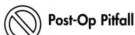 **Post-Op Pitfall**

Bariatric patients with an addiction to food may transfer their addiction to another substance, such as alcohol, with one study citing up to 25 percent of patients studied.

Margaret has seen patients who have started drinking more and more alcohol after surgery, and unfortunately, their weight loss numbers weren't good. Thankfully, they were typically seeing a therapist who was aware of their struggle and some of them sought treatment through AA and other supportive associations. If you suspect possible alcohol dependence, consider seeking professional treatment and support.

When to Seek Professional Help

Do seek professional help if you feel you may have an addiction transfer, such as alcohol, drugs, or gambling. In addition, if you find that you're slipping back into emotional eating or grazing, regardless of whether it's shown up on the scale or not, it's time to speak to a behavioral professional. In addition, it's generally a great time to touch base with your entire surgical team, including your dietitian, to get back on track with a healthy eating plan and lifestyle, especially before weight regain has become significant.

If you had the D/S, you may find that your weight loss and weight regain are fine, even with unhealthy lifestyle and behaviors. However, it's truly in your best interest to touch base with your team, including your behavioral provider, to ensure your diet and lifestyle are as healthy as they can be and you're sticking to your vitamin and mineral regimen.

Stress Can Deflate Your Success

Stress can certainly take its toll on your health and weight loss success, and this can't be underestimated in terms of long-term weight management. However, you can take steps to minimize your body's stress response. Among them is careful attention to your vitamin and mineral supplements prescribed by your center. Vitamin C, for example, is a potent antioxidant that can help combat stress, which can be a result not only of the surgery but higher weight itself. Antioxidants, as discussed in Chapter 8, help your body deal with oxidative stress and may also help fight off the effects of inflammation (seen with higher weight) and ultimately help diminish stress-related processes leading to premature aging.

Research has revealed that uncontrolled stress can increase your risk for decreased overall weight loss, increased weight regain, and addiction transfer, such as excessive alcohol intake. As discussed in Chapter 10, the hormones that produce stress, especially if chronic and unmanaged, typically increase your cravings for unhealthy carbs and fats, which could then leave your weight and energy flailing.

Check in with your team, including your dietitian, if you feel stress is deflating your success. Let's talk about some possible factors when you're stressed and how they can leave your weight loss in the lurch.

Sleep Deprivation

Studies looking at the relationship between weight and sleep have found that the less sleep you get, the more likely you are to have issues with higher weight.

According to research, people who sleep 6 hours a night had a 23 percent greater risk of obesity. The lowest risk for obesity occurs with people who sleep 7 or 8 hours a night, with amounts less than that resulting in corresponding increases in BMI. To add insult to injury, as far as sleep is concerned, obstructive sleep apnea (OSA) is very common when your weight is higher and is one of the last issues to go

> **Food for Thought**
>
> One large population study found that people who slept 4 hours or less were 73 percent more likely to be in the obese range than people who slept 7 to 8 hours a night.

away after surgery, if at all. Even if you're trying to get 8 hours of sleep a night, OSA can disrupt your sleep to such an extent that your body isn't getting adequate rest and isn't making the right amount of growth hormone—during sleep is the only time your body makes this weight friendly hormone. Therefore, you're more likely to have higher hunger hormones like ghrelin and greater cravings for sugar and fats, and not the healthy kinds either. In addition, you may have lower levels of leptin, which is weight friendly, thus adding more risk for weight regain or failed weight loss.

Even if you don't have OSA (or wear your CPAP mask [the breathing mask some people with sleep apnea are asked to wear to help regulate their breathing while they sleep] and have good control if you do), if you only get 5 hours of sleep a night, you are 50 percent more likely to have struggles with your weight. Sleep deprivation might just increase your risk for weight loss failure or higher weight regain.

Chronic sleep deprivation results in an increase in cortisol and decrease in adiponectin, resulting in greater cravings for sugar and fats and decreased oxidation of fat tissues, respectively. Adiponectin is a weight-friendly hormone that stimulates the oxidation of fat, decreases the likelihood of fat production in your body, helps improve insulin sensitivity, and helps decrease inflammatory markers in your body, possibly helping with blood sugar control and lowering risk for heart disease. Therefore, the fact that this hormone is decreased with sleep deprivation is another possible issue, especially if you find your sleep quality and time going down and your weight going up.

Speak with your surgical team if you feel you need help with your sleep and haven't been able to improve it or you feel you might need another sleep study to evaluate for OSA.

Skipped Meals or Poor Meal Planning

One of the most common red flags seen in bariatric nutrition practice is skipped meals or poor meal planning. Research has certainly revealed that skipped meals and irregular meal patterns (e.g., going several hours without eating) can signal weight issues or exacerbate existing weight issues.

One of the possible scenarios is that your brain essentially gets a message that you're in a famine-type situation and typically responds by lowering your body's caloric needs or decreasing your resting metabolic rate (RMR). Some of Margaret's patients are in a common pattern, at least they were pre-op, of skipping breakfast and lunch and then overeating at dinner and perhaps grazing throughout the evening or binge eating at night. Not surprisingly, when they awake they're typically not hungry. The process then repeats itself.

Although nutrition studies are conflicting on whether or not the "don't eat after 8 P.M." rule or similar strategies truly are effective or whether it's total calories and activity that count, skipping meals and increased night eating are often synonymous with lower weight loss and higher weight regain post-op bariatric surgery. It also leaves you at higher risk for low blood sugars and increased irritability and lower energy during the day, as well as higher risk for over-eating and possibly binge eating, particularly if you struggled with this pre-op. Always shoot for at least 3 meals a day, no more than 5 hours apart, and try to get protein with every meal.

Anxiety and Depression

Studies report that while severe depression is rare after bariatric surgery, mild depression is not uncommon, particularly if you had complications or hospital readmissions. In addition to keeping in close contact with your surgical team, including your psychologist, psychiatrist, or therapist, and taking medications for depression or anxiety, if prescribed, there's more you can do to help combat anxiety and depression. One is paying close attention to your vitamin and mineral supplements.

B vitamins, consisting of 11 different nutrients, may help your brain and nervous system run smoothly. You definitely want to take the vitamin regimen your doctor or dietitian has reviewed with you to minimize not only your risk of deficiencies, but also possibly "stressing out" your nervous system.

Some of the B vitamins, such as B_6, have been found to help with depression in menopausal women, although don't stop taking any of your meds, including antidepressants, in favor of B_6 or any other vitamin or mineral supplement. Vitamin B_{12} bathes your nerve cells in a type of sheath, protecting your cells from nerve damage. In addition, B_{12} deficiency, especially seen with gastric bypass, could lead to a kind of anemia called pernicious anemia. Low levels of niacin or vitamin B_3 have been tied to fear, depression, irritability, instability, and even memory impairment. Add to this the fact that your B vitamins could be depleted at a much faster rate with surgeries like gastric bypass and the D/S, and you have the "perfect storm" of vitamin B depletion and stress!

In addition to a healthful, balanced diet and close adherence to your prescribed vitamin and mineral regimen, proper sleep, regular physical activity, and a regular stress-management program can go a long way toward helping manage anxiety and depression. Good support and your A team (see Chapter 10) can also make a big difference.

However, if you find that even after doing all these things you're feeling blue, see your behavioral provider as soon as possible, especially if you're having thoughts of suicide, which is rare but a big red flag, or any of the following symptoms:

- Marked decreased interest or pleasure in almost all activities most of the day, nearly every day, especially if you no longer like the hobbies you used to love

- Depressed mood most of the day, nearly every day

- Insomnia or too much sleep nearly every day

- Feelings of worthlessness or guilt

- Repeated thoughts of death or suicide

- Increased irritability for no apparent reason

To help decrease your risks for depression after your surgery …

- Have a solid stress-management system in place.

- Find hobbies or activities that are healthy and will help fill the void if you previously used food as a pacifier or mood enhancer.

- Use positive self-affirmations to help with self-esteem issues.

- Enlist the help of a good therapist, psychologist, or psychiatrist to help you sort out your feelings.

- Enlist the support of your A team to help you feel stronger.

- Ask about medication to help you feel better and stay feeling better.

 Post-Op Pitfall

Some antidepressants are time-released, which may become poorly absorbed after gastric bypass and D/S, so be sure to check with the doctor who prescribed your medication to be sure yours is well absorbed.

Caution: Toxic Environments

A statement commonly recited within professional weight management circles is "genetics loads the gun and environment pulls the trigger."

While nutritional genomics certainly will come out with many important breakthroughs in the coming years and there's no doubt genetic tendencies toward higher weight exist, some have termed our society *obesigenic* in its promotion of higher calories and easy access to processed or fast foods all hours of the day and night. Add to this the decreased time and availability of exercise and increased stress, and you have the perfect atmosphere for weight gain and obesity.

def•i•ni•tion

Obesigenic is a term coined to suggest that in today's society, many things could increase one's chances for overweight or obesity, including availability of fast foods, increased stress, toxic environments, decreased sleep, and a sedentary lifestyle.

Quite a few studies have revealed that non-Western societies that adopt a Western lifestyle gain weight, partly due to increased animal fats and sugars and decreased fruits and vegetables in their diets. This has been found across many cultures, further adding fuel to the fire in terms of the obesigenic environment theory.

The Dangers of a Sedentary Lifestyle

A great deal of research has compared a healthy diet alone, exercise alone, and the combination of diet and exercise. The consistent finding was that the combination was the most successful in terms of long-term weight loss maintenance. Patients who embrace physical activity on a regular basis and a healthy diet along with it seem to not only lose the most weight, but keep it off with the greatest ease.

Food for Thought

New world syndrome is a phrase characterized by a lack of physical activity. Current research reveals that less than 10 percent of American women and men participate in regular and vigorous physical activity.

Decreased physical activity and the Western technologies available—elevators, garage door openers, various remote controls, etc.—may further add to weight issues, especially if your ancestors might have been preprogrammed to survive famines by holding on to more weight.

The National Weight Control Registry (NWCR) is an ongoing list of people who have maintained an average weight loss of about 60 pounds (going from a BMI of 36.3 to 24.9) and have kept off the weight for at least 6 years. Although many people with higher BMIs may have different genetics or challenges in weight loss and maintenance of weight loss after surgery, it's important to note that the NWCR noted physical activity equivalent to 60 to 90 minutes a day, or the equivalent of about 28,000 calories burned per week in physical activity, the equivalent of walking 4 miles per day, as the average exercise level reported. Certainly, not everyone who has had weight loss surgery must adhere to this level of exercise, but data seem to confirm the importance of physical activity, particularly daily for at least 60 minutes.

Friends, Family, and Other Possible Saboteurs

Friends and family may seem like the least likely saboteurs to your weight loss success, but Margaret has seen, on more than a few occasions, situations where a patient's significant other was jealous of their success or fearful they would leave them.

There might be some merit to that fear, as studies reveal that approximately 30 percent of divorces occur after weight loss surgery. The most typical reason seems to be that the weight loss surgery patient, upon losing a significant amount of weight and improving their self-esteem, realizes they were in a toxic situation at home and decides to leave. Therefore, in these cases, divorce may be the healthiest option for the patient, particularly if there was verbal abuse or any other kind of toxic component to the relationship.

If you find yourself in this situation, there is help. The first place to look may be your psychologist, psychiatrist, or mental health therapist associated with your surgical program. Perhaps you've been seeing a private therapist or know of a social worker who can help you work through the issues you're having at home. Know that you're not alone, and that seeking help is the first important step to getting out of a negative and potentially harmful situation, not only in terms of weight regain risk but overall emotional and physical health, since the stress of the situation alone could pack on the pounds and harm your health.

Also, be aware of seemingly well-meaning friends who may be jealous of your success and start asking you to join them at fast-food restaurants or previous unhealthy situations you might have participated in prior to your surgery. As hard as it may be, you might need to end unhealthy friendships and focus on being around people with healthier lifestyles. This is one of the many reasons why local post-op support groups may be helpful to reinforce positive lifestyles with like-minded people who support rather than sabotage your weight loss efforts.

Another possible saboteur of your weight loss is self-sabotage. Sometimes, it's hard to change your belief in your ability to be successful with your weight for life, especially when it's highly likely you've been on many diets, with nothing but failure to show for it. Of course, weight loss surgery is a wonderful tool, but your thoughts, both positive and negative, regarding your ability to be successful for life can strongly impact your long-term success. As mentioned previously, the average person has about 50,000 thoughts a day, many times the same thought, so it's important to monitor what you're thinking about on a daily basis.

If you find you're telling yourself it's the same old, same old and expecting you'll gain back all your weight after surgery, there may be a higher likelihood you'll at least regain more than the norm mentioned in Chapter 10. Seeking help from a trained behavioral therapist, ideally one from your center or who works extensively with weight loss surgery patients, can significantly improve your chances for long-term weight loss success.

Just Say No to Processed Foods

Fast foods have been implicated in America's sharp increase in weight issues and obesity. And it's understandable why: they're widely available, typically very high in fat and calories, and low in vitamins and minerals.

If you were a lover of fast foods prior to your surgery, chances are you may feel the temptation to indulge in them at least occasionally post-op, especially when the honeymoon is over, if you find yourself under stress, if you're at a weight plateau, or if you're struggling with emotional eating or temptation to return to some old unhealthy habits. Checking in with your center's psychologist and dietitian can make all the difference in the world and help you break through previous barriers that held you back.

Food for Thought

Research on fast-food restaurant clients revealed a higher incidence of overall poor diet and exercise habits and higher body mass index (BMI) compared to non-fast-food eaters.

Even if you find yourself at a fast-food restaurant with no other choice at a particular meal, opt for the healthier foods like a salad with grilled chicken and low-calorie dressing or the lower-fat, lower-calorie options offered. Keep in mind that processed foods typically leave you feeling sluggish and less likely to want to exercise. They may also leave you feeling guilty and defeated and, in the worst-case scenario, may increase your risk for higher-than-normal weight regain or weight loss failure overall.

Keeping in close touch with all your surgical team members, including your dietitian, psychologist, and behavioral provider, is key to staying on track or getting quickly and soundly back on track if you stray.

The Least You Need to Know

◆ Weight regain, at least to some extent, is normal after weight loss surgery, but it's important to identify red flags to asses if it's excessive.

◆ Common behavioral red flags post-op include grazing, emotional eating, binge eating, and substituting alcohol or other unhealthy habits for food.

◆ Stress can wreak havoc on your weight loss efforts and needs to be managed for ultimate success and health.

◆ Factors of a toxic environment include processed foods; a sedentary lifestyle; and saboteurs such as friends, family, and even you, if you're not thinking positive thoughts.

Part 4

Recipes for Eating Well After Weight Loss Surgery

Part 4 is the recipe section. Joe and I have put together tons of delicious and healthful recipes we're sure you and your family and friends will love. We've included everything from high-protein starters to get your day off right, to main dishes sure to please, to scrumptious desserts you won't believe are good for you—150 recipes in all!

If you're one who's intimidated in the kitchen, don't be with the following recipes in your arsenal. You'll find most are easy to prepare, the ingredients are readily available in your local stores, and the portions and nutritional information provided with each and every recipe help you eat well after your weight loss surgery. We know you can do this. Prove it to yourself by turning the page!

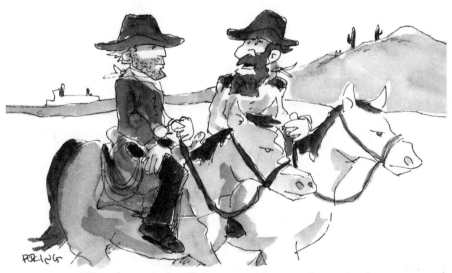

"How 'bout some scallion mini-quiches tonight, pardner?
To maintain our waistlines."

Chapter 12

High-Protein Starters

In This Chapter

- ◆ Good reasons to eat breakfast
- ◆ Delicious, high-protein cereals
- ◆ Protein-packed eggs and omelets
- ◆ Pancakes, scones, and muffins you'll love

Breakfast is one of the most important meals of the day. When you wake up in the morning, it's important to start your day off right with a healthful and nutritious meal because your body is already a little dehydrated from the night and yearning for some fuel. Eating breakfast also jump-starts your metabolism for the day, which can help you lose weight and keep it off.

After your surgery, breakfast is necessary. Because you can't eat a great deal at one time, and because of your dietary needs, it's important that you eat several small meals throughout the day. The recipes in this chapter have a lot of protein, many have a lot of antioxidants, and a few are portable, so you can take them with you for a healthful snack later in the day.

Pumpkin Pie Oatmeal

If you like pumpkin pie, you'll love this healthful and delicious oatmeal with hints of cinnamon, nutmeg, and maple.

Yield: 1 serving
Prep time: 2 minutes
Cook time: 16 minutes
Serving size: about ½ cup
Each serving has:
140 calories
19 g carbohydrate
5 g sugars
6.5 g protein
6 g fat
1 g saturated fat
3 g cholesterol
126 mg sodium
2.3 g fiber
25 IU vitamin D
170 mg potassium
170 mg calcium
3 mcg selenium

¼ **cup skim milk**
6 **TB. water**
¼ **cup quick-cooking oats**
½ **tsp. ground cinnamon**
½ **tsp. ground nutmeg**

4 **TB. canned pumpkin**
4 **TB. sliced almonds**
1 **TB. sugar-free maple syrup**
4 **TB. vanilla Greek yogurt**

1. In a medium saucepan over medium heat, bring skim milk and water to a gentle boil, about 10 minutes.

2. Add oats, cinnamon, and nutmeg, and stir to combine. Reduce heat low, and simmer for 5 minutes or until desired consistency is reached.

3. Stir in pumpkin, almonds, maple syrup, and Greek yogurt. Heat for 1 more minute, and serve immediately.

 Food for Thought _____

Why did we call for skim milk in this recipe over whole or even 2 percent? Here's why: for the amount of milk called for in Pumpkin Pie Oatmeal, skim milk has 34 calories and .1 gram fat, 2 percent has 47 calories and 1.6 grams fat, and whole milk has 66 calories and 3.9 grams fat.

Chilled Mixed Berry and Walnut Oatmeal

On hot summer mornings, you'll love this chilled oatmeal topped with sweet blueberries, raspberries, and blackberries.

½ cup old-fashioned rolled oats

¼ cup almond milk

¼ cup water

½ tsp. ground cinnamon

1 tsp. Splenda

1 TB. fresh blueberries

1 TB. fresh blackberries

1 TB. fresh raspberries

1 TB. walnuts, chopped

Yield: 1 serving
Prep time: 12 hours or overnight
Serving size: about ½ cup
Each serving has:
224 calories
35 g carbohydrate
7 g sugars
15 g protein
9 g fat
.4 g saturated fat
0 g cholesterol
38 mg sodium
9 g fiber
25 IU vitamin D
77 mg potassium
83 mg calcium
.4 mcg selenium

1. The night before, mix oats, almond milk, water, cinnamon, and Splenda in a cereal bowl. Cover with plastic wrap, and refrigerate overnight.

2. Before serving, add blueberries, blackberries, raspberries, and walnuts to top of oatmeal.

Food for Thought

Many kinds of milk are available, including almond, soy, oat, goat, cow, etc. In this recipe, we call for almond milk because it's slightly sweeter than the other milks, and it also gives a nice nutty flavor to the oatmeal.

Chai Craisin Oatmeal

This chai oatmeal will delight your taste buds with a hint of vanilla and a slight tartness from the dried craisins.

Yield: 1 serving
Prep time: 2 minutes
Cook time: 2 minutes
Serving size: ¼ cup
Each serving has:
255 calories
31 g carbohydrate
10 g sugars
28 g protein
4 g fat
.3 g saturated fat
0 g cholesterol
421 mg sodium
3 g fiber
25 IU vitamin D
170 mg potassium
175 mg calcium
0 mcg selenium

½ cup quick-cooking oats

2 tsp. instant chai mix

2 tsp. dried cranberries, chopped

2 tsp. Splenda

¼ cup light vanilla soy milk

¾ cup water

1 TB. vanilla protein powder

1. In a microwave-safe dish, combine oats, chai mix, dried cranberries, Splenda, soy milk, water, and protein powder.

2. Microwave, covered with a paper towel, for 2 minutes.

3. Stir and serve immediately.

 Food for Thought _____

Cranberries have been proven to help fight cancer, heart disease, and urinary tract infections. They've also been proven to be a probiotic.

Banana-Walnut Oatmeal

This delicious oatmeal with bananas and walnuts surprises with hints of vanilla, nutmeg, and cinnamon.

¼ cup light vanilla soy milk

1 cup water

½ cup quick-cooking oats

½ large banana, peeled and mashed (about ½ cup)

½ TB. sugar-free maple syrup

1 TB. vanilla protein powder

½ tsp. ground cinnamon

¼ tsp. ground nutmeg

½ TB. toasted walnuts

Yield: 1 serving
Prep time: 2 minutes
Cook time: 7 minutes
Serving size: ¼ cup
Each serving has:
349 calories
45 g carbohydrate
8 g sugars
32 g protein
6 g fat
.4 g saturated fat
0 g cholesterol
326 mg sodium
6 g fiber
0 IU vitamin D
241 mg potassium
36 mg calcium
.6 mcg selenium

1. In a medium saucepan over medium heat, heat soy milk and water for 5 minutes or until almost boiling.

2. Add oats and cook, stirring, for 1 or 2 minutes or until creamy.

3. Remove from heat and stir in mashed banana, maple syrup, protein powder, cinnamon, and nutmeg.

4. Pour into a serving bowl, top with walnuts, and serve.

Food for Thought

Bananas are a great source of potassium, and the walnuts in this recipe are a delicious source of healthy fats.

Creamy Wheat-Berry Cereal

This simple hot cereal features refreshing cranberries, delicious almonds, and the sweet taste of brown sugar.

Yield: 1 serving
Prep time: 2 minutes
Cook time: 20 minutes
Serving size: ¾ cup
Each serving has:
328 calories
37 g carbohydrate
6.5 g sugars
33 g protein
5 g fat
.4 g saturated fat
0 g cholesterol
351 mg sodium
5 g fiber
60 IU vitamin D
165 mg potassium
252 mg calcium
0 mcg selenium

¼ cup plus 1 tsp. old-fashioned rolled oats

1 TB. dried cranberries

¾ cup light vanilla soy milk

¼ cup plus 1 tsp. cooked wheat berries

½ tsp. brown sugar Splenda

1 TB. vanilla protein powder

½ tsp. ground cinnamon

1 tsp. slivered almonds, toasted

1. In a large, microwave-safe bowl, mix together oats, cranberries, and soy milk. Microwave on high, covered with a paper towel, for 3 minutes.

3. Stir in cooked wheat berries, and microwave 1 or 2 more minutes, or until heated through.

4. Let stand for 1 minute. Stir in brown sugar Splenda, protein powder, and cinnamon. Sprinkle with toasted almonds, and serve.

Cooking Tip

Cooking wheat berries is fairly simple. Using a 3½:1 water to wheat berries ratio (3½ cups water to 1 cup wheat berries), heat the water and wheat berries on high until the water comes to a boil, cover, reduce heat to low, and cook until the water has completely been absorbed. For this recipe, you need approximately 3 tablespoons wheat berries to ⅓ cup water. Cook for about 10 minutes.

Good-for-You Scrambled Eggs

This version of classic scrambled eggs uses liquid egg substitute and some tofu, accented by some hot pepper sauce and turmeric. The result is much lower in fat and is an excellent source of protein.

¼ cup liquid egg substitute

1 tsp. ground turmeric

½ tsp. hot pepper sauce

¼ tsp. salt

¼ tsp. freshly cracked black pepper

1 tsp. extra-virgin olive oil

2 TB. firm tofu

Yield: 1 serving
Prep time: 5 minutes
Cook time: 2 minutes
Serving size: about ¼ cup
Each serving has:
105 calories
2.5 g carbohydrate
1 g sugars
11 g protein
5 g fat
.7 g saturated fat
0 g cholesterol
766 mg sodium
.4 g fiber
65 IU vitamin D
119 mg potassium
136 mg calcium
0 mcg selenium

1. In a small bowl, and with a fork, blend egg substitute, turmeric, hot pepper sauce, salt, and pepper.

2. In a small, nonstick skillet over medium-low heat, heat olive oil.

3. Crumble tofu into the skillet and cook, stirring, for 20 to 30 seconds or until warmed through.

4. Add egg mixture to skillet, and stir for 1 minute or until egg is set but still creamy. Serve immediately.

Food for Thought

Turmeric is a spice with a slightly peppery flavor known as "Indian saffron" because of its golden yellow color.

Poached Eggs with Home Fries and Country Ham

This is a breakfast classic with Yukon gold potatoes, delicious country ham, and poached eggs, but with a healthy spin.

Yield: 8 servings
Prep time: 10 minutes
Cook time: 48 minutes
Serving size: 1 cup
Each serving has:
376 calories
40 g carbohydrate
3 g sugars
21 g protein
15 g fat
4 g saturated fat
236 g cholesterol
501 mg sodium
5 g fiber
30 IU vitamin D
1,234 mg potassium
60 mg calcium
25 mcg selenium

2 tsp. vinegar

8 medium Yukon gold potatoes, cubed

4 TB. extra-virgin olive oil

1 large Vidalia onion, diced small

2 cups button mushrooms, sliced

2 tsp. paprika

2 tsp. garlic powder

4 whole scallions (green and white parts), sliced

¼ tsp. salt

½ tsp. freshly cracked black pepper

1 (12-oz.) pkg. low-sodium, low-fat ham, sliced

8 large eggs

1. Fill a medium saucepan half full with water, add vinegar, and bring to a very light simmer over medium-low heat.

2. Fill another medium saucepan with water and potatoes, and set over high heat. When water boils, allow potatoes to cook for 5 minutes.

3. In a large sauté pan over medium-high heat, add olive oil, onion, and mushrooms, and sauté for 10 minutes or until onions are slightly translucent.

4. Add potatoes to the sauté pan, and cook for about 15 minutes or until potatoes are golden brown, stirring occasionally.

5. Add paprika, garlic powder, scallions, salt, and pepper to potato mixture.

6. Reduce heat to low, and arrange slices of ham over potatoes. Cover and cook for 3 or 4 minutes.

7. While ham is heating, poach eggs in vinegar water for 3 or 4 minutes or until eggs are cooked to your liking.

8. When eggs are finished, divide home fries and ham among 8 plates and top each with 1 poached egg. Serve immediately.

Cooking Tip

Poaching an egg can be tricky. The water has to be hot enough to cook the egg, but not so hot that the water boils. I like to crack the egg in a small cup, and gently pour the egg into the hot water. Give it a gentle stir in a circle motion so the egg white curls around itself, and let it sit and cook. The vinegar helps coagulate the proteins. Remove the cooked egg from the water using a slotted spoon.

Spinach, Tomato, Feta, and Basil Omelet

This delicious omelet—bright and colorful thanks to the green spinach and basil and vibrant red tomatoes—is sure to please.

Yield: 1 serving
Prep time: 2 minutes
Cook time: 7 minutes
Serving size: ½ cup
Each serving has:
165 calories
9 g carbohydrate
5 g sugars
19 g protein
6 g fat
2 g saturated fat
6 g cholesterol
822 mg sodium
2 g fiber
49 IU vitamin D
379 mg potassium
126 mg calcium
.6 mcg selenium

1 tsp. extra-virgin olive oil

5 cherry tomatoes, diced

1 whole scallion, sliced

1 cup fresh baby spinach

½ cup liquid egg substitute

1 TB. skim milk

1 TB. low-fat crumbled feta cheese

⅛ tsp. salt

⅛ tsp. freshly cracked black pepper

1 TB. fresh basil, chopped *chiffonade*

1. Spray a small, nonstick skillet with cooking spray. Add olive oil, and heat over medium-high heat.

2. Add tomatoes and scallion to the skillet, and cook, stirring once or twice, for 1 or 2 minutes or until vegetables are softened.

3. Arrange spinach on top, cover, and let spinach wilt for about 30 seconds. Stir to combine.

4. In a small bowl, combine egg substitute and skim milk.

5. Pour egg mixture into the skillet, reduce heat to medium-low, and continue cooking, stirring constantly with a heatproof rubber spatula, for about 20 seconds or until egg is starting to set. Continue cooking, lifting edges so uncooked egg flows underneath, for about 30 more seconds or until egg is mostly set.

6. Sprinkle feta cheese, salt, and pepper over omelet. Cover, reduce heat to low, and cook for about 2 minutes or until egg is completely set and cheese is melted. Fold omelet in half using the spatula. Garnish with chiffonade basil and serve.

def•i•ni•tion

Chiffonade means to cut leafy vegetables and herbs into thin strips. To do this, stack the leaves, largest to smallest, and roll them tightly, from stem to the tip of the leaf. Then simply cut across the rolled leaves with a sharp knife, producing fine ribbons.

Turkey-Bacon, Tomato, and Scallion Mini Quiches

These mini quiches are chock full of fresh tomatoes, scallions, and crispy turkey-bacon.

2¼ cups liquid egg substitute

1 cup skim milk

4 whole scallions, sliced

½ cup tomato, diced

1½ cups shredded low-fat Swiss cheese

½ cup turkey-bacon, chopped

1 tsp. freshly cracked black pepper

Yield: 8 servings
Prep time: 5 minutes
Cook time: 28 minutes
Serving size: 1 quiche
Each serving has:
147 calories
4 g carbohydrate
3 g sugars
498 g protein
.1 g fat
301 g saturated fat
16 g cholesterol
7 mg sodium
3 g fiber
24 IU vitamin D
202 mg potassium
189 mg calcium
4 mcg selenium

1. Preheat the oven to 350°F. Lightly coat a 12 (½-cup) nonstick muffin tin with cooking spray.

2. In a large bowl, whisk together egg substitute and skim milk. Stir in scallions, tomato, Swiss cheese, turkey-bacon, and pepper.

3. Divide egg mixture evenly among the prepared muffin cups, and bake for 25 to 28 minutes or until eggs are cooked and beginning to brown on top.

4. Run a knife around the edges to loosen quiches from the cups, and serve.

 Food for Thought

Here's two bits of good news: turkey-bacon has less fat than regular bacon, and the tomatoes in this recipe provide the antioxidant licopene, which can protect your body from many different types of cancer such as prostate cancer.

Cheesy Egg and Polenta Casserole

This is a great breakfast casserole with tons of flavor along with hearty polenta, creamy mozzarella cheese, rich Parmesan cheese, and Italian turkey sausage.

Yield: 8 servings
Prep time: 10 minutes
Cook time: 1 hour
Serving size: ¼ cup
Each serving has:
176 calories
15 g carbohydrate
1.4 g sugars
13 g protein
7 g fat
1.4 g saturated fat
18 g cholesterol
866 mg sodium
1.1 g fiber
11 IU vitamin D
119 mg potassium
189 mg calcium
.9 mcg selenium

1 TB. plus 2 tsp. extra-virgin olive oil

⅓ cup Spanish onion, diced

4 cups low-sodium, low-fat vegetable stock

1 cup yellow cornmeal

½ tsp. salt

½ tsp. freshly cracked black pepper

¾ cup Italian turkey sausage, casing removed

½ cup reduced-fat shredded mozzarella cheese

½ cup grated Parmesan cheese

1½ cups liquid egg substitute

1. In a large saucepan over medium heat, heat 1 tablespoon olive oil. Add onion and cook, stirring, for 2 to 3 minutes or until onion is softened but not browned.

2. Add vegetable stock, and bring to a boil. Gradually whisk in cornmeal. Add salt and pepper, and cook, whisking constantly, for 1 or 2 minutes or until polenta bubbles. Reduce heat to low, and cook, whisking frequently, for 10 to 15 minutes or until very thick.

3. Meanwhile, heat remaining 2 teaspoons oil in a large skillet over medium heat. Add sausage, and cook, stirring and breaking sausage into small pieces with a spoon, for about 4 minutes or until sausage is lightly browned and no longer pink. Drain if necessary and transfer to a cutting board; let cool. Finely chop when cool enough to handle.

4. Position oven rack in the upper third of the oven, and preheat the oven to 350°F. Coat a 9×13-inch casserole dish with cooking spray.

5. When polenta is done, stir in mozzarella cheese and ¼ cup Parmesan cheese. If polenta seems too stiff, add small amounts of water to thin it to a thick but not stiff consistency. Spread polenta in the prepared baking pan.

6. Make 6 (2-inch-wide) indentations in polenta with the back of a tablespoon. Fold egg substitute into polenta.

7. Scatter sausage over polenta and egg substitute, and sprinkle remaining ¼ cup Parmesan cheese evenly over top. Bake for 15 minutes, set the broiler on low, and broil for 2 to 4 minutes or until egg is set. Let stand for 5 minutes before serving.

def•i•ni•tion

Polenta, loosely translated, is "cornmeal mush." It's much like grits in a sense, but polenta can be served immediately as a mush or chilled, cut into shapes, and reheated. Polenta is one of those foods you can have a lot of fun with by adding different ingredients.

Blackberry-Ricotta Pancakes

These pancakes feature sweet blackberries, rich ricotta cheese, and hints of lemon and nutmeg.

Yield: 8 servings
Prep time: 5 minutes
Cook time: 12 minutes
Serving size: 2 small pancakes
Each serving has:
171 calories
21 g carbohydrate
5 g sugars
12 g protein
4.5 g fat
2 g saturated fat
10 g cholesterol
153 mg sodium
3 g fiber
61 IU vitamin D
228 mg potassium
158 mg calcium
17 mcg selenium

1 cup whole-wheat flour	**¾ cup part-skim ricotta cheese**
¼ cup plus 4 TB. all-purpose flour	**¾ cup vanilla Greek yogurt**
¼ cup vanilla protein powder	**¾ cup liquid egg substitute**
2 tsp. Splenda	**1 cup fat-free buttermilk**
2 tsp. baking powder	**2 tsp. lemon zest**
½ tsp. baking soda	**2 TB. fresh lemon juice**
1 tsp. ground nutmeg	**1½ cups frozen blackberries**

1. In a small bowl, whisk together whole-wheat flour, all-purpose flour, protein powder, Splenda, baking powder, baking soda, and nutmeg.

2. In a large bowl, whisk together ricotta, Greek yogurt, egg substitute, buttermilk, lemon zest, and lemon juice until smooth. Stir dry ingredients into wet ingredients until just combined.

3. Spray a nonstick skillet with cooking spray, and place over medium heat.

4. Using a ¼ cup measure, spoon batter for 2 pancakes into the hot skillet. Sprinkle a few blackberries on each pancake, and cook for about 2 minutes or until edges are dry and bubbles begin to form.

5. Flip over pancakes, and cook for about 2 minutes more or until golden brown. Repeat with batter and blackberries, adjusting heat as necessary to prevent burning. (To keep pancakes warm while the others are cooking, put them on a plate and flip another plate upside down on top.)

Cooking Tip
Greek yogurt, which is used in many of the recipes in this book, has more protein than regular yogurt. For even more benefits, you can use a fat-free or reduced-fat Greek yogurt instead.

Maple-Blueberry Muffins

These delicious maple and blueberry muffins are light and fluffy and sure to put your sweet tooth at ease.

2 TB. ground flaxseeds

¾ cup whole-wheat flour

¾ cup plus 2 TB. all-purpose flour

¼ cup vanilla protein powder

1½ tsp. baking powder

1 tsp. ground cinnamon

½ tsp. ground nutmeg

½ tsp. ground cloves

½ tsp. baking soda

¼ tsp. salt

1 TB. Splenda

¼ cup canned white beans, rinsed and drained

½ cup liquid egg substitute

½ cup sugar-free maple syrup

½ cup fat-free buttermilk

½ cup vanilla Greek yogurt

2 tsp. vegetable oil

2 tsp. orange zest

1 TB. fresh orange juice

½ tsp. vanilla extract

1½ cups fresh blueberries

Yield: 12 servings
Prep time: 8 minutes
Cook time: 25 minutes
Serving size: 1 muffin
Each serving has:
106 calories
18 g carbohydrate
3 g sugars
6 g protein
2 g fat
.3 g saturated fat
.6 g cholesterol
113 mg sodium
2 g fiber
3 IU vitamin D
98 mg potassium
36 mg calcium
8 mcg selenium

1. Preheat the oven to 400°F. Lightly coat a regular 12-cup muffin tin with cooking spray.

2. In a large bowl, whisk together ground flaxseeds, whole-wheat flour, all-purpose flour, protein powder, baking powder, cinnamon, nutmeg, cloves, baking soda, salt, and Splenda.

3. In a food processor fitted with a chopping blade or in a blender, purée white beans for 1 minute or until beans have made a smooth purée.

4. In a medium bowl, whisk together egg substitute and maple syrup until smooth. Add buttermilk, Greek yogurt, vegetable oil, white bean purée, orange zest, orange juice, and vanilla extract until blended.

5. Make a well in dry ingredients and stir in wet ingredients with a rubber spatula just until moistened. Be careful not to overmix batter.

6. Fold or gently stir in blueberries. Scoop batter into the prepared muffin cups.

7. Bake for 15 to 25 minutes or until muffin tops are golden brown and spring back when touched lightly.

8. Let cool in the pan for 5 minutes. Loosen edges with a knife and turn out muffins onto a wire rack to cool slightly.

Cooking Tip

The white beans in this recipe replace the fat and help the muffins retain moisture. When puréeing beans, if you want, run the purée through a fine sieve to remove the beans' outer cover. Or if you want to leave it, it is a good source of fiber.

Apple-Cinnamon Muffins

These apple and cinnamon muffins with a crisp oat topping and subtle hints of vanilla will remind you of fall.

¼ **cup brown sugar Splenda**

½ **cup whole-wheat flour**

Pinch plus ½ tsp. salt

⅛ **tsp. ground cinnamon**

2 TB. reduced-fat margarine

3 TB. old-fashioned rolled oats

2 TB. canned white beans, rinsed and drained

½ **cup Splenda**

2 tsp. vanilla extract

¼ **cup liquid egg substitute**

½ **cup all-purpose flour**

2 TB. vanilla protein powder

½ **tsp. baking powder**

½ **tsp. baking soda**

¼ **cup vanilla Greek yogurt**

2 TB. fat-free buttermilk

2 medium Granny Smith apples, peeled and diced

Yield: 12 servings
Prep time: 8 minutes
Cook time: 20 minutes
Serving size: 1 muffin
Each serving has:
82 calories
13 g carbohydrate
3 g sugars
3 g protein
2 g fat
.5 g saturated fat
.5 g cholesterol
140 mg sodium
2 g fiber
1.3 IU vitamin D
77 mg potassium
19 mg calcium
6 mcg selenium

1. Preheat the oven to 375°F. Line a regular 12-cup muffin tin with paper liners.

2. In a food processor fitted with a chopping blade or in a blender, purée white beans for 1 minute or until beans have made a smooth purée.

3. In a large mixing bowl, and with an electric mixer on low speed, beat brown sugar Splenda, ¼ cup whole-wheat flour, pinch salt, and cinnamon for 2 minutes or until mixture comes together.

4. Place margarine in a small bowl, cover with a paper towel, and microwave for about 30 seconds.

5. Add margarine and beat on low for 1 minute or until crumb mixture forms. Set mixer aside, and work in oats with your hands. Pour topping into a small bowl, and set aside.

6. In the large bowl, and with an electric mixer on low speed, beat puréed white beans, Splenda, and vanilla extract for 2 minutes or until light and fluffy. Add egg substitute, and beat to combine, scraping down the sides of the bowl.

7. In a medium bowl, whisk together all-purpose flour, remaining ¼ cup whole-wheat flour, protein powder, baking powder, baking soda, and ½ teaspoon salt.

8. Add flour mixture all at once to the mixing bowl with bean mixture, along with Greek yogurt and buttermilk. Beat on low speed for 1 minute, scraping down the sides of the bowl after 5 seconds, or just until blended. Stir in diced apples.

9. Spoon a slightly heaping ⅛ cup batter into each muffin cup. Sprinkle oat topping evenly over top of each muffin.

10. Bake for about 20 minutes or until muffins are lightly browned and tops spring back after being pushed.

11. Let cool in the pan for 5 minutes. Turn out muffins onto a wire rack to cool slightly.

Cooking Tip

When choosing an apple for baking, pick one that's crisp and tart such as Granny Smith, Gala, or honeycrisp.

Sun-Dried Tomato–Cottage Cheese Muffins

These muffins featuring sun-dried tomatoes, sweet basil, and creamy cottage cheese, will surprise you. And they won't hurt your waistline. *(Adapted from www.101cookbooks.com.)*

1 cup fat-free cottage cheese

½ cup grated Parmesan cheese

¼ cup whole-wheat flour

1 tsp. baking powder

¼ cup sun-dried tomatoes (dry), chopped

¼ cup fresh basil, chopped

¼ cup water

1 cup liquid egg substitute

½ tsp. salt

¼ tsp. freshly cracked black pepper

Yield: 9 servings
Prep time: 8 minutes
Cook time: 35 minutes
Serving size: 1 muffin
Each serving has:
65 calories
5 g carbohydrate
2 g sugars
8 g protein
1 g fat
1 g saturated fat
5 g cholesterol
376 mg sodium
.6 g fiber
71 IU vitamin D
106 mg potassium
74 mg calcium
3 mcg selenium

1. Preheat the oven to 400°F. Line a regular 12-cup muffin tin with paper liners; you'll only need 9 cups.

2. In a medium bowl, combine cottage cheese, all but 2 tablespoons Parmesan cheese, flour, baking powder, sun-dried tomatoes, basil, water, egg substitute, and salt and pepper until well mixed.

3. Divide batter among 9 muffin cups, filling each ¾ full. Scatter remaining Parmesan cheese over top.

4. Bake for 30 to 35 minutes or until muffins have risen and are golden brown. Serve hot or at room temperature.

 Food for Thought _____

Thanks to their vitamin C content, sun-dried tomatoes have been proven to lower the risk for heart disease, diabetes, and cancer.

Cherry-Pecan Scones

These scones—which taste like cherry pie but *better*—are a healthful and portable snack.

Yield: 16 servings
Prep time: 8 minutes
Cook time: 10 minutes
Serving size: 1 scone
Each serving has:
138 calories
22 g carbohydrate
3.5 g sugars
5 g protein
4 g fat
1 g saturated fat
1 g cholesterol
185 mg sodium
2 g fiber
1 IU vitamin D
63 mg potassium
24 mg calcium
17 mcg selenium

¼ cup liquid egg substitute

1 cup reduced-fat buttermilk

2 TB. canola oil

2 tsp. grated orange zest

½ cup old-fashioned rolled oats

1¼ cups whole-wheat flour

1½ cups all-purpose flour

¼ cup vanilla protein powder

⅓ cup Splenda

1 TB. baking powder

1 tsp. salt

½ cup dried cherries

¼ cup sliced pecans

1. Preheat the oven to 350°F. Lightly coat a cookie sheet with pan spray.

2. In a small bowl, combine egg substitute with buttermilk. Add canola oil and orange zest, and mix to combine.

3. In a large bowl, mix together oats, whole-wheat flour, all-purpose flour, protein powder, Splenda, baking powder, and salt.

4. Stir buttermilk mixture into dry ingredients, and mix just until dough comes together. Do not overmix.

5. Fold in cherries and pecans.

6. Scoop heaping tablespoons of dough onto the prepared cookie sheet, and bake 10 minutes or until scones are slightly golden on top.

 Food for Thought

Cherries are proven to be an anti-inflammatory and can help ease joint pain, even arthritis.

Chapter 13

Healthful Snacks

In This Chapter

- Tasty trail mixes
- Super salsas and relishes
- Sweet fruit treats
- Portable snacks to make and take

Two important factors in eating well after weight loss surgery—and keeping the weight off—are what you eat and how often you eat. That's where snacking comes in.

In this chapter, we give you more than a dozen healthful snack recipes, most of which are both quick and easy to prepare. Many are also suitable to make ahead of time, pack in zipper-lock bags or travel plastic containers, and take with you for a quick and satisfying snack throughout the day or week. With good and good-for-you snacks portioned and ready to go, you can grab a snack as you run out the door, eliminating the need to visit or even think about the vending machine later!

Although we give you plenty of party-worthy appetizers in Chapter 14, don't overlook this chapter when planning a party, as many of these recipes hold their own at parties. And beyond snacking, the salsas, dips, and relishes in this chapter are great accompaniments to many of the entrées in later chapters.

Classic Trail Mix

This classic trail mix features dried cranberries, almonds, and peanuts, with the additional twist of dried figs and a crispy crunchy protein bar.

Yield: 8 servings
Prep time: 5 minutes
Serving size: 4 tablespoons
Each serving has:
104 calories
12 g carbohydrate
3 g sugars
4 g protein
5 g fat
1 g saturated fat
0 g cholesterol
54 mg sodium
1 g fiber
0 IU vitamin D
118 mg potassium
53 mg calcium
3 mcg selenium

1 low-fat (less than 5 g) crunchy protein bar

¼ cup whole unsalted almonds

4 TB. unsalted peanuts

4 TB. dried cranberries

4 TB. dried, halved dates

1. Cut protein bars lengthwise into 3 equal pieces and then cut each of those into 6 equal parts.

2. In a small bowl, combine protein bar pieces, almonds, peanuts, cranberries, and dates.

3. Evenly divide mixture among 8 zipper-lock bags. Store in a cool, dry place for up to 2 weeks.

> **Cooking Tip**
>
> If you crave a chewier trail mix, use a chewy protein bar instead of a crunchy one. Just be sure it has less than 5 grams fat.

Off-the-Trail Mix

Not your typical trail mix, but equally delicious with feta cheese, succulent turkey, crisp walnuts, and delicious pumpkin seeds.

1 TB. cubed feta cheese

2 TB. low-sodium, low-fat turkey, diced

1 TB. walnuts

½ TB. unsalted pumpkin seeds

1 TB. unsweetened dried cranberries

1. In a zipper-lock bag, combine feta cheese, turkey, walnuts, pumpkin seeds, and cranberries.

2. Store in the refrigerator for up to 1 week.

Food for Thought

Unsweetened dried cranberries are delicious and have less sugar than some of the other dried fruits like dried cherries.

Yield: 1 serving
Prep time: 5 minutes
Serving size: 5½ table-spoons
Each serving has:
138 calories
9 g carbohydrate
5 g sugars
8 g protein
10 g fat
2 g saturated fat
12 g cholesterol
241 mg sodium
1 g fiber
0 IU vitamin D
132 mg potassium
23 mg calcium
6 mcg selenium

Fruity Peanut Protein Bars

These delicious peanut butter bars with tons of dried fruits and hints of apples will surely please your sweet tooth.

Yield: 16 servings
Prep time: 10 minutes
Cook time: 35 minutes
Serving size: 1 bar
Each serving has:
97 calories
14 g carbohydrate
4 g sugars
6 g protein
2 g fat
.5 g saturated fat
.3 g cholesterol
122 mg sodium
2 g fiber
15 IU vitamin D
33 mg potassium
41 mg calcium
3 mcg selenium

½ cup plain protein powder

¼ cup oat bran

½ cup whole-wheat flour

2 TB. wheat germ

¼ tsp. kosher salt

¼ cup unsweetened dried cherries

¼ cup unsweetened dried cranberries

¼ cup unsweetened dried blueberries

¼ cup unsweetened dried apricots

¾ cup silken tofu

¼ cup apple juice

¼ cup brown sugar Splenda

¼ cup liquid egg substitute

⅓ cup reduced-fat peanut butter

1. Preheat the oven to 350°F. Line the bottom of a 13×9-inch glass baking dish with parchment paper and lightly coat with canola oil.

2. In a large mixing bowl, combine protein powder, oat bran, flour, wheat germ, and salt. Set aside.

3. Coarsely chop cherries, cranberries, blueberries, and apricots, and place in a small bowl. Set aside.

4. In another medium mixing bowl, whisk tofu until smooth. Add apple juice, brown sugar Splenda, egg substitute, and peanut butter, whisking to combine after each addition. Add to protein powder mixture, and stir well to combine. Fold in dried fruit.

5. Spread batter evenly in the prepared baking dish, and bake for 35 minutes or until bars have firmed.

6. Remove from the oven and cool completely before cutting into 16 squares. Store in an airtight container at room temperature for up to 1 week.

 Food for Thought

You can mix things up in this recipe by using different nut butters other than peanut butter.

Mixed-Bean Salsa

Garbanzo beans, black beans, kidney beans, and cannellini beans star in this hearty four-bean salsa tossed with fresh garlic, lime juice, and cilantro.

1 (14.5-oz.) can black beans, drained and rinsed

1 (14.5-oz.) can kidney beans, drained and rinsed

1 (15-oz.) can garbanzo beans, drained and rinsed

1 (14.5-oz.) can cannellini beans, drained and rinsed

1 TB. vegetable oil

1 tsp. cumin

2 TB. chili powder

1 tsp. fresh lime juice

1 (8-oz.) jar low-sodium chunky salsa

2 tsp. fresh garlic (about 1 large clove), minced

1 TB. fresh parsley, chopped

Yield: 8 servings
Prep time: 45 minutes
Serving size: 3 table-spoons
Each serving has:
168 calories
29 g carbohydrate
4 g sugars
10 g protein
2 g fat
0 g saturated fat
0 g cholesterol
424 mg sodium
8 g fiber
0 IU vitamin D
297 mg potassium
56 mg calcium
0 mcg selenium

1. In a large mixing bowl, combine black beans, kidney beans, garbanzo beans, cannellini beans, vegetable oil, cumin, chili powder, lime juice, salsa, garlic, and parsley.

2. Chill in the refrigerator for at least 30 minutes before serving with sliced pita bread or chips.

Food for Thought

All the beans in this recipe amp up the protein. Beans are a good way to boost protein in any dish, even in some recipes you might not suspect beans to work well, such as in some of the muffin recipes in Chapter 12.

Corn and Black Bean Salsa

This sweet corn and black bean salsa with vibrant red bell peppers and delicious fresh herbs is a great addition to any table. (*Adapted from www.cooksrecipes.com.*)

Yield: 14 servings
Prep time: 40 minutes
Serving size: 2 table-spoons
Each serving has:
37 calories
7 g carbohydrate
.3 g sugars
1 g protein
1 g fat
.1 g saturated fat
0 g cholesterol
109 mg sodium
1 g fiber
0 IU vitamin D
83 mg potassium
5 mg calcium
0 mcg selenium

2 cups frozen corn kernels, thawed

½ cup black beans, rinsed

1 TB. vegetable oil

2 TB. diced red bell pepper

¼ cup diced red onion

1 clove garlic, minced

1 jalapeño pepper, ribs and seeds removed, and chopped

1 TB. fresh lime juice

½ tsp. salt

½ tsp. ground cumin

⅛ tsp. freshly cracked black pepper

1 TB. fresh cilantro, chopped

1 TB. fresh parsley, chopped

1. In a medium bowl, combine corn, black beans, vegetable oil, red bell pepper, onion, garlic, jalapeño, lime juice, salt, cumin, pepper, cilantro, and parsley.

2. Allow to sit for at least 30 minutes in the refrigerator before serving.

 Food for Thought

Not only is this salsa great with chips, but it's also terrific served with grilled chicken, pulled pork on soft tacos, quesadillas—you name it!

Fresh Mango Salsa

This delicious and healthful mango salsa is complemented by coconut, ginger, and cilantro.

2 mangoes

2 TB. fresh cilantro, chopped

1 TB. fresh ginger, peeled and minced

1 TB. unsweetened coconut flakes

½ tsp. salt

⅛ tsp. red pepper flakes

1 small red onion, sliced

½ tsp. white wine vinegar

Yield: 6 servings
Prep time: 10 minutes
Serving size: ¼ cup
Each serving has:
58 calories
14 g carbohydrate
.2 g sugars
.7 g protein
.3 g fat
0 g saturated fat
0 g cholesterol
197 mg sodium
1 g fiber
0 IU vitamin D
17 mg potassium
3 mg calcium
0 mcg selenium

1. Cut mangoes in half around the stone and then criss-cross flesh with a knife into ¼-inch squares. Push diced mango flesh outward, and slice off the squares from the skin into a bowl.

2. Add cilantro, ginger, coconut flakes, salt, red pepper flakes, onion, and white wine vinegar.

3. Allow to sit in the refrigerator for up to 30 minutes before serving with any number of foods such as chicken and fish.

Cooking Tip

A mango core is pretty big, so be careful when cutting around it. If you've never cut a mango before, first chop off one end so you have a level surface to do your cutting.

Fresh Corn Relish

This tangy sweet corn relish with bell peppers and sweet Vidalia onions would be great on chicken, fish, or even chips.

Yield: 8 servings
Prep time: 15 minutes
Cook time: 35 minutes
Serving size: 2 table-spoons
Each serving has:
189 calories
39 g carbohydrate
10 g sugars
4 g protein
1 g fat
0 g saturated fat
0 g cholesterol
883 mg sodium
5 g fiber
0 IU vitamin D
416 mg potassium
32 mg calcium
0 mcg selenium

4 cups fresh corn kernels

6 red bell peppers, ribs and seeds removed, and chopped (5 cups)

5 orange bell peppers, ribs and seeds removed, and chopped (4 cups)

2 small Vidalia onions, chopped (2 cups)

4 cups apple cider vinegar

2 cups Splenda

1 tsp. salt

1 TB. turmeric

1 bay leaf

1 tsp. freshly cracked black pepper

1 TB. mustard seed

1. In a large saucepan over medium heat, combine corn, red bell peppers, orange bell peppers, and onion. Add cider vinegar, Splenda, salt, turmeric, bay leaf, pepper, and mustard seed.

2. Bring to a boil, and simmer over low heat for 25 minutes or until vegetables are tender.

3. Remove bay leaf, and store in the refrigerator for up to 1 week. Serve with burgers, chips, even chicken.

 Post-Op Pitfall _____

Whenever you're cooking with a bay leaf, be sure to remove it before serving the food so no one mistakenly takes a bite of it because it's hard and really unpleasant to eat.

Apple-Orange Chutney

This sweet apple and orange chutney with hints of ginger is perfect to serve with toast in the morning or as a dip with cheese.

2 Gala apples, peeled, cored, and chopped

¼ cup fresh orange juice

2 TB. orange zest

½ small Vidalia onion, chopped (¼ cup)

2 TB. red wine vinegar

2 TB. brown sugar Splenda

1½ tsp. freshly grated ginger, peeled

½ tsp. allspice

¼ tsp. freshly cracked black pepper

Yield: 8 servings
Prep time: 10 minutes
Cook time: 1 hour
Serving size: 2 table-spoons
Each serving has:
21 calories
5 g carbohydrate
3 g sugars
.2 g protein
0 g fat
0 g saturated fat
0 g cholesterol
.3 mg sodium
.5 g fiber
0 IU vitamin D
51 mg potassium
4 mg calcium
0 mcg selenium

1. In a medium saucepan over medium heat, combine apples, orange juice, orange zest, onion, red wine vinegar, brown sugar Splenda, ginger, allspice, and black pepper.

2. Bring to a boil; reduce heat to low, and simmer, covered, for 50 minutes.

3. Uncover and simmer over low heat for 3 more minutes to cook off excess liquid. Let cool before serving over chicken or fish.

🚫 **Post-Op Pitfall** _____

When you zest citrus, be sure not to get any of the pith (the white part). It has a bitter flavor no one will find appealing. When zesting, it's important to only get the colorful skin on the outside because it carries a lot of flavor.

Papaya-Pomegranate Relish

This sweet and tart papaya pomegranate relish overflowing with antioxidants is good and good for you. *(Adapted from www. eatingwell.com.)*

Yield: 12 servings
Prep time: 15 minutes
Serving size: 2 table-spoons
Each serving has:
27 calories
7 g carbohydrate
5 g sugars
.3 g protein
0 g fat
0 g saturated fat
0 g cholesterol
105 mg sodium
.5 g fiber
0 IU vitamin D
50 mg potassium
11 mg calcium
.2 mcg selenium

2 cloves garlic, crushed and peeled

½ tsp. salt

3 TB. rice vinegar

2 tsp. Splenda

2 tsp. hot pepper sauce

1 papaya, peeled, seeded, and finely diced

1 pomegranate, fruit removed

½ cup diced red onion

¼ cup fresh cilantro, chopped

1. In a medium bowl, combine garlic, salt, rice vinegar, Splenda, hot pepper sauce, papaya, pomegranate, red onion, and cilantro.

2. Allow to sit in the refrigerator for 30 minutes before serving with chips or chicken.

 Food for Thought

Pomegranates might seem a little intimidating if you're buying a fresh one for the first time, but as soon as you break it open, removing the seeds is *so* simple! You just have to simply pluck them out.

Avocado and Grapefruit Relish

Fresh avocado and grapefruit pair with sweet honey and fresh mint in this relish you're sure to love.

1 large grapefruit, seeded, peeled, and segmented (without membrane)

½ avocado, peeled, seeded, and diced

1 small red onion, thinly sliced

1 TB. fresh mint, chopped

1 tsp. red wine vinegar

1 tsp. honey

½ tsp. red pepper flakes

Yield: 8 servings
Prep time: 10 minutes
Serving size: 2 tablespoons
Each serving has:
80 calories
12 g carbohydrate
8 g sugars
1 g protein
4 g fat
.6 g saturated fat
0 g cholesterol
3 mg sodium
3 g fiber
0 IU vitamin D
265 mg potassium
17 mg calcium
0 mcg selenium

1. In a medium bowl, combine grapefruit segments, avocado, red onion, mint, vinegar, honey, and red pepper flakes.

2. Toss well to combine, and serve over fish or chicken.

Cooking Tip

For a milder version of this recipe, feel free to omit the red pepper flakes.

Roasted Garlic and Goat Cheese Dip

This creamy roasted garlic goat cheese dip swirled with rich Parmesan cheese and topped with delicious chives is sure to please at your next party. *(Adapted from www.lowfatlifestyle.com.)*

Yield: 12 servings
Prep time: 15 minutes
Cook time: 45 minutes
Serving size: 2 table-spoons
Each serving has:
53 calories
3 g carbohydrate
.6 g sugars
5 g protein
3 g fat
1.5 g saturated fat
7 g cholesterol
157 mg sodium
0 g fiber
1.5 IU vitamin D
64 mg potassium
84 mg calcium
2 mcg selenium

1 head garlic

1 tsp. extra-virgin olive oil

1 (8-oz.) pkg. fat-free cream cheese, softened

2 TB. plain Greek yogurt

4 TB. goat cheese

¼ cup grated Parmesan cheese

¼ tsp. salt

½ tsp. freshly cracked black pepper

3 TB. skim milk

2 TB. fresh chives, chopped

1. Preheat the oven to 400°F.

2. Slice top off garlic bulb to reveal cloves. Drizzle olive oil over top, and wrap garlic head in aluminum foil. Bake for 45 minutes.

3. When cool, remove garlic cloves from their skins by gently squeezing into a medium bowl. Mash with a fork.

4. Add cream cheese, Greek yogurt, goat cheese, Parmesan cheese, salt, pepper, and milk, mixing well and adding extra milk if necessary to achieve a spreadable consistency.

5. Spoon into a serving bowl, and sprinkle with chopped chives.

 Food for Thought

This recipe can be used to create many variations of goat cheese dip such as cranberry goat cheese dip with dried cranberries, or tomato-basil goat cheese dip with sun-dried tomatoes and fresh chopped basil.

Antioxidant Fruit and Yogurt

This sweet treat not only provides protein, but also fills you up with healthy antioxidants. *(Adapted from www.foodnetwork.com.)*

2 TB. fresh mango, diced	**1 tsp. fresh lime juice**
1 TB. fresh blueberries	**¼ cup vanilla Greek yogurt**
2 TB. fresh pomegranate fruit	

1. In a small bowl, gently toss mango, blueberries, and pomegranate fruit with lime juice.

2. Spoon Greek yogurt into a serving dish, top with fruit mixture, and serve.

Cooking Tip

Feel free to mix and match different fruits to add to the yogurt. You can even try adding dried fruits. All of these have a ton of healthful antioxidants.

Yield: 1 serving
Prep time: 3 minutes
Serving size: ½ cup
Each serving has:
69 calories
12 g carbohydrate
11 g sugars
4 g protein
1 g fat
.6 g saturated fat
4 g cholesterol
43 mg sodium
1 g fiber
0 IU vitamin D
176 mg potassium
113 mg calcium
2 mcg selenium

Fresh Berries with Maple Yogurt

Here, fresh blueberries and raspberries are topped with sweet, maple-scented Greek yogurt.

Yield: 8 servings
Prep time: 5 minutes
Serving size: ½ cup
Each serving has:
50 calories
10 g carbohydrate
5 g sugars
2 g protein
1 g fat
.4 g saturated fat
2 g cholesterol
39 mg sodium
1 g fiber
0 IU vitamin D
111 mg potassium
74 mg calcium
1 mcg selenium

1¼ cups vanilla Greek yogurt	1½ cups fresh blueberries
¼ cup sugar-free maple syrup	1 cup fresh raspberries

1. In a small bowl, combine Greek yogurt and maple syrup.

2. Divide berries among 8 serving bowls.

3. Top each bowl of berries with maple syrup–yogurt mixture, and serve immediately. (If you're not using all 8 servings at once, store maple yogurt and berries separately until ready to serve.)

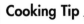

Cooking Tip

Swap out the berries if you like, or you could even try replacing them with some dried fruit and granola.

Baked Apples

This tastes just like apple pie and ice cream—but without the extra fat and calories (and the guilt)!

¼ cup dried cranberries

1 cup chopped walnuts

¾ cup brown sugar Splenda

¾ cup water

1½ tsp. ground cinnamon

¼ tsp. ground nutmeg

¼ tsp. ground cloves

5 honeycrisp apples, peeled, cored, and sliced

1¼ cups vanilla Greek yogurt

Yield: 16 servings
Prep time: 5 minutes
Cook time: 20 minutes
Serving size: ¼ cup
Each serving has:
101 calories
13 g carbohydrate
10 g sugars
2 g protein
5 g fat
1 g saturated fat
2 g cholesterol
14 mg sodium
2 g fiber
0 IU vitamin D
107 mg potassium
43 mg calcium
.4 mcg selenium

1. In a large, microwave-safe dish, combine dried cranberries, walnuts, brown sugar Splenda, water, cinnamon, nutmeg, cloves, and apples.

2. Microwave, covered, on high, stirring occasionally, for 20 minutes or until apples are soft.

3. Serve hot or chilled over Greek yogurt.

Food for Thought

This recipe would work equally well with any peaches or pears you might have lying around. Use the same number as the number of apples called for here.

Almond and Cranberry Biscotti

This tasty little almond and dried cranberry cookie goes great with coffee. *(Adapted from mayoclinic.com.)*

Yield: 24 servings
Prep time: 10 minutes
Cook time: 40 minutes
Serving size: 1 cookie
Each serving has:
54 calories
8 g carbohydrate
4 g sugars
3 g protein
1 g fat
0 g saturated fat
0 g cholesterol
31 mg sodium
0 g fiber
2 IU vitamin D
31 mg potassium
9 mg calcium
3 mcg selenium

¼ **cup whole-wheat flour**

¼ **cup all-purpose flour**

¼ **cup vanilla protein powder**

¼ **cup plain protein powder**

½ **cup Splenda**

1 **tsp. baking powder**

½ **cup liquid egg substitute**

¼ **cup low-fat milk**

2½ **TB. vegetable oil**

2 **TB. dark honey**

1 **tsp. almond extract**

¼ **cup chopped almonds**

⅔ **cup dried cranberries**

1. Preheat the oven to 350°F. Lightly coat a cookie sheet with cooking spray.

2. In a large bowl, combine whole-wheat flour, all-purpose flour, vanilla protein powder, plain protein powder, Splenda, and baking powder.

3. In a separate bowl, whisk together egg substitute, milk, vegetable oil, honey, and almond extract.

4. Add the dry ingredients to the liquid ingredients a little at a time, and mix until all ingredients are fully incorporated.

5. Add almonds and cranberries, and mix until ingredients are evenly distributed.

6. Pour out dough onto the prepared cookie sheet, and form into a log 12 inches long, 3 inches wide, and 1 inch thick.

7. Bake for 25 minutes or until lightly brown. Allow to cool slightly, and slice with a serrated knife into 24 (½-inch) slices.

8. Return cookies to oven for about 15 minutes or until they're crisp. Remove from the oven and let cool completely. Store in an airtight container.

 Food for Thought _____

Many honey varietals are available, depending on what flower is used. Dark honey is produced by chestnut, huckleberry, and avocado flowers. Lighter-colored honeys are made from lavender and clover.

Chapter 14

Appetizers That Really Please

In This Chapter

- ◆ Tasty chicken and seafood hors d'oeuvres
- ◆ Olé! Mexican appetizers
- ◆ Veggie noshes and nibbles
- ◆ Delicious dips and spreads

A few months after your weight loss surgery, you might be seeing amazing results, feeling pretty good, and wanting to celebrate your success. So why not throw a party? In this chapter, we give you recipes great for entertaining. From chicken dishes to seafood treats—even vegetarian options—we've got the whole party covered.

Another plus: the recipes in this chapter are easily adaptable. Try mixing and matching some of the flavors to come up with some new and interesting culinary creations of your own. There's a little something for everyone, so dig in!

Chicken Sate with Spicy Peanut Sauce

These delicious grilled chicken skewers feature spicy peanut sauce made with fresh ginger, coconut, lime, and peanut butter.

Yield: 8 servings
Prep time: 70 minutes
Cook time: 8 minutes
Serving size: about 3 skewers
Each serving has:
234 calories
10 g carbohydrate
2 g sugars
32 g protein
8.5 g fat
2 g saturated fat
71 g cholesterol
690 mg sodium
1 g fiber
0 IU vitamin D
19 mg potassium
4 mg calcium
0 mcg selenium

1¼ cups low-sodium chicken broth

1 cup plus 2 tsp. plus 3 TB. low-sodium soy sauce

1 cup light coconut milk

2 shallots, thinly sliced

3 cloves garlic, peeled and minced

4 tsp. brown sugar Splenda

1 tsp. lime zest

3½ TB. fresh ginger, peeled and minced

2 lb. low-fat chicken tenders, about 16 tenders

16 bamboo skewers, soaked in water for 20 minutes

½ cup low-fat creamy peanut butter

2 TB. fresh lime juice

¼ tsp. chili flakes

½ tsp. cayenne

1 shallot, chopped

¼ cup peanuts, chopped

4 TB. fresh cilantro, chopped

1. Preheat the grill to medium-high heat.

2. In a medium bowl, whisk together 1 cup chicken broth, 1 cup plus 2 teaspoons soy sauce, coconut milk, sliced shallots, 2 cloves minced garlic, 2 teaspoons brown sugar Splenda, lime zest, and 2 tablespoons ginger. Add chicken strips, and marinate in the refrigerator for 1 hour.

3. Remove chicken from marinade and discard marinade. Thread chicken strips onto the skewers, and set in refrigerator.

4. In a blender, blend peanut butter, remaining ¼ cup chicken broth, remaining 3 tablespoons soy sauce, remaining 2 teaspoons brown sugar Splenda, remaining 1½ tablespoons ginger, lime juice, remaining 1 teaspoon minced garlic, chili flakes, cayenne, and chopped shallot for 1 or 2 minutes or until smooth. Set aside.

5. Grill chicken on skewers for 3 or 4 minutes per side or until internal temperature reaches 165°F. Serve with dipping sauce, chopped peanuts, and cilantro.

Food for Thought

Capsacin, the ingredient that makes peppers hot and the red pepper flakes, also has some healthful benefits. It's been shown to provide pain relief, help fight prostate cancer, burn fat, help your heart by reducing cholesterol, and fight inflammation.

Tomato and Chicken Bruschetta with Goat Cheese and Chives

Here, crispy bruschetta bread is topped with fresh tomatoes, chicken, creamy goat cheese, and chives.

1 whole-grain baguette, cut diagonally into 16 (½-in.-thick) slices

1 medium tomato, diced small

6 oz. chicken tenders (about 3 tenders, ¾ cup chopped chicken), cooked, chopped small

2 TB. extra-virgin olive oil

3 cloves garlic, peeled and minced

1 TB. sherry vinegar

2 TB. water

¼ tsp. salt

¼ tsp. freshly cracked black pepper

2 TB. goat cheese

3 TB. fresh chives, chopped

Yield: 16 servings	
Prep time: 10 minutes	
Cook time: 14 minutes	
Serving size: 1 bruschetta	
Each serving has:	
85 calories	
9 g carbohydrate	
1 g sugars	
5 g protein	
3 g fat	
1 g saturated fat	
9 g cholesterol	
164 mg sodium	
.5 g fiber	
0 IU vitamin D	
45 mg potassium	
18 mg calcium	
4 mcg selenium	

1. Preheat the oven to 400°F.

2. Arrange baguette slices in a single layer on a large baking sheet. Bake, turning slices over halfway through, for about 14 minutes or until toasted but not browned.

3. In a medium bowl, combine tomatoes, chicken tenders, olive oil, garlic, vinegar, water, salt, and pepper.

4. Spread goat cheese on toasted baguette slices. Top with chicken-tomato mixture, sprinkle with chives, and serve.

Cooking Tip

If you allow the goat cheese to sit at room temperature for a few minutes before spreading it on the baguette, it will be easier to spread.

Mini Artichoke Crudités

Tasty hot artichokes with red onion and tofu are set over toasted pita slices in this sure-to-please appetizer.

Yield: 18 servings
Prep time: 10 minutes
Cook time: 2 minutes
Serving size: 1 crudité
Each serving has:
40 calories
7 g carbohydrate
.3 g sugars
2 g protein
.6 g fat
.2 g saturated fat
1 g cholesterol
110 mg sodium
1 g fiber
2.5 IU vitamin D
27 mg potassium
20 mg calcium
5 mcg selenium

1 (6.5-oz.) jar artichoke hearts, drained and chopped

¼ cup grated Parmesan cheese

⅓ cup red onion (about 1 medium), finely chopped

1 TB. low-fat mayonnaise

3 TB. silken tofu, puréed in a blender

¼ cup liquid egg substitute

2 (6½-in.) whole-wheat pitas, cut into 18 pieces

1. Preheat the broiler.

2. In a medium bowl, mix together artichoke hearts, Parmesan cheese, red onion, mayonnaise, tofu purée, and egg substitute.

3. Top pita slices with equal amounts of artichoke heart mixture, and arrange slices in a single layer on a large baking sheet.

4. Broil for 2 minutes or until topping is bubbly and lightly browned, and serve immediately.

Cooking Tip

If you like, you can use finely chopped chicken, seafood, beef, or pork instead of the tofu called for in this recipe. Be sure the protein you choose is lean, though.

Tuna Summer Rolls

These light and healthful sushi rolls feature fresh tuna, watercress, and soy sauce.

1 cup sushi rice, uncooked	3 TB. low-sodium soy sauce
1¼ cups water	¼ tsp. salt
2 TB. fresh ginger, peeled and minced	½ lb. tuna steak
2 TB. rice vinegar	8 (8-in.) rice paper sheets
3½ tsp. whole shallots, minced	2 cups *watercress,* trimmed and chopped
2 tsp. plus 1 TB. Splenda	¼ cup white vinegar
	¼ tsp. *wasabi* powder

Yield: 8 servings
Prep time: 30 minutes
Cook time: 23 minutes
Serving size: 1 roll
Each serving has:
160 calories
27 g carbohydrate
.4 g sugars
10 g protein
.6 g fat
.1 g saturated fat
13 g cholesterol
435 mg sodium
.1 g fiber
38 IU vitamin D
175 mg potassium
16 mg calcium
14 mcg selenium

1. Rinse rice thoroughly in a sieve under cold running water. Drain well.

2. In a medium saucepan over high heat, bring water to a boil and add rice. Cover, reduce heat to low, and simmer 20 minutes or until liquid is absorbed. Remove from heat and let stand 5 minutes.

3. Stir in ginger, rice vinegar, 2 teaspoons shallots, 1 teaspoon Splenda, 1 tablespoon soy sauce, and salt. Set aside.

4. In a small bowl, combine 1 tablespoon soy sauce and 1 teaspoon Splenda. Brush mixture evenly over tuna steak. Allow to marinate in the refrigerator for 10 minutes.

5. Heat a nonstick skillet over medium-high heat. Add tuna, and cook for 1½ minutes per side or until desired degree of doneness. Cut tuna into 8 (¼-inch-thick) slices.

6. Add 1 inch warm-hot water from the faucet to a large, shallow dish. Add 1 rice paper sheet to the dish, and let stand for 30 seconds or just until soft.

7. Place softened rice paper sheet on a flat surface. Arrange ¼ cup watercress on half of sheet, leaving a ½ inch border along the edge. Top with ⅓ cup rice mixture, and spread evenly. Arrange 1 tuna slice over rice. Fold sides of sheet over filling, and starting with filled side, roll up jelly-roll style. Repeat with remaining rice paper sheets, watercress, rice mixture, and tuna. Cut each roll in half diagonally.

8. To prepare sauce, combine white vinegar, remaining 1 tablespoon Splenda, remaining 1½ teaspoons shallots, and wasabi.

9. Arrange 2 roll halves on each of 8 plates, and serve 2¼ teaspoons sauce with each serving.

def•i•ni•tion

Watercress is an aquatic/semi-aquatic leafy green plant that has a peppery flavor. **Wasabi,** also known as Japanese horseradish, is sold in either root or powder form and has a spicy flavor. Wasabi is very spicy, so a little goes a long way.

Shrimp Cocktail

This classic shrimp cocktail is poached in lemon and Old Bay Seasoning with classic cocktail sauce.

2 TB. Old Bay Seasoning

2 bay leaves

1 tsp. salt

1 tsp. whole black pepper-corns

2 qt. water

2 whole lemons, cut in ½

1 lb. (21 to 30 count, about 24) shrimp, peeled and deveined

½ cup cocktail sauce

Yield: *8 servings*		
Prep time: 5 minutes		
Cook time: 20 minutes		
Serving size: 2 or 3 shrimp		
Each serving has:		
67 calories		
3 g carbohydrate		
2 g sugars		
12 g protein		
.7 g fat		
.1 g saturated fat		
111 g cholesterol		
520 mg sodium		
.4 g fiber		
0 IU vitamin D		
200 mg potassium		
25 mg calcium		
22 mcg selenium		

1. In a large saucepan over high heat, combine Old Bay Seasoning, bay leaves, salt, pepper, water, and lemons. Bring to a boil.

2. Add shrimp and cook for 5 to 10 minutes or until shrimp curls and "heads" nearly touch tails.

3. Pour cooked shrimp over ice and allow to cool. Remove shrimp from water.

4. Serve cold shrimp with cocktail sauce. (If you're cooking off more shrimp than called for here, reuse the cooking liquid, but instead of dumping the hot liquid over ice, remove shrimp individually with a spoon and put on ice.)

 Food for Thought

Seafood is a great way to include healthy fats such as omega-3 and omega-6 fatty acids into your diet and are also good sources of protein.

Shrimp and Crab Salad Crostinis

Chilled shrimp and crab salad with fresh herbs rests over crisp baguette slices in this surprising appetizer. *(Adapted from www. lowfatlifestyle.com.)*

Yield: *16 servings*
Prep time: 10 minutes
Cook time: 2 minutes
Serving size: 1 crostini
Each serving has:
153 calories
29 g carbohydrate
1 g sugars
6 g protein
1 g fat
0 g saturated fat
6 g cholesterol
380 mg sodium
1 g fiber
0 IU vitamin D
29 mg potassium
8 mg calcium
1 mcg selenium

16 (¼-in.-thick) whole-wheat baguette slices

¼ cup cooked salad shrimp, chopped

¼ cup canned lump crabmeat

½ large red bell pepper, ribs and seeds removed, and diced very finely

1½ TB. plain Greek yogurt

1 TB. fresh parsley, chopped, plus leaves for garnish

1½ tsp. fresh chives, chopped

1½ tsp. fresh lime juice

1½ tsp. Dijon mustard

1 tsp. Old Bay Seasoning

1 tsp. grated Parmesan cheese

2 dashes hot pepper sauce

¼ tsp. salt

½ tsp. freshly cracked black pepper

1. Lightly coat a large, nonstick skillet with cooking spray, and heat over medium-high heat. Add baguette slices, and grill for 1 or 2 minutes per side or until golden brown. Using a spatula, remove bread from the skillet and place on paper towels. (Bread can be toasted ahead of time and stored in an airtight container at room temperature for up to 2 days.)

2. In a medium bowl, combine shrimp, crabmeat, red bell pepper, Greek yogurt, chopped parsley, chives, lime juice, Dijon mustard, Old Bay Seasoning, Parmesan cheese, and hot pepper sauce. Season with salt and pepper.

3. Distribute seafood mixture evenly onto each slice of toasted baguette. Garnish with parsley leaves and serve.

 Food for Thought

Adding mustard is a great low-calorie way to up the flavor of many dishes.

Crab Quesadillas

These delicious crab quesadillas kick things up a notch with cilantro, cheddar cheese, jalapeño peppers, and Old Bay Seasoning.

1 cup reduced-fat shredded cheddar cheese

3 TB. reduced-fat cream cheese, softened

1 TB. plain Greek yogurt

1 TB. liquid egg substitute

2 tsp. Old Bay Seasoning

4 whole scallions, chopped

½ medium red bell pepper, ribs and seeds removed, and finely chopped (about ¼ cup)

⅓ cup fresh cilantro, chopped

2 TB. jalapeño peppers, ribs and seeds removed, and chopped

1 tsp. orange zest

1 TB. fresh orange juice

1 cup canned lump crabmeat

4 (6½-in.) whole-wheat tortillas

2 tsp. canola oil

Yield: 16 servings
Prep time: 15 minutes
Cook time: 8 minutes
Serving size: 4 wedges
Each serving has:
36 calories
1 g carbohydrate
.3 g sugars
6 g protein
1 g fat
0 g saturated fat
14 g cholesterol
114 mg sodium
0 g fiber
0 IU vitamin D
69 mg potassium
84 mg calcium
5 mcg selenium

1. In a medium bowl, combine cheddar cheese, cream cheese, Greek yogurt, egg substitute, Old Bay Seasoning, scallions, red bell pepper, cilantro, jalapeños, orange zest, and orange juice. Gently stir in crabmeat.

2. Lay out tortillas on a work surface. Spread ¼ of filling on ½ of each tortilla. Fold tortillas in half, pressing gently to flatten.

3. Heat 1 teaspoon canola oil in a large, nonstick skillet over medium heat. Place 2 quesadillas in the pan, and cook, turning once, for 3 or 4 minutes or until golden on both sides. Transfer to a cutting board, and loosely cover with foil to keep warm. Repeat with remaining 1 teaspoon canola oil and 2 quesadillas.

4. Cut each quesadilla into 4 wedges, and serve.

Cooking Tip

Because they're so easy to pull together, try making quesadillas with different proteins such as chicken and lean beef.

South-of-the-Border Beef Salsa

This Mexican-style beef salsa is chock full of fresh tomatoes, onions, delicious ground beef, and plenty of southwest flavor.

Yield: *16 servings*
Prep time: 15 minutes
Cook time: 20 minutes
Serving size: 1 tablespoon
Each serving has:
98 calories
12 g carbohydrate
1 g sugars
5 g protein
3 g fat
1 g saturated fat
11 g cholesterol
316 mg sodium
1 g fiber
0 IU vitamin D
126 mg potassium
26 mg calcium
5 mcg selenium

½ lb. 97 percent lean ground beef

3 tsp. chili powder

2 tsp. ground cumin

1 tsp. salt

½ tsp. freshly cracked black pepper

1 small red onion, diced

1 small yellow bell pepper, ribs and seeds removed, and diced

1 small red bell pepper, ribs and seeds removed, and diced

⅓ cup salsa

½ cup shredded reduced-fat cheddar jack cheese

2 TB. sliced jalapeño peppers

1. In a nonstick skillet over medium-high heat, add beef and brown for about 10 minutes. Drain well.

2. In the same skillet with beef, add chili powder, cumin, salt, pepper, onion, yellow bell pepper, and red bell pepper. Mix well and cook for 10 minutes or until onion and bell peppers begin to soften.

3. Pour beef-bell pepper mixture into a serving bowl, and top with salsa, cheese, and jalapeños. Serve with tortilla chips for dipping.

Cooking Tip

Try switching out the ground beef for ground turkey or sea-food, which will make this single simple recipe into many.

Taco Dip with Salsa

This quick and easy taco dip boasts refried beans, bell peppers, fresh lettuce and tomatoes, and creamy mozzarella cheese. *(Adapted from www.cdkitchen.com.)*

1 cup fat-free refried beans

1 cup fat-free sour cream

1 cup plain Greek yogurt

1 TB. garlic, peeled and minced

1 (1.25-oz.) pkg. taco seasoning

5 whole scallions, chopped

1½ cups reduced-fat mozza-rella cheese, shredded

1 cup lettuce, shredded

2 medium tomatoes, chopped (about 1 cup)

1 medium green bell pepper, ribs and seeds removed, and chopped (about ½ cup)

1 (14.5-oz.) jar salsa

Yield: 16 servings
Prep time: 70 minutes
Serving size: 1 tablespoon dip
Each serving has:
83 calories
10 g carbohydrate
4 g sugars
9 g protein
.5 g fat
.3 g saturated fat
6 g cholesterol
338 mg sodium
1 g fiber
0 IU vitamin D
174 mg potassium
236 mg calcium
.5 mcg selenium

1. Spread refried beans on the bottom of an 8-inch-square glass baking dish.

2. In a medium bowl, combine sour cream, Greek yogurt, garlic, and taco seasoning. Spread evenly on top of beans. Sprinkle scallions on top.

3. In a large bowl, combine cheese, lettuce, tomatoes, and green bell pepper. Sprinkle over onions, and chill for 1 hour.

4. Serve with salsa and maybe some tortilla chips.

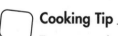

Cooking Tip

Try topping this with grilled chicken to add another layer of flavor to the dish, along with more protein.

Zucchini Fritters

These delicious zucchini fritters with fresh garlic and feta cheese go great with any number of dishes like grilled chicken and fish.

Yield: 8 servings
Prep time: 10 minutes
Cook time: 32 minutes
Serving size: 2 fritters
Each serving has:
162 calories
22 g carbohydrate
4 g sugars
8 g protein
5 g fat
1 g saturated fat
4 g cholesterol
130 mg sodium
4 g fiber
4 IU vitamin D
536 mg potassium
64 mg calcium
10 mcg selenium

3 lb. zucchini, coarsely grated and drained (about 6 cups)

1 large Spanish onion, chopped

2 cloves garlic, peeled and minced

4 whole scallions, sliced thin

2 TB. extra-virgin olive oil

½ cup crumbled feta cheese

½ cup liquid egg substitute

4 TB. fresh dill, chopped

¾ cup all-purpose flour

½ cup plus 2 TB. whole-wheat flour

2 TB. plain protein powder

1. In a large bowl, combine zucchini, onion, garlic, scallions, ½ tablespoon olive oil, feta cheese, egg substitute, dill, all-purpose flour, whole-wheat flour, and protein powder.

2. Lightly coat a large sauté pan with cooking spray, and place over medium heat. Add ½ tablespoon olive oil.

3. When the pan is hot, evenly spoon batter by about ¼ cup each, to make 16 mini fritters. (You may have to do this in batches. Use remaining olive oil for subsequent batches.) Cook for approximately 2 minutes per side. Serve immediately.

Cooking Tip

Make these fritters as if you were making pancakes. Pour the batter in the pan and wait until bubbles form on top, then flip them.

Onion Frittata Bites

These low-calorie onion frittata bites with Parmesan cheese and chives are perfect for a brunch party. *(Adapted from www.myrecipes. com.)*

1 tsp. extra-virgin olive oil

2 cups Vidalia onion, minced

1½ cups liquid egg substitute

4 TB. grated Parmesan cheese

½ tsp. salt

½ tsp. freshly cracked black pepper

¼ cup fat-free sour cream

48 (½-in.) pieces chives

Yield: 12 servings
Prep time: 10 minutes
Cook time: 20 minutes
Serving size: 2 frittata
Each serving has:
34 calories
2 g carbohydrate
1.5 g sugars
4 g protein
1 g fat
.3 g saturated fat
2 g cholesterol
189 mg sodium
0 g fiber
8 IU vitamin D
45 mg potassium
39 mg calcium
.3 mcg selenium

1. Preheat the oven to 350°F. Lightly coat an 11×7-inch baking dish with cooking spray.

2. In a nonstick skillet over medium heat, heat olive oil. Add onion, and cook for 15 minutes, stirring occasionally, or until golden brown. Spread onions in a single layer in the prepared baking dish.

3. In a medium bowl, combine egg substitute, 2 tablespoons Parmesan cheese, salt, and pepper. Pour egg mixture evenly over onions, and sprinkle remaining 2 tablespoons Parmesan cheese over top.

4. Bake for 20 minutes or until set. Cool slightly before cutting into 24 pieces. Top each piece with ½ teaspoon sour cream and 2 chive pieces. Serve immediately.

 Food for Thought

Frittatas are an easy way to do eggs. Hop out of bed, throw some random veggies in a pan with some eggs, and pop it in the oven. While you finish getting ready for the day, the eggs cook and will be all set by the time you're ready to eat.

Vegetable and Ricotta–Stuffed Mushrooms

Creamy ricotta cheese and delicious fresh carrot and zucchini star in these stuffed mushrooms.

Yield: 18 servings
Prep time: 10 minutes
Cook time: 24 minutes
Serving size: 1 mushroom
Each serving has:
37 calories
2 g carbohydrate
1 g sugars
3 g protein
2 g fat
1 g saturated fat
4 g cholesterol
183 mg sodium
.6 g fiber
5 IU vitamin D
129 mg potassium
73 mg calcium
4 mcg selenium

18 large button mushrooms, stems removed

1 (10-oz.) pkg. chopped frozen spinach, thawed and drained

1 TB. extra-virgin olive oil

1 medium zucchini, shredded

1 large carrot, peeled and shredded

¾ cup low-fat ricotta cheese

¼ cup silken tofu, puréed

1 tsp. fresh chives, chopped

¼ cup liquid egg substitute

1 tsp. salt

1 tsp. freshly ground black pepper

¼ cup grated Parmesan cheese

¼ cup low-sodium vegetable broth

1. Preheat the oven to 350°F. Generously coat a 9×13-inch baking dish with cooking spray.

2. Wipe mushrooms with a clean paper towel. Remove and discard stems.

3. Place spinach in a large bowl.

4. In a small frying pan over medium heat, heat olive oil. Squeeze out as much water as possible from zucchini, and add it to the frying pan along with carrot. Cook for 2 to 4 minutes or until vegetables are softened.

5. Add vegetables to spinach in the bowl, and mix well. Fold in ricotta cheese, tofu, chives, egg substitute, salt, and pepper.

6. Place mushroom caps cavity side up in the prepared baking dish. Spoon vegetables into mushroom caps, and top with Parmesan cheese. Pour vegetable broth into the bottom of the baking dish around mushrooms. Bake, uncovered, for 15 to 20 minutes or until cheese is bubbly and mushrooms are cooked.

 Food for Thought

Ricotta cheese can be used in many culinary dishes, such as cheesecakes, cannoli cream, and even pizza.

Yogurt "Cheese" and Herb Torte

Refreshing yogurt "cheese" dip combines with fresh sage, thyme, rosemary, and other herbs in this lovely concoction. *(Adapted from www.myrecipes.com.)*

6 cups plain Greek yogurt

2 TB. garlic, sliced (about 2 or 3 cloves)

2 TB. fresh basil, chopped

1 TB. fresh rosemary, chopped

1 TB. fresh thyme, chopped

1 TB. fresh sage, chopped

1 TB. whole shallots, minced

3 TB. extra-virgin olive oil

1 tsp. fresh lemon zest

½ tsp. salt

¼ tsp. freshly cracked black pepper

¼ tsp. crushed red pepper flakes

Yield: *32 servings*
Prep time: 24 hours, 20 minutes
Serving size: 1 spoonful dip
Each serving has:
40 calories
3 g carbohydrate
3 g sugars
2 g protein
2 g fat
.6 g saturated fat
3 g cholesterol
69 mg sodium
0 g fiber
0 IU vitamin D
108 mg potassium
84 mg calcium
1.5 mcg selenium

1. Place a colander in a large bowl. Line the colander with 4 layers of cheesecloth, allowing the cheesecloth to extend over the outside edges of the colander.

2. Spoon yogurt into the cheesecloth-lined colander. Cover loosely with plastic wrap, and refrigerate for 12 hours. Spoon yogurt cheese from the cheesecloth into a medium bowl, cover, and refrigerate for 3 hours. Discard liquid from the large bowl.

3. In a small bowl, combine garlic, basil, rosemary, thyme, sage, shallots, olive oil, lemon zest, salt, pepper, and crushed red pepper flakes.

4. Place ½ of yogurt cheese in a serving bowl, and spread ½ of herb mixture on top. Repeat with remaining cheese and herb mixture. Cover and refrigerate for at least 12 hours and up to 1 week. Serve at room temperature.

Food for Thought

Although *torte* is the word for "cake" in central Europe, we've referred to this recipe as a torte because of the layering of the ingredients. The yogurt serves as the "cake" and the herb spread serves as the "icing."

Roasted Tomato and Garlic Hummus

This light and healthful hummus made with roasted garlic and tahini is great as a dip or as a sandwich spread.

Yield: 8 servings
Prep time: 10 minutes
Serving size: 1 tablespoon
Each serving has:
96 calories
12 g carbohydrate
7 g sugars
7 g protein
3 g fat
.4 g saturated fat
.5 g cholesterol
118 mg sodium
2 g fiber
0 IU vitamin D
142 mg potassium
38 mg calcium
2 mcg selenium

2 (14.5-oz.) cans canned garbanzo beans, rinsed and drained

2 TB. *tahini*

4 TB. fresh lemon juice

5 cloves garlic, roasted

4 TB. cumin

¼ tsp. salt

1 tsp. freshly cracked black pepper

¼ cup plain Greek yogurt

¼ cup low-sodium roasted tomatoes, drained

1 TB. plain protein powder

1. In a food processor fitted with a chopping blade, combine garbanzo beans, tahini, lemon juice, garlic, cumin, salt, black pepper, Greek yogurt, tomatoes, and protein powder for 2 minutes or until smooth.

2. Serve with pita bread, sliced vegetables, or chips.

def•i•ni•tion

Tahini is a paste made from ground sesame seeds that is used in many Middle Eastern foods, including hummus.

Roasted Eggplant Dip

Delicious oven-roasted eggplant, roasted garlic, tomatoes, onion, and fresh herbs star in this tasty dip.

1 head garlic

1 (1-lb.) eggplant, peeled and halved lengthwise

1 small red onion, cut into ½-in.-thick slices

1 medium tomato, cut in ½ and seeds removed

¼ cup silken tofu

2 TB. plain protein powder

3 TB. fresh lemon juice

2 TB. fresh chives, chopped

2 TB. fresh cilantro, chopped

1 TB. extra-virgin olive oil

½ tsp. salt

¼ tsp. freshly cracked black pepper

Yield: 8 servings
Prep time: 10 minutes
Cook time: 55 minutes
Serving size: 1 tablespoon
Each serving has:
78 calories
7 g carbohydrate
2 g sugars
10 g protein
2 g fat
0 g saturated fat
0 g cholesterol
252 mg sodium
2 g fiber
9 IU vitamin D
205 mg potassium
41 mg calcium
1 mcg selenium

1. Preheat the oven to 450°F.

2. Cut off top of garlic bulb, and wrap loosely in foil. Bake for 30 minutes or until garlic is soft. Let cool slightly.

3. Reduce oven temperature to 400°F. Coat a baking sheet with cooking spray.

4. Place eggplant halves, cut side down, on the prepared baking sheet. Roast for 10 minutes.

5. Add onion slices and tomato halves to the baking sheet with eggplant, and roast for 10 to 15 more minutes or until all vegetables are soft. Let cool slightly.

6. Separate garlic cloves, and squeeze pulp into a blender. Add roasted vegetables, tofu, protein powder, lemon juice, chives, cilantro, olive oil, salt, and pepper, and blend for 3 or 4 minutes or until smooth.

Food for Thought

Eggplants are a great source of antioxidants. They come in many different colors such as white, purple, and green and are a great addition to many different recipes.

Chapter 15

Super Sandwiches and Pizzas

In This Chapter

◆ Scrumptious sandwiches

◆ Burgers you'll crave

◆ Pizzas with pizzazz

If you're one of the many people who think of pizza, burgers, and other sandwiches as the ultimate gotta-have-it comfort food, you've come to the right place. In this chapter, you'll find nearly a dozen recipes for some classics … and some classics with new twists. Also included are new recipes you may not have thought of. But rest assured, all the recipes in this chapter are light and healthful and fit in well with your post-op eating plan.

And speaking of pizza, few foods are so suited to personalization. Maybe you like pepperoni on yours, but your spouse or children prefer all-veggies. With this chapter's Basic Pizza Dough recipe in your culinary arsenal, and your favorite toppings, you can make it DIY pizza night any night! And don't forget the calzones, flatbreads, and more you also can make with the pizza dough.

Buffalo Chicken Wrap

These moist chicken tenders are coated in a zesty cayenne sauce and finished with crumbled blue cheese.

Yield: 8 servings
Prep time: 8 minutes
Cook time: 10 minutes
Serving size: ½ wrap
Each serving has:
306 calories
27 g carbohydrate
2 g sugars
26 g protein
11 g fat
3.5 g saturated fat
57 g cholesterol
558 mg sodium
2 g fiber
0 IU vitamin D
127 mg potassium
66 mg calcium
1.6 mcg selenium

3 TB. hot pepper sauce

5 TB. white vinegar

½ tsp. cayenne

3 tsp. extra-virgin olive oil

1½ lb. reduced-fat chicken tenders (about 12 tenders)

3 TB. reduced-fat mayonnaise

5 TB. plain Greek yogurt

¼ tsp. freshly cracked black pepper

½ cup crumbled blue cheese

4 (6½-in.) whole-wheat tortillas

2 cups mixed greens

1½ cups sliced celery

2 medium vine ripe tomatoes, chopped

1. In a medium bowl, whisk together hot pepper sauce, 4 tablespoons vinegar, and cayenne.

2. In a large, nonstick skillet over medium-high heat, heat olive oil. Add chicken tenders, and cook for 3 or 4 minutes per side or until cooked through and no longer pink in the middle. Add chicken to the bowl with hot sauce mixture, and toss to coat well.

3. In a small bowl, whisk together mayonnaise, Greek yogurt, pepper, and remaining 1 tablespoon vinegar. Stir in blue cheese.

4. To assemble wraps, lay 1 tortilla on your work surface or a plate. Spread 1 tablespoon blue cheese sauce over tortilla, and top with ¼ of chicken, mixed greens, celery, and tomato. Drizzle with some hot sauce remaining in the bowl, and roll tortilla into wrap. Repeat with remaining ingredients.

5. Cut wraps in half, and serve with remaining blue cheese sauce for dipping.

Cooking Tip

Try using different flavors of wraps for a change of pace. A number of delicious flavors are available, such as roasted red pepper and spinach.

Turkey, Tomato, and Arugula Pita Panini

These delicious panini feature oven-roasted turkey, Parmesan cheese, and fresh tomato and arugula.

3 TB. reduced-fat mayonnaise	4 (6½-in.) whole-wheat pitas, sliced in ½
5 TB. plain Greek yogurt	16 oz. low-fat, low-sodium sliced turkey
4 TB. grated Parmesan cheese	2 cups arugula
4 TB. chopped fresh basil	4 tomatoes, cut into 16 slices
2 tsp. fresh lemon juice	4 tsp. extra-virgin olive oil
¼ tsp. freshly cracked black pepper	

Yield: *8 servings*
Prep time: 8 minutes
Cook time: 20 minutes
Serving size: ½ pita panino
Each serving has:
207 calories
23 g carbohydrate
3 g sugars
16 g protein
6.5 g fat
2 g saturated fat
41 g cholesterol
855 mg sodium
3 g fiber
5 IU vitamin D
418 mg potassium
67 mg calcium
36 mcg selenium

1. In a small bowl, combine mayonnaise, Greek yogurt, Parmesan cheese, basil, lemon juice, and pepper. Spread about 2 teaspoons inside each pita half.

2. Divide turkey, arugula, and tomato slices among pita pockets.

3. Lightly coat a sauté pan with cooking spray and set over medium heat. Add 1½ teaspoons vegetable oil.

4. When oil is hot, place 2 panini in the pan. Using a spatula, press down on the panini. Cook for about 2 minutes or until panini are golden. Reduce heat to medium-low, flip over panini, apply pressure to the other sides, and cook for 1 to 3 more minutes or until second side is golden.

5. Repeat process until all panini are cooked.

 Food for Thought _____

To reduce some of the fat in this recipe, you can substitute mustard, nonfat yogurt, or fat-free mayonnaise for the mayonnaise.

Chicken and Asparagus Pita Sandwiches

Zesty stone-ground mustard and tomatoes complement the chicken and asparagus in these pita sandwiches.

Yield: 8 servings
Prep time: 8 minutes
Cook time: 12 minutes
Serving size: ½ pita
Each serving has:
196 calories
25 g carbohydrate
6 g sugars
20 g protein
3 g fat
1 g saturated fat
35 g cholesterol
392 mg sodium
4 g fiber
0 IU vitamin D
530 mg potassium
114 mg calcium
17 mcg selenium

1 lb. fresh asparagus, trimmed and cut into 3-in. pieces

1½ cups plain Greek yogurt

2 tsp. lemon juice

1½ tsp. stone-ground mustard

½ tsp. salt

1 lb. cooked chicken breast, cubed (about 2 cups)

3 medium tomatoes, sliced into 16 slices

2 cups salad greens

4 (6½-in.) whole-wheat pitas, sliced in ½

1. Place asparagus in a small saucepan and cover with water. Set over high heat and bring to a boil. Cover and cook for 2 minutes or until crisp-tender. Drain and set aside.

2. In the same pan over low heat, combine Greek yogurt, lemon juice, mustard, and salt. Cook for 1 or 2 minutes or until heated through. Remove from heat.

3. Place chicken on a microwave-safe plate, and microwave on high for 45 to 60 seconds or until warmed.

4. Evenly distribute chicken, sauce, asparagus, tomatoes, and greens among pita pockets, and serve.

Cooking Tip

The bottom of the asparagus spear is woody and hard to chew. To find the perfect place to cut the asparagus, hold a spear at both the bottom and top and bend it until it breaks in half. Line up that asparagus with the rest of the spears, and cut straight across. Discard the bottoms, and use the tops.

Falafel Pita Burgers with Lemon Yogurt Sauce

Even meat eaters will love these vegetarian garbanzo bean burgers with delicious herbs and spices served with a creamy lemon sauce.

2 (14.5-oz.) cans garbanzo beans, rinsed and drained

8 whole scallions, chopped

½ cup liquid egg substitute

3 TB. whole-wheat flour

1 TB. plain protein powder

2 TB. chopped fresh oregano

1 tsp. ground cumin

¾ tsp. salt

3 TB. extra-virgin olive oil

½ cup plain Greek yogurt

1 TB. lemon juice

⅓ cup chopped fresh parsley

4 (6½-in.) whole-wheat pitas, sliced in ½

2 medium tomatoes, sliced

2 cups mixed greens

Yield: 8 servings
Prep time: 10 minutes
Cook time: 9 minutes
Serving size: 1 pita burger plus 2 tablespoons yogurt sauce

Each serving has:
268 calories
39 g carbohydrate
6 g sugars
13 g protein
8 g fat
1 g saturated fat
1 g cholesterol
789 mg sodium
7 g fiber
4 IU vitamin D
197 mg potassium
83 mg calcium
17 mcg selenium

1. In a food processor fitted with a chopping blade, add garbanzo beans, scallions, egg substitute, flour, protein powder, oregano, cumin, and ½ teaspoon salt. Pulse, stopping once or twice to scrape down the sides, until a coarse mixture forms that holds together when pressed. (The mixture will be moist.)

2. Form into 8 patties.

3. In a large, nonstick skillet over medium-high heat, heat olive oil. Add garbanzo bean patties, and cook for 4 or 5 minutes or until golden and beginning to crisp. Carefully flip over patties, and cook for 2 to 4 more minutes or until golden brown.

4. In a medium bowl, combine Greek yogurt, remaining ¼ teaspoon salt, lemon juice, and parsley.

5. Divide patties among pitas along with tomatoes and mixed greens. Top with yogurt sauce, and serve.

Food for Thought

When using scallions, or green onions, you can use the green part or the white part—or a combination. Both are edible and tasty, but the green part has a stronger onion flavor than the white. I always use both ends.

Black Bean Burgers

These simple and delicious black bean burgers are highlighted with fresh garlic and fruity extra-virgin olive oil.

Yield: 8 servings
Prep time: 65 minutes
Cook time: 5 minutes
Serving size: 1 burger
Each serving has:
93 calories
15 g carbohydrate
1 g sugars
4 g protein
4 g fat
.5 g saturated fat
0 g cholesterol
368 mg sodium
5 g fiber
0 IU vitamin D
295 mg potassium
36 mg calcium
.4 mcg selenium

2 (14.5-oz.) cans black beans, drained and rinsed

8 cloves garlic, peeled and minced

½ cup fresh cilantro, chopped

½ tsp. salt

¼ tsp. freshly cracked black pepper

2 TB. whole-wheat bread-crumbs

2 TB. extra-virgin olive oil

1. In a large bowl, mash together beans and garlic. Stir in cilantro and salt, freshly cracked black pepper, and breadcrumbs. Form mixture into 8 patties. Transfer patties to a plate, and refrigerate for about 1 hour.

2. In a large, nonstick frying pan over medium heat, heat olive oil. Add patties and cook, turning over once, for about 5 minutes or until warmed and outsides are slightly crisp.

3. Serve immediately on a low-fat bun of your choice.

 Food for Thought _____

These burgers are a great way to get a little extra fiber in your diet because beans are full of fiber. Also, beans are high in protein, so try adding them to a number of different dishes.

Turkey Burgers

Moist and delicious, these turkey burgers feature fresh chopped onions, herbs, and spices.

⅔ cup couscous

1 cup water

4 tsp. canola oil

1 large red bell pepper, ribs and seeds removed, and diced (1 cup)

1 large Vidalia onion, diced

4 cloves garlic, peeled and minced

2 tsp. dried thyme

1 tsp. salt

½ tsp. black pepper

½ tsp. paprika

1½ lb. ground turkey

8 whole-wheat hamburger buns, lightly toasted

2 tomatoes, cut into 8 slices

8 leaves romaine lettuce

Yield: 4 servings
Prep time: 35 minutes
Cook time: 10 minutes
Serving size: 1 burger
Each serving has:
275 calories
33 g carbohydrate
5 g sugars
26 g protein
6 g fat
.7 g saturated fat
34 g cholesterol
549 mg sodium
4 g fiber
0 IU vitamin D
220 mg potassium
55 mg calcium
21 mcg selenium

1. In a small saucepan over high heat, bring water to a boil. Add couscous, reduce heat to low, and cook for 5 minutes. Cover and allow to sit for about 15 minutes or until all water has been absorbed.

2. Meanwhile, in a small, nonstick skillet over low heat, heat canola oil. Add bell pepper, onion, garlic, thyme, salt, pepper, and paprika. Cook, stirring, for 1 or 2 minutes or until bell pepper and onion are slightly softened. Let cool.

3. Prepare a grill or preheat the broiler to low. Oil the grill rack or broiler pan.

4. In a medium bowl, combine turkey, couscous, and bell pepper mixture, and mix thoroughly but lightly. Shape into 8 (¾-inch-thick) patties.

5. Grill or broil patties for about 5 minutes per side or until browned and no longer pink inside. Place on whole-wheat buns, and garnish with 1 tomato slice and 1 lettuce leaf.

Food for Thought

Turkey burgers have less fat than traditional beef burgers. This recipe is easily adaptable if you want to customize the ingredients such as adding caramelized onions and sautéed mushrooms, or maybe even serving the burger over a salad.

Salmon Patties

These fresh salmon burgers might surprise you, with their zesty lemon, fresh garlic, and a little help from Mrs. Dash served over a crisp radicchio lettuce slaw.

Yield: 8 servings
Prep time: 35 minutes
Cook time: 12 minutes
Serving size: 1 burger
Each serving has:
158 calories
6 g carbohydrate
.7 g sugars
14 g protein
9 g fat
2 g saturated fat
14 g cholesterol
226 mg sodium
.3 g fiber
288 IU vitamin D
219 mg potassium
148 mg calcium
20 mcg selenium

1 (14-oz.) can Alaskan salmon, drained, picked over for bones, and flaked

2 egg whites, lightly beaten

¼ cup fresh parsley, chopped

Zest of 2 medium lemons

Juice of 2 medium lemons

3 cloves garlic, peeled and finely chopped

½ cup plain breadcrumbs

1 TB. plain protein powder

2 tsp. Mrs. Dash Italian Seasoning

2 tsp. Dijon mustard

1 TB. Worcestershire sauce

5 TB. extra-virgin olive oil

¼ cup grated Parmesan cheese

2 hearts romaine lettuce, shredded

1 head radicchio, shredded

1. In a large bowl, combine salmon, egg whites, parsley, zest of 1 lemon, juice of 1 lemon, ⅔ of chopped garlic, breadcrumbs, protein powder, and Mrs. Dash Italian Seasoning. Form mixture into 8 mini patties.

2. In a salad bowl, add remaining zest of 1 lemon, remaining juice of 1 lemon, remaining garlic, Dijon mustard, and Worcestershire sauce. Whisk in 4 tablespoons olive oil and Parmesan cheese. Add black pepper, and no salt. Add lettuce and radicchio, and toss to coat.

3. In a nonstick sauté pan over medium-high heat, heat remaining 1 tablespoon olive oil. Add salmon patties, and cook for 2 or 3 minutes on each side. (This may take 2 batches.)

4. Serve salmon patties atop lettuce-radicchio slaw.

 Food for Thought

Salmon is an excellent source of omega-3 fatty acids, which is considered a good fat.

Basic Pizza Dough

This basic high-protein, whole-wheat pizza dough can be used as a base for all sorts of pizzas.

3 tsp. *active dry yeast*

1⅓ cups plus 4 TB. warm water

2¼ cups all-purpose flour

1½ cups whole-wheat flour

½ cup plain protein powder

2 tsp. salt

1½ TB. extra-virgin olive oil

Yield: 8 servings
Prep time: 70 minutes
Cook time: 10 minutes
Serving size: ⅛ slice pizza dough
Each serving has:
251 calories
44 g carbohydrate
.2 g sugars
12 g protein
4 g fat
.5 g saturated fat
0 g cholesterol
644 mg sodium
4 g fiber
0 IU vitamin D
159 mg potassium
14 mg calcium
28 mcg selenium

1. In a small bowl, dissolve yeast in 4 tablespoons water. Let stand for 5 minutes. (After sitting, top of water and yeast should be bubbly. If not, yeast is no longer active and you'll need fresh yeast.)

2. In a medium mixing bowl, combine all-purpose flour, whole-wheat flour, protein powder, and salt.

3. Work in the yeast and remaining 1⅓ cups of water and mix until dough forms a ball.

4. Turn out dough onto a lightly floured work surface, and knead for about 3 minutes or until dough is smooth and elastic.

5. Transfer dough to a large bowl sprayed with pan spray. Coat dough with extra-virgin olive oil, cover with plastic wrap, and set aside in a warm place to allow dough to rise for 1 hour or until double in size.

6. After dough has risen, roll out to about 8 inches in diameter, top with your favorite toppings, and bake for approximately 10 minutes or until crust is crispy.

def•i•ni•tion

Active dry yeast is a common form of yeast that are alive but dormant because of the lack of moisture.

Pear, Walnut, and Arugula Pizza with Feta

Sweet pears and salty feta cheese combine on this pizza that's sure to satisfy your pallet.

Yield: 8 servings
Prep time: 10 minutes
Cook time: 45 minutes
Serving size: 1 pizza
Each serving has:
340 calories
57 g carbohydrate
8 g sugars
15 g protein
7 g fat
1.4 g saturated fat
2.5 g cholesterol
754 mg sodium
6 g fiber
0 IU vitamin D
303 mg potassium
49 mg calcium
29 mcg selenium

1 batch Basic Pizza Dough (recipe earlier in this chapter)

1 TB. extra-virgin olive oil

2 large Vidalia onions, sliced

2 medium pears, peeled, cored, and sliced

3 TB. balsamic vinegar

½ tsp. freshly cracked black pepper

2 cups arugula

½ cup feta cheese

¼ cup chopped walnuts

1. Preheat the oven to 450°F.

2. Form Basic Pizza Dough into 8 (4-inch) pizza crusts, and bake for 4 or 5 minutes. Remove from the oven and set aside.

3. Meanwhile, in a large, nonstick skillet over medium-high heat, heat olive oil. Add onions and cook, stirring often, for about 7 minutes or until onions are soft and golden.

4. Stir in sliced pears, and cook, stirring often, for 1 or 2 minutes or until pears are slightly soft and heated through.

5. Add vinegar and pepper, and continue cooking, stirring often, for about 2 more minutes or until liquid has evaporated and onion is tender and coated with a dark glaze.

6. Divide arugula among baked pizza crusts, approximately ¼ cup each. Evenly distribute onion-pear mixture among the pizzas, and sprinkle with feta cheese and walnuts.

7. Transfer pizzas to a large baking sheet, and bake for 5 to 10 minutes or until crispy. Allow to cool for 5 minutes and serve.

Cooking Tip

Consider investing in a baking stone for your oven. They promote even heating and produce a crisp crust to pizzas.

Margarita Pizza

You can't get much better than this classic tomato and mozzarella pizza sprinkled with fresh chopped basil.

1 batch **Basic Pizza Dough** (recipe earlier in this chapter)

2 cloves garlic, minced

1½ TB. extra-virgin olive oil

6 TB. plain Greek yogurt

8 cups (about 10) sliced tomatoes

¼ tsp. salt

¼ tsp. freshly cracked black pepper

1 cup low-fat shredded mozzarella cheese

½ cup fresh basil, chopped

Yield: 8 servings
Prep time: 5 minutes
Cook time: 15 to 20 minutes
Serving size: 1 pizza
Each serving has:
74 calories
7 g carbohydrate
4 g sugars
7 g protein
3 g fat
.5 g saturated fat
3 g cholesterol
151 mg sodium
1.5 g fiber
0 IU vitamin D
318 mg potassium
159 mg calcium
.4 mcg selenium

1. Preheat the oven to 350°F.

2. Form Basic Pizza Dough into 8 (4-inch) pizza crusts, and bake for 4 or 5 minutes.

3. In a small bowl, combine garlic, olive oil, and yogurt. Spread over pizza crusts.

4. Arrange sliced tomatoes evenly over pizzas. Season with salt and pepper, and evenly distribute mozzarella cheese over top of each.

5. Bake for 10 to 15 minutes or until cheese is melted and crust is crisp.

6. Remove from the oven, and sprinkle with basil. Allow to sit for 5 minutes and serve.

Food for Thought

Basil is sometimes used in desserts and can be used as a dessert garnish much like mint. Both are easily found in the produce section in your local grocery store, or if you have a green thumb, you can easily grow them yourself.

Grilled Mexican-Style Corn and Black Bean Pizza

Sweet corn, black beans, and creamy mozzarella cheese top this south-of-the-border pizza.

Yield: 8 servings	
Prep time: 8 minutes	
Cook time: 15 minutes	
Serving size: 1 slice	
Each serving has:	
326 calories	
50 g carbohydrate	
4 g sugars	
18 g protein	
7 g fat	
1 g saturated fat	
3 g cholesterol	
795 mg sodium	
6 g fiber	
0 IU vitamin D	
477 mg potassium	
173 mg calcium	
29 mcg selenium	

2 plum tomatoes, diced

1 (14.5-oz.) can black beans, drained and rinsed

2 cups frozen corn kernels, thawed

4 TB. cornmeal

1 batch Basic Pizza Dough (recipe earlier in this chapter)

⅔ cup low-sodium barbecue sauce

1 cup low-fat shredded mozzarella cheese

1. Preheat the grill to medium.

2. In a medium bowl, combine tomatoes, beans, and corn.

3. Sprinkle cornmeal onto a large baking sheet. Stretch dough into about a 12-inch-diameter circle, and lay it on top of cornmeal, coating entire underside of dough.

4. Transfer crust from the baking sheet to the grill. Close the lid, and cook for 4 or 5 minutes or until crust is puffed and lightly browned on the bottom.

5. Using a large spatula, flip over crust. Spread barbecue sauce over crust, and quickly sprinkle tomato mixture and mozzarella cheese over sauce. Close the lid, and grill for 4 or 5 more minutes or until cheese is melted and bottom of crust is browned. Cut into 8 slices and serve.

Cooking Tip

Always rinse and strain canned beans because there's a lot of salt in the liquid. That liquid also contains oligosaccharides from the beans. (Oligosaccharides are sugar chains the body has to work hard to break down. The result: gas.)

Chapter 16

Satisfying Soups

In This Chapter

◆ Versatile vegetable-based soups

◆ Yummy creamed soups

◆ Bold bisques

◆ Hearty chilies

Sometimes, nothing hits the spot like soup. Whether you're looking for a smooth, broth-based soup to sip and slurp when you're not feeling 100 percent or a hearty chili or creamy soup to warm you on a chilly fall day, this chapter has what you want to fill your soup bowl. Many of the recipes in this chapter are extremely high in protein, too, and in the following pages we give you a few fat- and calorie-cutting tricks you'll be able to apply to many of your favorite recipes.

An added bonus: most soups are perfect for making now and freezing for later meals. Try making a large batch of one soup—or two or three different kinds of soups—at a time and freeze them for meals throughout the week or for individual grab-and-go portions for when you're rushing out the door for work. (Soups that contain pastas and cream soups don't freeze as well. However, with the pasta soups, you can make and freeze the base and add the pasta later when you thaw it.)

Southeast Asian Salmon and Tofu Soup

Delicious Asian salmon, tofu, and bean thread noodles star in this soup that's light, healthful, and high in protein. *(Adapted from www. eatingwell.com.)*

Yield: 8 servings
Prep time: 30 minutes
Cook time: 32 minutes
Serving size: about ¾ cup
Each serving has:
248 calories
13 g carbohydrate
3 g sugars
25 g protein
9 g fat
2 g saturated fat
75 g cholesterol
486 mg sodium
1 g fiber
238 IU vitamin D
418 mg potassium
94 mg calcium
31 mcg selenium

½ cup **bean thread noodles**

1 TB. vegetable oil

4 TB. garlic (about 4 or 5 cloves), peeled and sliced

9 cups low-fat, low-sodium chicken broth

1½ (15-oz.) cans diced tomatoes, with juice

1½ TB. low-sodium soy sauce

1½ TB. **chili garlic sauce**

1½ lb. wild salmon fillet, skinned and cubed

¾ cup extra-firm tofu, cubed

1 cup whole scallions, chopped

½ cup chopped fresh cilantro

1 whole lime, cut into 8 wedges

1. Place noodles in a large bowl, cover with hot tap water, and soak for 20 to 25 minutes or until softened. Drain.

2. Meanwhile, in a medium saucepan over medium heat, heat vegetable oil. Add garlic and cook, stirring often, for about 3 minutes or until golden brown. Using a slotted spoon, transfer garlic to a paper towel.

3. Carefully pour broth into the pan, bring to a boil, and cook for about 15 minutes. Stir in tomatoes and their juice, soy sauce, and chili garlic sauce.

4. Stir in salmon and tofu, reduce heat to low, and cook for about 2 minutes or until salmon is nearly cooked through.

5. Stir in drained noodles and scallions, and simmer for 1 more minute.

6. Top with cilantro and crispy garlic, and serve with lime wedges.

def•i•ni•tion

Bean thread noodles are an Asian-style noodle made from a starch such as mung bean starch and water. They are also known as cellophane noodles. **Chili garlic sauce** is an Asian sauce made from fresh garlic and chili flakes.

Vegetarian Hot Pot

Here, a tasty array of colorful vegetables such as snow peas, bok choy, and carrots simmer in a light vegetable soy broth. *(Adapted from www.eatingwell.com.)*

7½ **cups low-fat, low-sodium vegetable broth**

2 TB. **fresh ginger, peeled and grated**

4 **cloves garlic, peeled and chopped**

3 tsp. **vegetable oil**

2 **cups shiitake mushrooms, sliced**

½ **cup snow peas**

½ tsp. **crushed red pepper flakes**

2 **small heads** *bok choy,* **stems and leaves chopped separately**

1 (4½-oz.) **pkg. Chinese wheat noodles**

2 (14-oz.) **pkg. firm tofu**

1½ **cups carrots, peeled and cut into strips**

5 tsp. **rice vinegar or to taste**

3 tsp. **low-sodium soy sauce**

1½ tsp. **toasted sesame oil**

¼ **cup chopped fresh chives**

Yield: 8 servings
Prep time: 15 minutes
Cook time: 45 minutes
Serving size: ¾ cup
Each serving has:
227 calories
23 g carbohydrate
2 g sugars
11 g protein
10 g fat
1 g saturated fat
0 g cholesterol
554 mg sodium
3 g fiber
169 IU vitamin D
124 mg potassium
392 mg calcium
11 mcg selenium

1. In a stock pot pan over high heat, bring broth, ginger, and garlic to a simmer. Reduce heat to medium-low and simmer, partially covered, for 15 minutes. Discard ginger and garlic.

2. Meanwhile, in a large, nonstick skillet over medium-high heat, heat vegetable oil. Add mushrooms, snow peas, and crushed red pepper flakes. Cook, stirring often, for 3 to 5 minutes or until vegetables are tender.

3. Add bok choy stems, and cook, stirring often, for 3 or 4 minutes or until bok choy is tender.

4. Add mushroom mixture to broth. Add noodles, and simmer for 3 minutes.

5. Add chopped bok choy greens and tofu, and simmer for about 2 minutes or until heated through. Stir in carrots, vinegar, soy sauce, and sesame oil. Serve immediately, garnished with chives.

def•i•ni•tion

Bok choy is Chinese cabbage. To cut the bok choy, cut off the bottom "nub" and discard. Then, cut the bok choy in quarters lengthwise and separate the white and greens.

Chicken Tortilla Soup

This quick and easy chicken tortilla soup features a zesty tomato broth and mixed vegetables and is topped with shredded cheddar cheese and toasted tortilla strips. (*Adapted from www.eatingwell.com.*)

Yield: 8 servings
Prep time: 15 minutes
Cook time: 1 hour
Serving size: ¾ cup
Each serving has:
205 calories
19 g carbohydrate
4 g sugars
27 g protein
3 g fat
0 g saturated fat
52 g cholesterol
656 mg sodium
4 g fiber
0 IU vitamin D
343 mg potassium
135 mg calcium
.5 mcg selenium

 Food for Thought

If you're watching your salt intake, here's some good news: citrus juices can be used in many recipes as a flavor enhancer in lieu of adding more salt.

4 (6½-in.) corn tortillas

Cooking spray

2 tsp. vegetable oil

5 poblano peppers, ribs and seeds removed, and diced

2 medium onions (about 1½ cups), diced

½ cup diced zucchini

½ cup diced yellow squash

2 tsp. ground cumin

2 lb. low-fat chicken tenders, cut into 1-in. cubes (about 4 cups)

8 cups low-fat, low-sodium chicken broth

2 (14-oz.) cans diced tomatoes, with liquid

4 TB. fresh lime juice

¾ cup low-fat shredded cheddar cheese

¼ cup chopped fresh cilantro

1. Preheat the oven to 400°F.

2. Slice tortillas in half and then cut into thin strips ⅛ inch wide. Spread tortilla strips in an even layer on a baking sheet and spray with cooking spray. Bake for 12 to 15 minutes or until browned and crispy.

3. Meanwhile, in a large saucepan over medium heat, heat vegetable oil. Add poblano peppers, onions, zucchini, and squash, and cook, stirring, for 3 to 5 minutes or until onions begin to soften.

4. Add cumin and cook, stirring, for 1 minute.

5. Add chicken, chicken broth, and tomatoes and their liquid. Bring to a boil, reduce heat to medium-low, and simmer for 12 to 15 minutes or until chicken is cooked through. Remove from heat, and stir in lime juice.

6. Serve topped with baked tortilla strips, cheddar cheese, and cilantro.

Creamy Broccoli and Cheddar Soup

This creamy broccoli and cheddar soup features fresh garlic, hearty potatoes, and a hint of ground mustard seeds.

1 TB. extra-virgin olive oil

1½ medium Vidalia onions, diced (about 1¼ cups)

1 large carrot, peeled and diced

2 large celery stalks, diced

1 large potato, diced

4 tsp. minced garlic (about 5 cloves)

1½ TB. whole-wheat flour

1 tsp. powdered mustard

¼ tsp. cayenne

10 cups low-fat, low-sodium vegetable broth

1¼ cups broccoli stems and florets

1¼ cups low-fat silken tofu, puréed in a blender

2 medium tomatoes, diced

1½ cups low-fat shredded cheddar cheese

¼ tsp. kosher salt

½ tsp. freshly cracked black pepper

Yield: *8 servings*	
Prep time: 10 minutes	
Cook time: 35 minutes	
Serving size: ¾ cup	
Each serving has:	
153 calories	
23 g carbohydrate	
5 g sugars	
12 g protein	
2 g fat	
.3 g saturated fat	
4 g cholesterol	
675 mg sodium	
3 g fiber	
47 IU vitamin D	
454 mg potassium	
368 mg calcium	
2 mcg selenium	

1. In a large pot over medium heat, combine olive oil, onions, carrot, and celery. Cook, stirring often, for 5 minutes.

2. Add potato and garlic, and cook, stirring occasionally, for 2 minutes.

3. Stir in flour, powdered mustard, and cayenne. Cook for 2 minutes.

4. Add vegetable broth and broccoli stems and florets. Bring to a light simmer. Cover, reduce heat to medium-low, and simmer, stirring occasionally, for 10 minutes.

5. Pour into soup, along with salt and pepper and cook, stirring constantly, for 2 more minutes.

6. Reduce heat to low, add tomatoes and cheese, and cook for 5 minutes or until cheese is incorporated. Serve immediately.

Food for Thought

In this recipe, tofu replaces the cream that would normally be used to make cream soup. This increases the amount of protein and lowers the fat and cholesterol.

Creamy Mushroom Soup

Fresh garlic and red wine highlight this delicious earthy mushroom soup.

Yield: 10 servings
Prep time: 15 minutes
Cook time: 90 minutes
Serving size: ½ cup
Each serving has:
140 calories
21 g carbohydrate
7 g sugars
1 g protein
0 g fat
0 g saturated fat
0 g cholesterol
634 mg sodium
1 g fiber
37 IU vitamin D
1,154 mg potassium
121 mg calcium
23 mcg selenium

5 small red onions, peeled and sliced

4 tsp. fresh minced garlic (about 5 cloves)

1½ cups nonalcoholic red wine

1 tsp. brown sugar Splenda

2 (8-oz.) pkg. button mushrooms

2 (8-oz.) pkg. shiitake mushrooms

1 (8-oz.) pkg. crimini mushrooms

1½ tsp. dried sage

1½ tsp. dried thyme

1½ tsp. dried tarragon

⅓ tsp. ground nutmeg

10 cups low-sodium vegetable broth

3 TB. low-sodium soy sauce

1½ TB. balsamic vinegar

1¼ cups silken tofu

½ tsp. kosher salt

¼ tsp. freshly cracked black pepper

1. In a large pot over medium heat, combine onions, garlic, red wine, and brown sugar Splenda. Cook, stirring often, for 20 minutes or until onions are reddish brown.

2. Add button mushrooms, shiitake mushrooms, and crimini mushrooms. Cook, stirring constantly, for 10 minutes.

3. Add sage, thyme, tarragon, nutmeg, and vegetable broth. Simmer for 40 minutes.

4. Add soy sauce and vinegar.

5. In a blender, blend soup and tofu until smooth in multiple batches. (Be sure to only fill the blender to about ¼ full or soup may pop the lid.)

6. Season with salt and pepper and serve.

Cooking Tip

This recipe calls for nonalcoholic wine, but you can use wine with alcohol if you have some. The alcohol will cook off. Also, when choosing a wine to cook with, choose a wine you would drink.

Quick and Easy White Bean Soup

Fresh oregano and Parmesan cheese complement this quick white bean soup. *(Adapted from www.marthastewart.com.)*

2 TB. plus 2 tsp. extra-virgin olive oil

16 whole scallions, sliced

8 cloves garlic, peeled and minced

4 tsp. fresh oregano, chopped

7 cups low-fat, low-sodium vegetable broth

6½ (19-oz.) cans white beans, drained and rinsed

4 tsp. fresh lemon juice

¼ tsp. kosher salt

½ tsp. freshly cracked black pepper

8 TB. grated Parmesan cheese

Yield: 8 servings
Prep time: 15 minutes
Cook time: 45 minutes
Serving size: ¾ cup
Each serving has:
275 calories
38 g carbohydrate
3 g sugars
14 g protein
8 g fat
1.5 g saturated fat
4 g cholesterol
428 mg sodium
10 g fiber
0 IU vitamin D
500 mg potassium
132 mg calcium
1 mcg selenium

1. In a medium saucepan over medium heat, heat olive oil. Add scallions, garlic, and oregano, and cook, stirring frequently, for about 3 minutes or until scallions begin to soften.

2. Stir in vegetable broth and beans, and bring to a boil. Cook for about 10 minutes or until heated through. Using a wooden spoon or potato masher, lightly mash some beans to thicken soup. Stir in lemon juice, and season with salt and pepper.

3. Sprinkle with Parmesan cheese and serve.

Food for Thought

Garlic is an excellent anti-inflammatory and has been proven to be antiviral, antibacterial, and antifungal. The antioxidants found in garlic make it a powerful immune booster, too.

Roasted Pear and Butternut Squash Soup

This hearty soup features creamy butternut squash and sweet pears and is topped with crumbled Gorgonzola cheese.

Yield: 8 servings
Prep time: 25 minutes
Cook time: 65 minutes
Serving size: ½ cup
Each serving has:
217 calories
29 g carbohydrate
10 g sugars
17 g protein
5 g fat
3 g saturated fat
27 g cholesterol
633 mg sodium
6 g fiber
14 IU vitamin D
701 mg potassium
175 mg calcium
1 mcg selenium

2 Bartlett pears, peeled, quartered, and cored

6 cups butternut squash, peeled, seeded, and cut into 2-in. chunks

3 medium tomatoes, cored and quartered

2 leeks, pale green and white parts only, sliced and washed

3 cloves garlic, paper removed and cloves crushed

2 TB. extra-virgin olive oil

1 tsp. salt

¼ tsp. freshly cracked black pepper

6 cups low-fat, low-sodium chicken broth

¼ cup silken tofu

3 TB. plain protein powder

1 tsp. ground cinnamon

½ tsp. ground nutmeg

½ tsp. ground cloves

2 tsp. fresh sage, chopped

⅔ cup crumbled *Gorgonzola* cheese

2 TB. fresh chives, thinly sliced

1. Preheat the oven to 400°F.

2. In a large bowl, combine pears, squash, tomatoes, leeks, garlic, olive oil, ¼ teaspoon salt, and pepper. Spread evenly on a large, rimmed baking sheet. Roast, stirring occasionally, for 40 to 55 minutes or until vegetables are tender. Let cool slightly.

3. Place ½ of vegetables and 3 cups broth in a blender, and purée until smooth. Transfer to a large saucepan over medium-low heat. Purée remaining vegetables and 2 cups broth, and add to the saucepan. Finally, purée remaining 1 cup broth, tofu, and protein powder, and add to the saucepan.

4. Stir in remaining ¾ teaspoon salt, cinnamon, nutmeg, cloves, and sage. Cook, stirring, for about 10 minutes or until hot. Garnish with cheese and chives, and serve.

def•i•ni•tion

Gorgonzola is a form of hard blue cheese that's easily crumbled. If you can't find Gorgonzola, you can substitute blue cheese or Parmesano Reggiano instead.

Smoky Curried Corn Bisque

Here, oven-roasted sweet corn bisque melds with creamy smoked tofu, sweet Vidalia onions, and fresh cilantro.

2 (16-oz.) pkg. frozen corn, thawed	2 cups low-fat, low-sodium chicken broth
2 tsp. vegetable oil	2 cups low-fat, low-sodium vegetable broth
1 medium Vidalia onion, chopped (about 1 cup)	½ cup smoked silken tofu
1 TB. curry powder	3 TB. plain protein powder
½ tsp. hot pepper sauce	1 cup light coconut milk
¼ tsp. kosher salt	1 TB. fresh cilantro, chopped
¼ tsp. freshly cracked black pepper	

Yield: 8 servings
Prep time: 15 minutes
Cook time: 80 minutes
Serving size: ½ cup
Each serving has:
186 calories
25 g carbohydrate
5 g sugars
13 g protein
6 g fat
3 g saturated fat
0 g cholesterol
367 mg sodium
3 g fiber
19 IU vitamin D
333 mg potassium
57 mg calcium
2 mcg selenium

1. Preheat the oven to 350°F. Spray a baking sheet with cooking spray.

2. Arrange corn on the prepared baking sheet and roast for 10 minutes or until golden brown.

3. Meanwhile, in a large saucepan over medium-high heat, heat vegetable oil. Add onion and cook, stirring occasionally, for about 3 minutes or until soft.

4. Add curry powder, roasted corn, hot pepper sauce, salt, and pepper, and stir to coat onions. Stir in corn, chicken broth, and vegetable broth. Increase heat to high, bring mixture to a boil, and cook for about 20 minutes.

5. Remove from heat and purée, with tofu and protein powder, in batches in a blender or food processor fitted with a chopping blade until everything is combined but still has a slightly lumpy texture. (Only fill the blender or food processor to ¼ full.)

6. Pour soup into a clean saucepan, add coconut milk, and cook over low heat for about 7 minutes. Serve in a bowl topped with chopped cilantro.

Cooking Tip

Coconut milk can be found in the grocery store in the canned goods or ethnic sections. It comes in regular fat or reduced fat.

Fresh Corn and Red Pepper Bisque

Roasted red peppers, sweet Vidalia onions, and fresh cilantro star in this delicious sweet corn bisque.

Yield: 8 servings
Prep time: 15 minutes
Cook time: 50 minutes
Serving size: ½ cup
Each serving has:
133 calories
24 g carbohydrate
7 g sugars
5 g protein
3 g fat
.5 g saturated fat
1 g cholesterol
568 mg sodium
3 g fiber
9 IU vitamin D
294 mg potassium
67 mg calcium
1 mcg selenium

4 tsp. extra-virgin olive oil

2 medium Vidalia onions, chopped (about 2 cups)

3 cups fresh corn kernels

2 large cloves garlic, peeled and minced

7 cups low-fat, low-sodium chicken broth

½ tsp. kosher salt

¼ tsp. freshly cracked black pepper

½ cup plain Greek yogurt

3 TB. plain protein powder

2 TB. cornmeal

2 red bell peppers, ribs and seeds removed, and diced

4 whole scallions, chopped

4 TB. fresh cilantro, chopped

2 tsp. hot pepper sauce

2 limes, cut into wedges

¼ cup puréed silken tofu

1. In a large, heavy saucepan over medium-high heat, heat olive oil. Add onions and cook, stirring often, for 6 or 7 minutes or until lightly browned.

2. Add corn and garlic, and cook, stirring often, for about 5 minutes or until corn is lightly browned.

3. Add chicken broth, and simmer for 12 to 15 minutes or until corn is tender. Stir in salt and pepper.

4. Using a slotted spoon, transfer 1½ cups corn mixture to a blender or food processor fitted with a chopping blade. Add Greek yogurt, protein powder, and ½ cup broth to the blender or food processor, and process for about 2 minutes or until mixture is smooth. Return purée to the pan.

5. Whisk in cornmeal, and bring to a boil over medium-high heat. Cook, whisking constantly, for 5 minutes or until soup thickens. Add bell peppers, scallions, cilantro, hot pepper sauce, and puréed tofu. Bring back up to a simmer and remove from heat. Serve with lime wedges.

 Food for Thought

Citrus fruits such as limes and lemons are a great way to add another layer of flavor to a dish. Try squeezing a little bit on your next chicken or seafood dish.

Chunky Turkey Chili

This tasty, high-protein chili is chock full of peppers, onions, and delicious ground turkey.

1½ lb. ground turkey

1 medium Vidalia onion, diced (about 1 cup)

3 (14.5-oz.) cans diced tomatoes, with juice

2 (16-oz.) cans pinto beans, rinsed and drained

2 cups low-fat, low-sodium vegetable broth

2 small yellow bell peppers, ribs and seeds removed, and diced (about 1 cup)

2 small red bell peppers, ribs and seeds removed, and diced (about 1 cup)

3 cloves garlic, peeled and minced

½ cup chunky salsa

4 tsp. chili powder

3 tsp. ground cumin

¼ tsp. kosher salt

¼ tsp. freshly cracked black pepper

2 bay leaves

½ cup low-fat shredded cheddar cheese

Yield: 8 servings
Prep time: 10 minutes
Cook time: 6 or 7 hours
Serving size: ½ cup
Each serving has:
274 calories
32 g carbohydrate
10 g sugars
32 g protein
2 g fat
0 g saturated fat
35 g cholesterol
616 mg sodium
9 g fiber
0 IU vitamin D
226 mg potassium
132 mg calcium
.4 mcg selenium

1. In a 3- or 4-quart slow cooker, combine turkey, onion, tomatoes, pinto beans, vegetable broth, yellow bell peppers, red bell peppers, garlic, salsa, chili powder, cumin, salt, pepper, and bay leaves. Stir occasionally, breaking up turkey.

2. Cover and cook on low for 6 or 7 hours.

3. Remove bay leaves. Serve topped with cheddar cheese.

Cooking Tip

Everyone likes his or her chili a certain way—and a certain spiciness. Use this recipe as a base, and make it spicier or milder, depending on your taste.

Black Bean Chili

This quick and easy chili stars tons of veggies, black beans, and a variety of herbs and spices such as thyme, oregano, and paprika.

Yield: 8 servings
Prep time: 10 minutes
Cook time: 8 hours
Serving size: ½ cup
Each serving has:
124 calories
23 g carbohydrate
5 g sugars
12 g protein
.2 g fat
0 g saturated fat
4 g cholesterol
618 mg sodium
6.5 g fiber
0 IU vitamin D
464 mg potassium
236 mg calcium
0 mcg selenium

2 cups water

½ cup apple juice

1½ cups low-fat, low-sodium vegetable broth

1 tsp. dried oregano

1 tsp. dried thyme

3 TB. low-sodium tomato sauce

1 tsp. ground cumin

⅛ tsp. cayenne

¼ tsp. paprika

¼ tsp. salt

¼ tsp. freshly cracked black pepper

2 medium Vidalia onions, diced

4 cloves garlic, peeled and minced

2 (4-oz.) cans green chilies, drained and chopped

2 (15-oz.) cans black beans, rinsed and drained

2 small red bell peppers, ribs and seeds removed, and diced (about 1 cup)

¼ cup chopped fresh cilantro

1½ cups low-fat shredded cheddar cheese

1. In a 3- or 4-quart slow cooker, combine water, apple juice, vegetable broth, oregano, thyme, tomato sauce, cumin, cayenne, paprika, salt, black pepper, onions, garlic, green chilies, black beans, and red bell peppers.

2. Cover and cook on low for 8 hours.

3. Stir in cilantro just before serving, and serve with cheddar cheese for topping.

Cooking Tip

Try adding different beans to this recipe to bring in more flavors and colors. Mixing beans such as kidney, black, and cannellini gives this chili a little more eye appeal.

Chilled Spiced Blueberry Soup

This refreshing fresh blueberry soup features hints of ginger and cinnamon.

4 cups fresh blueberries	**½ tsp. ground cardamom**
2½ cups water	**2 TB. cornstarch**
1 small cinnamon stick	**3 TB. vanilla protein powder**
1 TB. honey	**⅓ cup skim milk**
2 tsp. Splenda	**1 cup vanilla Greek yogurt**
1 TB. fresh ginger, peeled and grated	

Yield: 16 servings
Prep time: 10 minutes
Cook time: 20 minutes
Serving size: ¼ cup
Each serving has:
51 calories
10 g carbohydrate
8 g sugars
2 g protein
.6 g fat
.1 g saturated fat
1 g cholesterol
25 mg sodium
1 g fiber
2 IU vitamin D
40 mg potassium
23 mg calcium
.2 mcg selenium

1. In a large saucepan over high heat, combine blueberries, water, cinnamon stick, honey, Splenda, ginger, and cardamom. Bring to a boil, stirring occasionally. Reduce heat to medium-low, and simmer, stirring, for 1 or 2 minutes or until most of the blueberries have burst.

2. Remove and discard cinnamon stick, and purée soup in a blender until smooth. (You might have to do this in batches; only fill the blender ¼ full when puréeing hot liquids.) Place a fine sieve over the pan, and pour soup through it back into the pan, straining out any solids. Discard solids.

3. In a measuring cup, whisk cornstarch, protein powder, and milk until smooth. Whisk into blueberry mixture. Bring soup to a boil over medium heat, stirring. Boil, stirring constantly, for 1 more minute or until soup thickens slightly.

4. Remove from heat, and let cool for 10 minutes. Transfer to a bowl, loosely cover, and chill for at least 5 hours, or until cold, or up to 2 days.

5. Just before serving, whisk ¾ cup Greek yogurt into soup, and ladle into bowls.

6. Top each serving with ½ teaspoon Greek yogurt, and swirl decoratively into soup. Garnish with additional blueberries, if desired.

Cooking Tip

When puréeing hot liquids in a blender, the pressure from the steam can shoot the lid right off. Only fill the blender ¼ full, and place the lid tightly on the blender before puréeing.

Chapter 17

Sensational Salads

In This Chapter

- ◆ Tasty chicken and seafood salads
- ◆ Perfect pasta salads
- ◆ Delicious tofu salads
- ◆ Flavorful marinated salads

For a healthful lunch or a light dinner, a salad is just what the doctor ordered. In this chapter, we offer a dozen satisfying and tasty recipes that prove salads don't have to be plain or boring. In the following pages, you'll find some interesting new takes on some of your favorite salads, such as tuna salad and pasta salad, and a few new salads you might not have thought of, like smoked tofu and quinoa salad. Also in this chapter we give you a number of healthful salad dressing recipes that are lower in fat and calories than most store-bought dressings.

   Although you're certainly welcome to follow our recipes to the letter, we do encourage you to mix and match the ingredients in our recipes to make new and exciting salads with your own special twist.

Grilled Chicken Mixed Green Salad with Honey-Mustard Vinaigrette

This tasty mixed green salad is tossed with sliced apples, walnuts, and grilled chicken and drizzled with a light honey-mustard vinaigrette.

Yield: 8 servings
Prep time: 15 minutes
Cook time: 10 minutes
Serving size: about ¾ cup
Each serving has:
203 calories
37 g carbohydrate
12 g sugars
8 g protein
10 g fat
1 g saturated fat
44 g cholesterol
56 mg sodium
2 g fiber
.5 IU vitamin D
77 mg potassium
8 mg calcium
0 mcg selenium

8 (about 3-oz.) boneless, skinless chicken breasts

4½ TB. extra-virgin olive oil

3 TB. Mrs. Dash Chicken Seasoning

1½ TB. apple cider vinegar

½ tsp. honey

¾ cup water

1 small bulb garlic, peeled and chopped

½ tsp. freshly cracked black pepper

3 tsp. mustard powder

1 tsp. dry white wine

1 TB. liquid egg substitute

2 cups mixed field greens

4 Granny Smith apples, sliced

½ cup walnuts

¼ cup crumbled feta cheese

1. Preheat the grill to medium-high heat.

2. Coat chicken breasts with 3 tablespoons olive oil and Mrs. Dash Chicken Seasoning. Place chicken on the grill, and cook for about 5 minutes per side or until chicken reaches 165°F.

3. In a blender, add cider vinegar, honey, remaining 1½ tablespoons olive oil, water, garlic, pepper, dry mustard, white wine, and egg substitute, and blend on high for 2 minutes or until combined.

4. In a serving bowl, combine mixed greens, apple slices, walnuts, and feta cheese. Toss with dressing.

5. Slice chicken breasts, and serve over salad.

 Food for Thought

No-salt seasoning mixes such as Mrs. Dash are a great way to add flavor to many dishes without adding the extra sodium.

Kickin' Tuna Salad

This classic tuna salad features pickle relish, celery, and chives—plus egg whites for a little extra protein.

2 large hard-boiled eggs, peeled, yolks discarded, and whites chopped

5 (6-oz.) cans tuna, drained and flaked

2 TB. reduced-fat mayonnaise

¼ cup plain Greek yogurt

2 tsp. yellow mustard

4 stalks celery, chopped

¼ cup dill pickle relish

1 tsp. freshly cracked black pepper

½ tsp. kosher salt

1 tsp. fresh chives, chopped

Yield: 8 servings
Prep time: 20 minutes
Cook time: 7 minutes
Serving size: ½ cup
Each serving has:
146 calories
3 g carbohydrate
1 g sugars
29 g protein
2 g fat
.5 g saturated fat
32 g cholesterol
336 mg sodium
0 g fiber
0 IU vitamin D
295 mg potassium
28 mg calcium
87 mcg selenium

1. In a large bowl, combine egg whites, tuna, mayonnaise, Greek yogurt, mustard, celery, pickle relish, pepper, salt, and chives.

2. Serve on bread, with salad greens, or with crackers.

 Food for Thought _____

Tuna is a great fish to include in your diet because it's high in protein; omega-3 fatty acids; and important minerals such as selenium, magnesium, and potassium.

Shrimp Salad with Creamy Lime and Chili Dressing

This succulent shrimp salad features zesty lime and a hint of spice.

Yield: 8 servings
Prep time: 23 minutes
Serving size: ½ cup
Each serving has:
169 calories
10 g carbohydrate
3 g sugars
13 g protein
9 g fat
1.4 g saturated fat
119 g cholesterol
902 mg sodium
4 g fiber
0 IU vitamin D
402 mg potassium
88 mg calcium
1 mcg selenium

1 lb. (31 to 40 count, about 32) cooked shrimp, peeled and deveined

2 tsp. orange zest

1 tsp. lime zest

¾ tsp. salt

¾ tsp. freshly cracked black pepper

1 small sliced red onion (about ¼ cup)

6 TB. plain Greek yogurt

4 TB. fresh lime juice

1 tsp. chili powder

1 tsp. Splenda

½ tsp. crushed red pepper flakes

2 romaine lettuce hearts, chopped (4 cups)

2 medium heads endive, cored and torn into pieces

1 orange, peeled and cut into segments

2 avocados, peeled, pitted, and cut into ½-in. cubes

1 TB. extra-virgin olive oil

1 lime, cut into 8 wedges

1. In a medium bowl, toss together shrimp, orange zest, lime zest, salt, and pepper. Cover and marinate in the refrigerator for 10 minutes.

2. Place onion in a small bowl, cover with cold water and some ice, and let stand for at least 10 minutes. (This cuts down on the onion's bite.)

3. Meanwhile, in a medium bowl, whisk together Greek yogurt, 3 tablespoons lime juice, chili powder, Splenda, and crushed red pepper flakes.

4. In a large bowl, toss together romaine lettuce, endive, orange segments, and drained onion (squeeze dry to release any extra liquid). Add dressing, and toss to coat. Divide salad among 8 plates.

5. In a small bowl, toss avocados with remaining 1 tablespoon lime juice. Divide among salads.

6. Drain shrimp, reserving marinade.

7. In a large skillet over medium heat, heat olive oil. Add shrimp, and sauté for 2 or 3 minutes or until pink and firm. Divide shrimp among salads, and serve with lime wedges.

 Food for Thought

Incorporating avocados in your diet can lower your LDL cholesterol (the bad cholesterol) and raise your HDL cholesterol (the good cholesterol).

Egg White Salad

This classic egg salad, with fresh tomatoes and crisp celery, has no added fat and cholesterol from the yolks. *(Adapted from food. realsimple.com.)*

3 large eggs

1 plum tomato, diced

1 TB. fresh parsley, chopped

1 stalk celery, chopped

1 tsp. extra-virgin olive oil

⅛ tsp. salt

⅛ tsp. freshly cracked black pepper

Yield: 1 serving
Prep time: 15 minutes
Cook time: 35 minutes
Serving size: ½ cup
Each serving has:
104 calories
4 g carbohydrate
3 g sugars
12 g protein
5 g fat
.6 g saturated fat
0 g cholesterol
879 mg sodium
1 g fiber
0 IU vitamin D
362 mg potassium
40 mg calcium
20 mcg selenium

1. Place eggs in a small saucepan, fill with enough cold water to cover them by 3 inches, and set over high heat. Bring to a boil, cover, and remove from heat. Let stand for 15 minutes.

2. Remove eggs to a bowl of ice water to cool. When cool, peel eggs and separate whites from yolks. Chop whites, and save yolks for another use.

3. In a small bowl, combine egg whites, tomato, parsley, celery, olive oil, salt, and pepper.

4. Serve with sliced bread or crackers or over greens.

 Food for Thought _____

The egg white contains 87 percent water and 13 percent protein, while the egg yolk contains mostly fat and cholesterol.

Mediterranean Orzo-Artichoke Salad with Feta Cheese

This Mediterranean-style orzo artichoke salad features delicious crumbled feta cheese, baby spinach, red onions, and kalamata olives.

Yield: 8 servings
Prep time: 15 minutes
Cook time: 35 minutes
Serving size: ½ cup
Each serving has:
178 calories
32 g carbohydrate
2 g sugars
6 g protein
5 g fat
2 g saturated fat
8 g cholesterol
415 mg sodium
2 g fiber
0 IU vitamin D
168 mg potassium
63 mg calcium
2 mcg selenium

1 cup uncooked orzo pasta

2 cups fresh baby spinach, chopped

½ cup sun-dried tomatoes (dry), chopped

3 TB. chopped red onion

9 kalamata olives, pitted and chopped

½ tsp. freshly cracked black pepper

2 whole scallions, chopped

2 cloves garlic, peeled and minced

¼ tsp. kosher salt

1 (6-oz.) can artichoke hearts, drained and chopped

8 TB. reduced-fat Greek dressing

½ cup crumbled feta cheese

1. Cook orzo according to package directions, omitting salt and fat. Drain, and rinse with cold water.

2. In a large bowl, combine orzo, spinach, sun-dried tomatoes, red onion, kalamata olives, pepper, scallion, garlic, and salt.

3. Add artichoke hearts, Greek dressing, and ¼ cup feta cheese to orzo, and toss gently to coat.

4. Divide salad among 8 serving plates, and sprinkle each serving with remaining feta cheese.

 Food for Thought

In Italian, *orzo* means "barley," but in America, orzo is commonly thought of as rice-shaped pasta.

Smoked Tofu and Quinoa Salad

This yummy smoked tofu and quinoa salad features fresh herbs and refreshing lemon.

3 cups water

1 tsp. kosher salt

1½ cups quinoa, rinsed well

¼ cup fresh lemon juice

3 TB. extra-virgin olive oil

3 cloves garlic, minced

½ tsp. freshly cracked black pepper

2 (6-oz.) pkg. smoked firm tofu, cubed

1½ small red bell peppers, ribs and seeds removed, and diced

1½ cups yellow grape tomatoes, halved

1 small red onion, diced

1½ cups cucumber, diced

¾ cup fresh parsley, chopped

4 TB. fresh chives, chopped

¾ cup fresh mint, chopped

Yield: *8 servings*	
Prep time: 20 minutes	
Cook time: 25 to 30 minutes	
Serving size: ¼ cup	
Each serving has:	
211 calories	
26 g carbohydrate	
2 g sugars	
9 g protein	
8 g fat	
1 g saturated fat	
0 g cholesterol	
311 mg sodium	
4 g fiber	
65 IU vitamin D	
314 mg potassium	
185 mg calcium	
3 mcg selenium	

1. In a medium saucepan over high heat, bring water and ½ teaspoon salt to a boil. Add quinoa, and return to a boil.

2. Reduce heat to low, cover, and cook for 15 to 20 minutes or until water is absorbed. Spread quinoa on a baking sheet, and cool in the refrigerator for 10 minutes.

3. Meanwhile, in a large bowl, whisk together lemon juice, olive oil, garlic, remaining ½ teaspoon salt, and pepper. Add cooled quinoa, tofu, red bell peppers, tomatoes, red onion, cucumber, parsley, chives, and mint. Toss well to combine, and serve.

 Food for Thought

Quinoa isn't a grain (it's a seed), but it's used as a substitute for grains because of the covered simmering method used to cook it. Quinoa is also a complete protein, which means it contains all nine essential amino acids.

Greek Tofu Salad

In this salad, tofu is tossed with fresh herbs, olives, tomatoes, and feta cheese and flavored with a light citrus marinade. (*Adapted from www.eatingwell.com.*)

Yield: 8 servings
Prep time: 30 minutes
Serving size: ¼ cup
Each serving has:
98 calories
8 g carbohydrate
3 g sugars
7 g protein
5 g fat
1 g saturated fat
6 g cholesterol
127 mg sodium
2 g fiber
75 IU vitamin D
106 mg potassium
244 mg calcium
1 mcg selenium

⅓ cup crumbled feta cheese

1 small red onion, chopped

4 TB. whole scallions, chopped

12 kalamata olives, pitted and chopped

6 TB. fresh lemon juice

1 TB. extra-virgin olive oil

2 cloves garlic, peeled and minced

2 tsp. chopped fresh oregano

1 (14-oz.) pkg. firm tofu, crumbled

¼ tsp. kosher salt

¼ tsp. freshly cracked black pepper

2 medium tomatoes, coarsely chopped

2 small cucumbers, coarsely chopped

4 TB. fresh parsley, chopped

1. In a medium bowl, stir together feta cheese, red onion, scallions, olives, lemon juice, olive oil, garlic, and oregano.

2. Add tofu, and mash together with a fork. Season with salt and pepper. Cover and refrigerate for 20 minutes.

3. Add tomatoes, cucumbers, and parsley, add more salt and pepper as necessary, and serve.

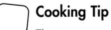

Cooking Tip

This is a great recipe to prepare early in the week and portion out so you can grab it when you're on the go.

Asian-Inspired Tofu Salad

Soy sauce, rice vinegar, honey, and fresh ginger form the marinade for this tofu salad.

3 TB. canola oil

3 TB. rice vinegar

2 TB. honey

3 tsp. low-sodium soy sauce

½ tsp. sesame oil

2 tsp. fresh ginger, peeled and minced

½ tsp. salt

1 tsp. freshly cracked black pepper

½ tsp. red pepper flakes

1 clove garlic, minced

1½ (14-oz.) pkg. extra-firm tofu, cut into 1-in. cubes

8 cups mixed salad greens

3 medium carrots, peeled, halved lengthwise, and sliced

2 large cucumbers, chopped

Yield: 8 servings
Prep time: 10 minutes
Cook time: 12 to 15 minutes
Serving size: ¼ cup
Each serving has:
150 calories
13 g carbohydrate
7 g sugars
8 g protein
7 g fat
.4 g saturated fat
0 g cholesterol
211 mg sodium
3 g fiber
113 IU vitamin D
167 mg potassium
300 mg calcium
0 mcg selenium

1. In a medium bowl, whisk together canola oil, rice vinegar, honey, soy sauce, sesame oil, ginger, salt, pepper, red pepper flakes, and garlic.

2. Place tofu and ¼ cup dressing in a large, nonstick skillet. Set over medium-high heat, and cook, turning every 2 or 3 minutes, for 12 to 15 minutes total or until golden brown. Remove from heat, add 2 tablespoons dressing to the skillet, and stir to coat.

3. Toss greens, carrots, and cucumbers with remaining dressing. Serve immediately, topped with warm tofu.

Cooking Tip

The marinade used for the tofu can also be used on other proteins such as shrimp and chicken.

Marinated Beefsteak Tomato and Tofu Salad

Low-fat, low-cholesterol beefsteak tomatoes and tofu star in this salad marinated in a simple red wine vinaigrette.

Yield: 8 servings
Prep time: 35 to 40 minutes
Serving size: 6 tomato wedges plus ¼ cup tofu
Each serving has:
107 calories
8 g carbohydrate
5 g sugars
4 g protein
8 g fat
1 g saturated fat
0 g cholesterol
66 mg sodium
2 g fiber
32 IU vitamin D
279 mg potassium
99 mg calcium
.6 mcg selenium

6 TB. red wine vinegar

4 TB. extra-virgin olive oil

2 shallots, minced

2 cloves garlic, peeled and minced

3 tsp. *capers*, rinsed and coarsely chopped

¼ tsp. salt

2 tsp. freshly cracked black pepper

¾ cup firm tofu, diced into ¼-in. cubes

6 beefsteak tomatoes

2 TB. fresh parsley, chopped

1. In a small bowl, whisk together red wine vinegar and olive oil. Stir in shallots, garlic, capers, salt, and pepper.

2. Pour marinade into a medium bowl with tofu, and toss to coat. Cover bowl with plastic wrap, and allow to marinate in the refrigerator for 15 to 20 minutes.

3. Core tomatoes, cut each into 8 wedges, and mix with tofu and marinade. Serve immediately sprinkled with parsley for garnish.

def•i•ni•tion

A **caper** is the pickled bud of a caper bush. They have a salty flavor and go great in many salads, chicken, and seafood dishes.

Marinated Mushroom and Tofu Salad

This mushroom and tofu salad is tossed with red bell pepper, scallions, and garlic and marinated in a classic Italian dressing.

2 (8-oz.) pkg. sliced button mushrooms

1 (14-oz.) pkg. firm tofu, cubed

4 whole scallions, chopped

1 medium Vidalia onion, sliced thin

1 clove garlic, peeled and minced

1 red bell pepper, ribs and seeds removed, and diced small

1 (8-oz.) bottle low-fat Italian dressing

Yield: 8 servings
Prep time: 8 to 10 hours
Serving size: ¼ cup
Each serving has:
61 calories
7 g carbohydrate
5 g sugars
6 g protein
1 g fat
.2 g saturated fat
.6 g cholesterol
342 mg sodium
1 g fiber
78 IU vitamin D
306 mg potassium
108 mg calcium
6 mcg selenium

1. In a large bowl, combine mushrooms, tofu, scallions, onion, garlic, bell pepper, and Italian dressing.

2. Marinate overnight, covered, in the refrigerator. Stir before serving.

Cooking Tip

This marinade also works well on a number of other foods. Try it on chopped vegetables such as tomatoes and cucumbers.

Sugar Snap Pea, Cherry Tomato, and Garbanzo Bean Pasta Salad

This light vegetable salad features fresh herbs and zesty citrus and is loaded with protein.

Yield: 8 servings
Prep time: 15 minutes
Cook time: 11 minutes
Serving size: ¼ cup
Each serving has:
222 calories
37 g carbohydrate
8 g sugars
10 g protein
3 g fat
1 g saturated fat
4 g cholesterol
150 mg sodium
3 g fiber
0 IU vitamin D
263 mg potassium
107 mg calcium
.4 mcg selenium

¾ cup low-fat cottage cheese

½ cup reduced-fat buttermilk

1 TB. extra-virgin olive oil

2½ TB. fresh dill, chopped

2½ TB. fresh parsley, chopped

2½ TB. grated Parmesan cheese

1½ tsp. lemon zest

1½ tsp. fresh lemon juice

½ tsp. kosher salt

¼ tsp. freshly cracked black pepper

1¼ cups uncooked whole-wheat bowtie pasta

1 cup fresh sugar snap peas

3 cups cherry tomatoes, halved

¼ cup canned garbanzo beans, drained and rinsed

1 yellow bell pepper, ribs and seeds removed, and sliced

1 red onion, sliced

6 whole scallions, sliced

1. In a large pot over high heat, bring water to a boil for cooking pasta.

2. Meanwhile, in a blender or in a food processor fitted with a chopping blade, purée cottage cheese for about 2 minutes or until smooth.

3. Add buttermilk and olive oil, and process for about 30 seconds or until smooth. Pour into a medium bowl, and stir in dill, parsley, Parmesan cheese, lemon zest, and lemon juice. Season with salt and pepper. Cover and refrigerate.

4. Add pasta to boiling water, and cook for about 10 minutes or until just *al dente.*

5. Add peas and cook for about 1 minute or until crisp-tender. Drain and rinse under cold running water.

6. Place pasta and peas in a medium bowl, and toss with tomatoes, garbanzo beans, bell pepper, red onion, and scallions. Season with more salt and pepper as necessary.

7. Just before serving, toss salad with dressing.

def•i•ni•tion

Al dente in Italian means "to the tooth" or "to the bite." So when you see *al dente* in a recipe, it basically means to cook the pasta, rice, vegetables, etc., to a tender state but so it still has a little bite.

Tabbouleh Salad with Garbanzo Beans

Garbanzo beans, juicy tomatoes, and bulgur star in this fresh mixed-herb salad highlighted with hints of fresh lemon. *(Adapted from mayoclinic.com.)*

1 cup low-fat, low-sodium vegetable broth	2 whole scallions, chopped	
1 cup fine-grind *bulgur*	1 TB. lemon zest	
2 cups cherry tomatoes, halved	1 clove garlic, peeled and minced	
½ cucumber, peeled, seeded, and diced	¾ tsp. kosher salt	
¼ cup fresh lemon juice	¼ tsp. freshly cracked black pepper	
¼ cup fresh parsley, chopped	¼ tsp. ground allspice	
3 TB. fresh mint, chopped	2 cups *garbanzo beans*	
2 TB. extra-virgin olive oil	½ small Vidalia onion, diced (about ¼ cup)	

Yield: 8 servings
Prep time: 30 minutes
Cook time: 8½ hours
Serving size: ¼ cup
Each serving has:
131 calories
19 g carbohydrate
4 g sugars
5 g protein
5 g fat
.6 g saturated fat
0 g cholesterol
266 mg sodium
3 g fiber
0 IU vitamin D
257 mg potassium
30 mg calcium
2 mcg selenium

1. In a medium saucepan over high heat, bring vegetable stock to a boil. Add bulgur, remove from heat, cover, and set aside for 15 minutes or until stock has absorbed.

2. In a large bowl, toss together cherry tomatoes, cucumber, lemon juice, parsley, mint, olive oil, scallions, lemon zest, garlic, salt, pepper, allspice, garbanzo beans, and onion.

3. Cover and let sit overnight in the refrigerator for best flavor.

def•i•ni•tion

Bulgur is a combination of several different wheat species and is a common ingredient in Turkish, Middle Eastern, and Mediterranean dishes. Because of its high nutritional value, bulgur is often used as a substitute for rice and couscous. Garbanzo beans are a member of the legume family and are high in protein.

Chapter 18

Delicious Main Dishes

In This Chapter

- ◆ Perfect poultry dishes
- ◆ Hearty pork and savory beef recipes
- ◆ Succulent seafood entrées

You've probably heard the question more times than you can count—and likely asked it yourself a time or two: "What's for dinner?" This chapter has your answer. Whether you're craving poultry, pork, or seafood, you'll find a tableful of delicious main dishes in this chapter.

Many of these dishes can serve as your main entrée, especially when served with some of the side dishes found in Chapter 20 or with a salad from Chapter 17.

Orange Chicken Fingers

These crispy chicken fingers are coated in cereal and drizzled with a sweet sesame-orange sauce.

Yield: 8 servings
Prep time: 15 minutes
Cook time: 25 minutes
Serving size: about 2 chicken fingers and 1 tablespoon sauce
Each serving has:
271 calories
36 g carbohydrate
8 g sugars
28 g protein
3 g fat
.3 g saturated fat
50 g cholesterol
291 mg sodium
4 g fiber
21 IU vitamin D
198 mg potassium
31 mg calcium
26 mcg selenium

3 TB. Dijon mustard

3 TB. frozen orange juice concentrate, thawed

3 TB. honey

2 tsp. sesame oil

1 tsp. freshly cracked black pepper

2 tsp. toasted sesame seeds

1½ lb. low-fat chicken tenders (about 16)

2 cups whole-wheat flour

1 cup liquid egg substitute

2 cups high-protein rice-and-wheat cereal, coarsely ground

1. In a medium bowl, whisk together Dijon mustard, orange juice concentrate, honey, sesame oil, and pepper until smooth.

2. Pour ½ of sauce into a small medium bowl, and stir in sesame seeds. Set aside.

3. Add chicken to remaining sauce, and marinate, covered, in the refrigerator for about 15 minutes.

4. Preheat the oven to 350°F. Lightly coat a baking sheet with cooking spray.

5. Add flour to a shallow bowl. Add egg substitute to another shallow bowl. Add cereal to a third shallow bowl.

6. Remove chicken from marinade, and discard marinade. Coat chicken in flour, dip in egg substitute, and dip in ground cereal. Place chicken on the prepared baking sheet, and repeat with remaining pieces. Bake for 25 minutes or until tenders reach 165°F.

7. Serve chicken drizzled with orange-sesame sauce.

 Food for Thought _____

Ground cereals make an excellent coating for all types of things from poultry to seafood.

Oven-Roasted Beer Can Chicken

Here, a whole roasted chicken is rubbed with an array of delicious spices such as garlic, coriander, and cumin along with sweet brown sugar.

1 (4-lb.) whole chicken

¼ cup firmly packed brown sugar

1 TB. chili powder

2 TB. paprika

1 TB. cumin

½ tsp. coriander

¼ tsp. cayenne

2 tsp. garlic powder

3 tsp. mustard powder

2 tsp. kosher salt

2 tsp. freshly cracked black pepper

½ to ¾ (12-oz.) can beer

Yield: 16 servings
Prep time: 15 minutes
Cook time: 35 to 40 minutes
Serving size: about a size of a deck of cards
Each serving has:
148 calories
3 g carbohydrate
3 g sugars
24 g protein
4 g fat
1 g saturated fat
79 g cholesterol
378 mg sodium
0 g fiber
0 IU vitamin D
18 mg potassium
17 mg calcium
18 mcg selenium

1. Move oven rack to the lowest position in oven, and preheat the oven to 400°F.

2. Rinse chicken in the sink and remove the insides. Pat dry with a paper towel.

3. In a small bowl, combine brown sugar, chili powder, paprika, cumin, coriander, cayenne, garlic powder, mustard powder, salt, and black pepper. Rub on skin of chicken.

4. Set chicken upright on an open beer can in a roasting pan, and place in the oven.

5. Bake for 35 to 40 minutes or until chicken reaches an internal temperature of 165°F. Before serving, discard beer can along with any liquid that may remain.

 Food for Thought _____

> The beer in this recipe is used to keep the chicken moist as it cooks by creating steam inside the chicken. Try using this same recipe and technique on the grill or smoker.

Southern-Style Chicken and Biscuits

A prime example of southern comfort food, here, chicken and biscuits pair with carrots, pearl onions, and thyme.

Yield: 8 servings
Prep time: 15 minutes
Cook time: 23 minutes
Serving size: ½ cup chicken and 1 biscuit
Each serving has:
271 calories
25 g carbohydrate
8 g sugars
23 g protein
9 g fat
2 g saturated fat
36 g cholesterol
260 mg sodium
4 g fiber
25 IU vitamin D
474 mg potassium
152 mg calcium
14 mcg selenium

⅔ cup whole-wheat flour

⅓ cup plus 4 TB. all-purpose flour

⅓ cup plain protein powder

2 TB. baking powder

1 tsp. kosher salt

¼ tsp. freshly cracked black pepper

2 egg whites

4 TB. plus 2 tsp. vegetable oil

2 cups skim milk

10 medium carrots, peeled and chopped

10 small stalks celery, chopped

2 (10-oz.) boxes frozen pearl onions, thawed

¾ cup plain Greek yogurt

½ cup water

½ tsp. dried thyme

1 lb. low-fat chicken tenders (about 12), cut into cubes

1. Preheat the oven to 450°F.

2. In a medium bowl, whisk together whole-wheat flour, ⅓ cup all-purpose flour, protein powder, baking powder, salt, and pepper. Set aside.

3. In a separate small bowl, whisk together egg whites, 4 tablespoons oil, and milk. Add to flour mixture, and stir until moistened.

4. Drop 8 (¼ cup) scoops dough onto a baking sheet, at least 2 inches apart. Bake for 12 to 14 minutes or until golden.

5. Meanwhile, in a large, heavy pot, heat remaining 2 teaspoons oil over medium-high heat. Add carrots, celery, and onions, and season with salt and pepper. Cook, stirring frequently, for 7 to 10 minutes or until vegetables are tender.

6. Sprinkle vegetables with remaining 4 tablespoons all-purpose flour, and stir in Greek yogurt, water, and thyme. Simmer, stirring occasionally, for 2 or 3 minutes or until liquid is thickened.

7. Add chicken, and simmer for 5 to 10 minutes or until cooked through. Serve chicken stew with biscuits.

🚫 **Post-Op Pitfall**

Beware of lumps! Use a whisk to stir in the flour so you lower the risk of lumps forming in the sauce.

Sweet and Sour Chicken Breasts

This new take on sweet and sour chicken with zesty orange and fresh mint will surely be a hit.

½ tsp. orange zest

¼ cup orange juice

¼ cup water

2 TB. honey

1 TB. Splenda

1 TB. plus 1 tsp. cider vinegar

½ tsp. salt

¼ tsp. ground *coriander*

1 tsp. cornstarch

¼ cup chopped fresh mint

8 (2-oz.) boneless, skinless chicken breasts

¼ tsp. freshly cracked black pepper

Yield: 8 servings
Prep time: 10 minutes
Cook time: 46 minutes
Serving size: 1 chicken breast and about 1 tablespoon sauce
Each serving has:
150 calories
5 g carbohydrate
4 g sugars
27 g protein
1.5 g fat
0 g saturated fat
68 g cholesterol
222 mg sodium
0 g fiber
0 IU vitamin D
318 mg potassium
14 mg calcium
21 mcg selenium

1. Spray the grill rack with cooking spray. Preheat the grill to medium heat.

2. In a small saucepan over medium-high heat, combine orange zest, orange juice, water, honey, Splenda, 1 tablespoon vinegar, ¼ teaspoon salt, and coriander. Bring to a boil.

3. In a small bowl, whisk together cornstarch and remaining 1 teaspoon vinegar until smooth. Add to the saucepan and return to a boil, whisking until thickened, for 30 seconds to 1 minute. Remove from heat, and stir in mint.

4. Sprinkle chicken with remaining ¼ teaspoon salt and pepper. Grill for about 15 minutes, turning to cook both sides, until an instant-read thermometer inserted into the thickest part reaches 165°F.

5. Serve chicken with orange dipping sauce on the side.

def•i•ni•tion

Coriander is a lemony-flavored spice commonly used in Mediterranean and Middle Eastern cooking. Coriander is the fruit of the plant, or the seeds. The leaves are called cilantro.

Braised Chicken Breasts

These succulent and juicy chicken breasts are *braised* in a creamy tomato sauce.

Yield: 8 servings
Prep time: 15 minutes
Cook time: 55 minutes
Serving size: 1 chicken breast and ¼ cup sauce
Each serving has:
207 calories
12 g carbohydrate
6 g sugars
30 g protein
4 g fat
1 g saturated fat
73 g cholesterol
329 mg sodium
2 g fiber
0 IU vitamin D
516 mg potassium
62 mg calcium
23 mcg selenium

8 (2-oz.) boneless, skinless chicken breasts

¾ tsp. salt

½ tsp. freshly cracked black pepper

1 TB. canola oil

4 cups diced Spanish onion (about 3 onions)

2 cloves garlic, minced

2 bay leaves

¼ tsp. Splenda

1 medium red bell pepper, ribs and seeds removed, and diced (1 cup)

1 small yellow bell pepper, ribs and seeds removed, and diced (½ cup)

2 TB. tomato paste

2 TB. paprika

1 tsp. crushed red pepper flakes

1 tsp. dried marjoram

1 cup low-sodium, reduced-fat chicken broth

½ cup plain Greek yogurt

1 TB. whole-wheat flour

2 TB. chopped fresh parsley

1. Pat chicken breasts dry with paper towels, and season with ½ teaspoon salt and pepper.

2. In a large, heavy large pot over medium heat, heat canola oil. Add onions, garlic, and bay leaves, and sprinkle with Splenda. Cook, stirring frequently, for 10 to 15 minutes or until onions are very soft and light brown.

3. Stir in red bell pepper, yellow bell pepper, tomato paste, paprika, and crushed red pepper flakes. Add chicken, and stir gently. Sprinkle with marjoram, and pour in chicken broth. Cover and simmer over medium-low heat for about 20 minutes or until chicken is very tender.

4. Meanwhile, in a small bowl, whisk together Greek yogurt, flour, and remaining ¼ teaspoon salt until smooth.

5. Remove chicken to a plate. Stir Greek yogurt mixture into sauce, return to a simmer, and cook, stirring, for about 10 minutes or until sauce coats the spoon. Reduce heat to low, return chicken to sauce, and reheat for about 1 minute. Remove bay leaves, and serve garnished with parsley.

def•i•ni•tion

Braising is the act of slowly cooking a protein in liquid on low temperature for hours at a time. The braising liquid in this recipe is also tasty on seafood. Simply replace the chicken broth with seafood broth, and add a few capers.

Turkey Meatloaf

This classic meatloaf with a twist features sweet tomatoes, ground turkey, fresh garlic, and onions but with less fat.

1½ lb. lean ground turkey

¾ cup old-fashioned rolled oats

½ cup liquid egg substitute

½ cup diced Spanish onion (about 1 small onion)

½ cup canned low-sodium diced tomatoes, drained

2 TB. wheat germ

1 TB. chopped garlic

Yield: 8 servings
Prep time: 15 minutes
Cook time: 25 minutes
Serving size: about ½-inch slice
Each serving has:
137 calories
7 g carbohydrate
1 g sugars
24 g protein
2 g fat
0 g saturated fat
34 g cholesterol
76 mg sodium
1 g fiber
3 IU vitamin D
15 mg potassium
7 mg calcium
0 mcg selenium

1. Preheat the oven to 350°F. Lightly coat a baking dish with cooking spray.

2. In a large bowl, combine turkey, rolled oats, egg substitute, onion, tomatoes, wheat germ, and garlic. Using your hands, form mixture into a loaf.

3. Place loaf in the prepared baking dish, and bake for 25 minutes or until the internal temperature reaches 165°F.

4. Allow to sit for 2 or 3 minutes before serving. Slice into ½-inch slices, and serve.

Cooking Tip

This is a basic meatloaf recipe, perfect for playing with and adding different spices and ingredients to suit your taste.

Spaghetti Squash and Turkey Meatballs

Here, spaghetti squash "pasta" and turkey meatballs are seasoned with oregano and thyme.

Yield: 8 servings
Prep time: 15 minutes
Cook time: 42 minutes
Serving size: ½ cup spaghetti squash, 1 meatball, and ¼ cup sauce
Each serving has:
210 calories
19 g carbohydrate
7 g sugars
31 g protein
2 g fat
0 g saturated fat
45 g cholesterol
185 mg sodium
2 g fiber
0 IU vitamin D
100 mg potassium
49 mg calcium
3 mcg selenium

½ cup chopped Vidalia onion (about 1 small onion)

⅔ cup whole-wheat breadcrumbs

1 TB. liquid egg substitute

2 tsp. dried oregano

⅔ cup scallions, chopped

4 cloves garlic, minced

2 lb. lean ground turkey

2 tsp. dried thyme

1 (12- to 16-oz.) spaghetti squash

½ cup low-fat, low-sodium chicken broth

1 (26- to 28-oz.) can low-sodium tomato sauce

5 TB. chopped fresh parsley

1. Preheat the oven to 400°F. Lightly coat a cookie sheet with cooking spray.

2. In a large bowl, combine onion, breadcrumbs, egg substitute, oregano, scallions, garlic, turkey, and thyme.

3. Form mixture into 40 (½-inch-thick) balls, and place on the prepared cookie sheet. Bake for 15 to 20 minutes or until internal temperature reaches 165°F.

4. Meanwhile, cut spaghetti squash in half, remove seeds, and place squash halves cut side down in a microwave-safe dish. Add chicken broth. Cover and microwave on high for about 15 minutes or until squash is fork-tender.

5. While squash is cooking, in a saucepan over low heat, heat tomato sauce for 5 to 7 minutes or until hot.

6. Using a fork, scrape baked squash into strands onto a large serving plate. Top with turkey meatballs and tomato sauce, and serve, garnished with chopped parsley.

Cooking Tip

Spaghetti squash has a mild flavor that works well for all types of "pasta" dishes. Try it with your favorite pasta sauce.

Stuffed Bell Peppers

This Italian favorite features ground turkey, rice, tomatoes, fresh garlic, and herbs.

5 TB. extra-virgin olive oil

1½ lb. lean ground turkey

2 medium Vidalia onions, chopped (about 4 cups)

4 cloves garlic, minced

4 tsp. Mrs. Dash Italian Seasoning

4 cups cooked wild rice

2 TB. fresh oregano

2 tsp. freshly cracked black pepper

4 cups canned low-sodium roasted tomatoes, drained

1 tsp. Worcestershire sauce

8 small bell peppers, tops and seeds removed

Yield: 8 servings
Prep time: 10 minutes
Cook time: 75 minutes
Serving size: 1 pepper
Each serving has:
132 calories
53 g carbohydrate
9 g sugars
27 g protein
12 g fat
2 g saturated fat
34 g cholesterol
112 mg sodium
7 g fiber
0 IU vitamin D
297 mg potassium
15 mg calcium
0 mcg selenium

1. Preheat the oven to 350°F. Lightly coat a baking dish with cooking spray.

2. In a sauté pan over medium-high heat, heat olive oil. Add ground turkey, and cook for 5 to 10 minutes or until brown.

3. Add onions and garlic, and sauté for about 10 minutes or until onions are translucent.

4. Add Mrs. Dash, wild rice, oregano, pepper, tomatoes, and Worcestershire sauce, and stir to combine. Cook for 2-3 minutes.

5. Stuff peppers with turkey and rice filling, place peppers in the prepared baking dish, and cook for about 45 minutes or until peppers are tender.

Cooking Tip

When cooking rice, use a 3-to-1 ratio: 3 liquid to 1 rice. For this recipe, use 4 cups rice and 12 cups liquid (or 3 quarts). Bring liquid and rice to a boil, turn down the heat to the lowest setting, and cover. Continue to cook rice until the liquid is absorbed, and fluff with a fork.

Apricot and Dried Cranberry Chutney Pork Chops

These delicious oven-roasted pork chops lightly seasoned with salt and freshly cracked black pepper are topped with a sweet apricot and dried cranberry chutney.

Yield: 8 servings
Prep time: 15 minutes
Cook time: 20 minutes
Serving size: 1 pork chop and about 2 tablespoons chutney
Each serving has:
169 calories
9 g carbohydrate
3 g sugars
24 g protein
4 g fat
1 g saturated fat
74 g cholesterol
207 mg sodium
.6 g fiber
0 IU vitamin D
457 mg potassium
10 mg calcium
35 mcg selenium

8 (3-oz.) center-cut pork loin chops

½ tsp. kosher salt

¼ tsp. freshly cracked black pepper

2 tsp. extra-virgin olive oil

¼ cup dried cranberries

½ cup dried apricots, chopped

2 TB. lemon juice

¼ tsp. crushed red pepper flakes

2 TB. chopped fresh mint

1. Preheat the oven to 350°F. Lightly coat a large skillet with cooking spray.

2. Sprinkle pork chops with salt and pepper.

3. Set skillet over medium heat, and add olive oil. Add pork chops, and cook for 1 or 2 minutes per side or until browned. Transfer chops to a 12-inch-square glass baking dish.

4. Add dried cranberries, dried apricots, lemon juice, and crushed red pepper flakes to the skillet, and increase heat to medium-high. Bring to a boil and cook, scraping up any browned bits, for 4 or 5 minutes or until sauce thickens into chutney. Pour cranberry-apricot chutney over pork chops.

5. Bake pork chops for 8 to 10 minutes or until just cooked through, about 145°F.

6. Divide chops and chutney among 8 plates, sprinkle with mint, and serve.

 Food for Thought _____

Dried fruits are great to have on hand for a quick snack when you need something sweet. Some of our personal favorites are dried cherries, apricots, and golden raisins. Be careful of the serving size because dried fruits tend to pack a lot of sugar.

Grilled Garlic-Maple Pork Tenderloin

The sweet taste of maple and garlic is infused in this pork tenderloin.

2 lb. pork tenderloin	1¼ tsp. sesame oil
1 cup sliced Vidalia onion (about 1 medium onion)	4 cloves garlic, chopped
3 tsp. ground mustard	½ tsp. freshly cracked black pepper
1 tsp. white wine	1 cup sugar-free maple syrup
1½ TB. apple cider vinegar	

1. In a large zipper-lock bag, combine pork tenderloin, onion, ground mustard, white wine, vinegar, sesame oil, garlic, black pepper, and maple syrup. Cover and allow to marinate for at least 2 hours in the refrigerator.

2. Preheat the grill to medium-low.

3. Remove pork tenderloin from marinade, discard marinade, and cook for 20 minutes or until internal temperature has reached 145°F.

4. Slice *on the bias* and serve.

def•i•ni•tion

On the bias basically means to cut on an angle as opposed to an up-and-down motion. It gives the item a nice presentation, and you have the appearance of getting more food.

Yield: 8 servings

Prep time: 2 hours, 15 minutes

Cook time: 20 minutes

Serving size: about the size of a deck of cards

Each serving has:

156 calories

8 g carbohydrate

1 g sugars

24 g protein

3 g fat

1 g saturated fat

74 g cholesterol

103 mg sodium

.4 g fiber

0 IU vitamin D

108 mg potassium

10 mg calcium

34 mcg selenium

Herb and Mustard Roasted Pork Loin

This zesty mustard and herb–encrusted oven roasted pork loin has fresh honey and garlic highlights.

Yield: 8 servings
Prep time: 15 minutes
Cook time: 1½ hours
Serving size: about the size of a deck of cards
Each serving has:
102 calories
2.5 g carbohydrate
1 g sugars
18 g protein
2 g fat
.6 g saturated fat
55 g cholesterol
143 mg sodium
0 g fiber
0 IU vitamin D
340 mg potassium
4 mg calcium
26 mcg selenium

¼ tsp. dried sage

¼ tsp. kosher salt

¼ tsp. freshly cracked black pepper

1 clove garlic, minced

1 (1½-lb.) boneless pork tenderloin

2 TB. Splenda

1 TB. cornstarch

¼ cup cider vinegar

¼ cup *stone-ground mustard*

1 TB. honey

1. Preheat the oven to 325°F.

2. In a small bowl, combine sage, salt, pepper, and garlic. Rub mixture thoroughly over pork loin.

3. Place pork in an uncovered roasting pan and place on the middle oven rack. Bake for 1½ hours or until the internal temperature reaches at least 150°F.

4. Meanwhile, in a small saucepan over medium heat, combine Splenda, cornstarch, vinegar, stone-ground mustard, and honey. Heat, stirring constantly, for 5 to 10 minutes or until mixture begins to bubble and thicken slightly.

5. Brush roast with glaze 3 or 4 times during the last ½ hour of cooking. Pour remaining glaze over roast before serving.

def•i•ni•tion

Stone-ground mustard is mustard seeds that are ground with a stone mill to a coarse texture. The flavor is slightly spicier than that of regular mustard.

Lamb and Vegetable Stew

Tons of fresh vegetables and herbs star in this delicious and hearty lamb stew that's low in saturated fat.

1 lb. boneless leg of lamb

1¼ tsp. kosher salt

1¼ tsp. freshly cracked black pepper

1½ TB. extra-virgin olive oil

2 large Vidalia onions, chopped

4 cloves garlic, minced

½ tsp. dried oregano

¼ tsp. dried rosemary

¼ tsp. dried thyme

1 (14-oz.) can low-sodium diced tomatoes, with liquid

1 large baking potato, peeled and diced

2 medium carrots, peeled and sliced

1 cup green beans

1 small eggplant, diced

1 medium zucchini, diced

6 bay leaves

3 TB. chopped fresh parsley

Yield: 8 servings
Prep time: 15 minutes
Cook time: 4 hours, 20 minutes
Serving size: ½ cup
Each serving has:
276 calories
26 g carbohydrate
6 g sugars
24 g protein
9 g fat
2 g saturated fat
52 g cholesterol
443 mg sodium
8 g fiber
0 IU vitamin D
852 mg potassium
63 mg calcium
17 mcg selenium

1. Season lamb with ¼ teaspoon salt and pepper.

2. In a large, heavy skillet over medium-high heat, heat 1 tablespoon olive oil. Add lamb, and *sear*, turning, for 2 to 4 minutes or until well browned. Transfer to a 4-quart slow cooker. Add to slow cooker.

3. Add remaining ½ tablespoon oil to the skillet, and reduce heat to medium. Add onions and cook, stirring, for 3 to 5 minutes or until softened. Add garlic, oregano, rosemary, and thyme, and cook, stirring, for 1 more minute. Add tomatoes and bring to a simmer, mashing with a potato masher or fork. Remove from heat, and spoon ½ of mixture over lamb.

4. Arrange potato in a layer in the slow cooker, and season with ¼ teaspoon salt and pepper. Add carrots, followed by green beans, followed by eggplant and zucchini, seasoning each layer with ¼ teaspoon salt and pepper. Spread remaining tomato-onion mixture over vegetables. Top with bay leaves.

5. Cover and cook on high for about 4 hours, or until lamb and vegetables are very tender, stirring occasionally. Discard bay leaves. Serve stew hot, garnished with parsley.

def•i•ni•tion

To **sear** is to cook a food at high temperature until a caramelized crust forms.

Grilled Filet Mignon and Veggie Kabobs

Tender beef tenderloin and a variety of summery vegetables like cherry tomatoes and zucchini tossed with fresh herbs and garlic and are grilled to perfection.

Yield: 6 servings
Prep time: 20 minutes
Cook time: 15 to 20 minutes
Serving size: 2 kabobs
Each serving has:
284 calories
8 g carbohydrate
4 g sugars
33 g protein
12 g fat
5 g saturated fat
95 g cholesterol
467 mg sodium
2.5 g fiber
0 IU vitamin D
911 mg potassium
45 mg calcium
36 mcg selenium

2 TB. extra-virgin olive oil

1 TB. chopped fresh thyme

½ TB. chopped fresh rosemary

2 cloves garlic, minced

½ tsp. kosher salt

¼ tsp. freshly cracked black pepper

12 cherry tomatoes

10 oz. small button mushrooms

2 medium zucchini, cut in ½ and sliced

2 small red onions, cut into wedges

1½ lb. beef tenderloin, trimmed of fat and cut into ½-in. cubes

12 (10-in.) bamboo skewers, soaked in water

1. Preheat the grill to medium-high.

2. In a large bowl, combine olive oil, thyme, rosemary, garlic, salt, pepper, cherry tomatoes, button mushrooms, zucchini, red onions, and beef cubes. Mix until vegetables and beef are coated in seasonings and oil.

3. Alternately thread equal amounts of vegetables and beef on each skewer.

4. Grill skewers, turning occasionally, for 15 to 20 minutes or until beef has reached an internal temperature of 130°F and vegetables are cooked.

Cooking Tip

When making kabobs on bamboo skewers, soak the skewers in water for at least 30 minutes before using them on the grill. You don't want the skewers to burn when the food is being cooked!

Seared Halibut with White Beans and Fennel

This delicious high-protein entrée features white beans, fresh tomatoes, and fennel.

2 TB. olive oil	1 cup dry white wine
4 small bulbs fennel, sliced	2 TB. Dijon mustard
4 TB. fennel fronds, chopped	1 tsp. freshly cracked black pepper
4 (15-oz.) cans white beans, rinsed and drained	
4 medium tomatoes, diced	4 tsp. fennel seed
	8 (4-oz.) halibut fillets (about 1½ lb.)

Yield: 8 servings
Prep time: 10 minutes
Cook time: 25 minutes
Serving size: 1 fillet and about ¼ cup bean mixture
Each serving has:
363 calories
40 g carbohydrate
4 g sugars
30 g protein
7 g fat
1 g saturated fat
27 g cholesterol
267 mg sodium
13 g fiber
128 IU vitamin D
1,443 mg potassium
170 mg calcium
32 mcg selenium

1. Spray a large, nonstick skillet with cooking spray, and set over medium heat. Add 1 tablespoon olive oil. Add sliced fennel, and cook, stirring occasionally, for about 6 minutes or until lightly browned.

2. Stir in beans, tomatoes, and wine. Cook, stirring occasionally, for about 3 minutes or until tomato begins to break down. Transfer to a bowl, and stir in chopped fennel fronds, Dijon mustard, and ½ teaspoon pepper. Cover to keep warm.

3. Rinse and dry the skillet, and set over medium-high heat. Add remaining 1 tablespoon olive oil, and heat until shimmering but not smoking.

4. In a small bowl, combine fennel seed and remaining ½ teaspoon pepper. Sprinkle evenly on both sides of halibut. Add halibut to the skillet, skinned side up, and cook for 3 to 6 minutes or until golden brown. Turn over halibut, cover, and remove from heat.

5. Allow halibut to finish cooking off heat for 3 to 6 more minutes or until just cooked through. Serve with bean mixture.

Food for Thought

When using whole fennel, cut off the green fronds from the top, and remove the green stalks. Cut the bulb in half, remove the bottom, slice the bulb thinly, and rinse.

Grilled Salmon Fillet with Lemon and Chive Crème Fraîche

Here, delicious grilled salmon is topped with lemon and chive *crème fraîche* made from puréed cashews and *miso*.

Yield: 8 servings
Prep time: 10 minutes
Cook time: 6 minutes
Serving size: about the size of a deck of cards and 2 tablespoons crème fraîche
Each serving has:
200 calories
3 g carbohydrate
1 g sugars
19 g protein
12 g fat
2 g saturated fat
47 g cholesterol
246 mg sodium
.3 g fiber
205 IU vitamin D
486 mg potassium
14 mg calcium
33 mcg selenium

1 TB. Mrs. Dash Lemon Pepper

½ cup raw cashews

2 tsp. light miso

¼ cup fresh lemon juice

¼ tsp. ground nutmeg

1 cup plus ½ tsp. water

2 TB. chopped fresh chives

8 (3-oz.) fillets fresh Atlantic salmon

2 TB. extra-virgin olive oil

¼ tsp. kosher salt

¼ tsp. freshly ground black pepper

1. Preheat the grill to medium.

2. In a blender, combine Mrs. Dash Lemon Pepper, cashews, light miso, lemon juice, nutmeg, and water. Blend on high speed for 3 to 5 minutes or until mixture is smooth and the consistency of sour cream.

3. Transfer mixture into a bowl, and stir in chopped chives. Cover with plastic wrap, and refrigerate until ready to serve.

4. Cut salmon fillet into 8 (3-ounce) portions (about the size of a deck of cards). Brush with extra-virgin olive oil, and sprinkle with salt and pepper.

5. Grill salmon for about 3 minutes on each side or until salmon reaches an internal temperature of 140°F.

6. Serve topped with crème fraîche.

def•i•ni•tion

Miso is a traditional Japanese food typically produced by fermenting soybeans. It's very salty, so use it sparingly. It can be found in plastic containers or jars in the refrigerator section of the grocery store. **Crème fraîche** is a thinner, French version of American sour cream.

Honey-Soy-Glazed Salmon

This honey and soy–glazed salmon is accentuated with fresh garlic and ginger.

2 whole scallions, sliced

3 TB. low-sodium soy sauce

2 TB. rice vinegar

2 TB. honey

2 cloves garlic, minced

2 tsp. fresh ginger, peeled and minced

8 (3-oz.) salmon fillets (about 1½ lb.)

2 tsp. sesame seeds, toasted

Yield: 8 servings
Prep time: 20 minutes
Cook time: 6 to 10 minutes
Serving size: 1 fillet
Each serving has:
144 calories
4 g carbohydrate
4 g sugars
17 g protein
6 g fat
1 g saturated fat
47 g cholesterol
375 mg sodium
0 g fiber
205 IU vitamin D
423 mg potassium
18 mg calcium
31 mcg selenium

1. In a medium bowl, whisk scallions, soy sauce, vinegar, honey, garlic, and ginger until honey is incorporated.

2. Place salmon in a zipper-lock bag. Add ¼ cup sauce, and let marinate in the refrigerator for 15 minutes. Reserve remaining sauce.

3. Preheat the broiler to low. Line a small baking pan with aluminum foil, and lightly coat with cooking spray.

4. Remove salmon from marinade, and add to the pan, skinned side down. Discard marinade. Broil salmon 4 to 6 inches from the heat source for 6 to 10 minutes or until cooked through. Drizzle with reserved sauce, garnish with sesame seeds, and serve.

 Food for Thought

Ginger causes the increased production of saliva, which helps relieve stomach aches, indigestion, and stomach cramping.

Grilled Tuna Steak Salad with Cucumber-Mint Yogurt Sauce

This grilled lemon-pepper tuna salad is both healthy and delicious and finished with a fresh cucumber-mint yogurt sauce.

Yield: 8 servings
Prep time: 10 minutes
Cook time: 34 minutes
Serving size: ½ pita about ¼ cup tuna salad
Each serving has:
280 calories
20 g carbohydrate
2 g sugars
30 g protein
8 g fat
2 g saturated fat
43 g cholesterol
207 mg sodium
1.5 g fiber
0 IU vitamin D
350 mg potassium
59 mg calcium
50 mcg selenium

8 (4-oz.) tuna steaks

4 TB. fresh lemon juice

4 tsp. extra-virgin olive oil

2 tsp. freshly cracked black pepper

2 medium cucumbers, peeled, seeded, and sliced

1⅓ cup plain Greek yogurt

3 TB. fresh mint, chopped

2 tsp. garlic, mashed

4 (6½-in.) whole-wheat pitas

2 cups *arugula*

2 lemons, cut into 8 wedges

1. Preheat the grill to medium.

2. Brush tuna with lemon juice and olive oil, and sprinkle with black pepper. Grill tuna for 4 minutes or until cooked through, being careful not to overcook it. Chill in refrigerator for at least 10 minutes.

3. In a blender, combine cucumbers, Greek yogurt, mint, and garlic.

4. In a medium bowl, flake tuna with a fork, and combine with blended yogurt sauce.

5. Slice pitas in ½, fill each with ¼ cup arugula, and evenly distribute tuna salad. Serve immediately with lemon wedges for garnish.

def•i•ni•tion

Arugula is a small leafy green that has a peppery-mustard taste. It's a delicious green to add to any salad, pizza, etc.

Shrimp Scampi

Yummy garlic shrimp.

2½ lb. (21 to 25 count, about 24) shrimp, peeled and deveined

1½ TB. olive oil

4 cloves garlic, minced

¼ tsp. kosher salt

¼ tsp. freshly cracked black pepper

2 tsp. Old Bay Seasoning

4 TB. fresh lemon juice

4 TB. chopped fresh parsley

8 lemon wedges

4 TB. chopped fresh chives

Yield: 8 servings
Prep time: 15 minutes
Cook time: 3 or 4 minutes
Serving size: about 3 shrimp
Each serving has:
178 calories
2 g carbohydrate
0 g sugars
29 g protein
5 g fat
1 g saturated fat
215 g cholesterol
283 mg sodium
0 g fiber
215 IU vitamin D
272 mg potassium
74 mg calcium
54 mcg selenium

1. Preheat the broiler to low. Position the rack 4 inches from the heat source.

2. Place shrimp on a large, rimmed baking sheet. Drizzle with olive oil; sprinkle with garlic; season with salt, pepper, and Old Bay Seasoning; and toss to coat. Rearrange in a single layer. Broil for 3 or 4 minutes or until opaque throughout.

3. Sprinkle with lemon juice and parsley, and toss to combine. Serve immediately, garnished with lemon wedges and chives.

Cooking Tip

Here's a simple test to see if shrimp is cooked through: when the head touches the tail, it's done.

Baked Shrimp with Crab and Spinach Stuffing

One taste of these shrimp stuffed with lump crabmeat and steamed spinach will transport you to the eastern shore.

Yield: 8 servings
Prep time: 10 minutes
Cook time: 20 minutes
Serving size: about 2 shrimp
Each serving has:
189 calories
20 g carbohydrate
2 g sugars
18 g protein
3 g fat
.7 g saturated fat
102 g cholesterol
378 mg sodium
1 g fiber
45 IU vitamin D
275 mg potassium
115 mg calcium
36 mcg selenium

3 lb. (21 to 25 count, about 32) shrimp, peeled and deveined

¼ cup spinach, steamed

2 cups whole-wheat breadcrumbs

2 tsp. butter, melted

½ tsp. salt

½ tsp. freshly cracked black pepper

3 TB. dry white wine

1 large egg

2 (6-oz.) cans lump blue crabmeat

1. Preheat the oven to 400°F. Lightly coat a cookie sheet with cooking spray.

3. Slice shrimp on the inside of the curve halfway through meat. Set aside.

4. Press spinach to extract as much liquid as possible. Add spinach to a large bowl along with breadcrumbs, butter, salt, pepper, white wine, and egg, and mix well. (If stuffing seems too wet, cut back on the amount of wine and/or adjust the amount of breadcrumbs used.)

5. Lightly fold in crabmeat so lumps of crabmeat stay intact.

6. Roll stuffing into ½-inch balls, and mold shrimp around it so shrimp sits flat on the cookie sheet and tail is resting on top. Bake for about 20 minutes, and serve immediately.

Cooking Tip

Cut down on the saturated fat in this recipe by using spray butter or a vegetable oil instead of the spreadable butter.

Broiled Scallops with Sweet Lime Glaze

Here, delicious sea scallops are tossed in a sweet and tangy lime glaze and broiled until golden brown.

4 TB. honey

1 tsp. Splenda

4 TB. fresh lime juice

1 TB. water

1½ TB. olive oil

1½ lb. (about 18) *sea scallops*

4 tsp. lime zest

2 fresh limes, cut into 8 wedges

Yield: 8 servings
Prep time: 15 minutes
Cook time: 6 minutes
Serving size: about 3 scallops
Each serving has:
132 calories
11 g carbohydrate
8 g sugars
14 g protein
3 g fat
.4 g saturated fat
28 g cholesterol
138 mg sodium
0 g fiber
0 IU vitamin D
258 mg potassium
22 mg calcium
19 mcg selenium

1. Preheat the broiler to low. Position the rack 4 inches from the heat source. Cover a broiler pan or cookie sheet with aluminum foil, and spray generously with cooking spray.

2. In a large bowl, whisk together honey, Splenda, lime juice, water, and olive oil. Add scallops, and toss gently to coat.

3. Arrange scallops in a single layer on the prepared broiler pan or baking sheet. Broil for about 5 minutes or until opaque throughout when tested with a tip of a knife. Turn over scallops, and broil for 1 more minute.

4. Divide scallops among 8 warmed plates. Pour any juices from the broiler pan or baking sheet over scallops. Sprinkle with lime zest, and serve with 1 lime wedge.

def•i•ni•tion

Sea scallops are the larger scallops while **bay scallops** are tiny. Bay scallops are slightly sweeter than sea scallops.

Seafood Risotto

Here, a medley of seafood swims in a creamy Arborio rice risotto.

Yield: 8 servings
Prep time: 15 minutes
Cook time: 90 minutes
Serving size: ½ cup
Each serving has:
347 calories
42 g carbohydrate
1.5 g sugars
26 g protein
7 g fat
1 g saturated fat
70 g cholesterol
612 mg sodium
2 g fiber
18 IU vitamin D
506 mg potassium
52 mg calcium
32 mcg selenium

2⅔ cups canned clam liquid

6⅔ cups water

2 (6.5-oz.) cans chopped clams, liquid reserved

2 small Vidalia onions, diced (about 1½ cups)

3 TB. extra-virgin olive oil

2⅔ cups Arborio rice

1 cup white wine

½ lb. (31 to 40 count, about 18) medium shrimp, peeled and deveined

1 lb. bay scallops

¾ tsp. saffron

1 tsp. freshly cracked black pepper

1 lb. fresh haddock

1¼ tsp. chopped fresh basil

1. In a medium saucepan over high heat, heat canned clam juice, water, and clam juice reserved from canned chopped clams.

2. In a medium sauté pan over medium-high heat, sauté onions with olive oil for 10 minutes or until translucent.

3. Add rice and white wine to sauté pan with onions. Cook, continuously stirring, for 15 to 20 minutes or until liquid is almost gone. Ladle more liquid from the saucepan into rice. Continue until liquid is gone.

4. When approximately 2 cups liquid remain, add shrimp, scallops, chopped clams, saffron, and black pepper to saucepan with rice. Gently stir in cooked haddock, and cook until remaining liquid is absorbed.

5. Final product should be creamy and Arborio rice should be cooked fully. If more liquid is needed, add more wine, water, or clam juice. (The whole process should take about 30 to 45 minutes.) Serve immediately.

Cooking Tip

The haddock in this recipe is added cooked. You can cook the haddock ahead of time in the oven, steam it, or simply cut it into bite-size pieces and add it raw a little earlier in the cooking process (step 3).

Vegetarian Delights

In This Chapter

- ◆ Asian-inspired vegetable and tofu dishes
- ◆ Rice, pasta, and lentil recipes
- ◆ Tasty vegetarian sandwiches

Part of eating well, after weight loss surgery or not, is eating your daily requirement of vegetables. In this chapter, we offer over a dozen great vegetarian dishes that make it easy to eat your veggies.

Vegetables provide your body with a number of vitamins and minerals it cannot live without. They also supply phytochemicals that help protect your body from cancer-causing free radicals.

And whether you're a vegetarian or not, it never hurts to include a combination of nuts, seeds, grains, legumes, and vegetables at every meal.

Vegetarian Stir-Fry

This delicious and healthful vegetarian stir-fry features a medley of fresh vegetables, tofu, fresh garlic, and soy sauce.

Yield: 8 servings
Prep time: 15 minutes
Cook time: 30 minutes
Serving size: ½ cup
Each serving has:
90 calories
8 g carbohydrate
.6 g sugars
7 g protein
3 g fat
0 g saturated fat
0 g cholesterol
478 mg sodium
2 g fiber
86 IU vitamin D
134 mg potassium
234 mg calcium
2 mcg selenium

1 TB. vegetable oil

1 (14-oz.) pkg. extra-firm tofu, cut into ½-in. cubes

1 small Vidalia onion, diced (about ½ cup)

1 TB. ginger, freshly grated

2 cloves garlic, minced

1 cup broccoli, chopped into ¼-in. florets

½ cup sliced water chestnuts

1 can baby corn cobs, rinsed and drained

½ cup bean sprouts

½ cup sliced shiitake mushrooms

1 cup snow peas

¼ cup water

¼ cup low-sodium soy sauce

1. In a medium saucepan over high heat, heat vegetable oil. Add tofu, and cook for 10 minutes or until golden brown on all sides. Remove tofu from the pan, and set aside.

2. Add onion, ginger, garlic, broccoli, water chestnuts, baby corn, bean sprouts, mushrooms, and snow peas to the pan, and sauté for about 5 minutes or until vegetables start to get some golden-brown color.

3. Add water and soy sauce to the pan, and cook for 10 to 15 minutes or until vegetables are tender. Add tofu back to the pot before serving.

Cooking Tip

When you sear tofu, be sure the pan is really hot or the tofu will stick to it. Also, it's easier to use a metal or hard plastic spatula to move the tofu around in the pan (scrape the bottom of the pan with the spatula) because the tofu tends to crumble if you use a spoon.

Asian-Inspired Baked Tofu and Bok Choy

Tasty and healthful baked tofu marinated in soy and sesame oil pairs with steamed bok choy.

1½ (14-oz.) pkg. firm tofu

4 TB. low-sodium soy sauce

4 TB. rice vinegar

2 TB. low-fat, low-sodium vegetable broth

2 TB. brown sugar Splenda

2 tsp. Dijon mustard

1 tsp. garlic chili sauce

2 cloves garlic, minced

4 heads bok choy, bottom nub removed, and cut in ½ lengthwise

1 medium carrot, peeled and sliced into matchsticks

2 tsp. sesame oil

¼ tsp. kosher salt

½ tsp. freshly cracked black pepper

2 TB. whole scallions, chopped

1 TB. sesame seeds

Yield: 8 servings		
Prep time: 15 minutes		
Cook time: 33 minutes		
Serving size: 2 tofu triangles and ½ bok choy		
Each serving has:		
133 calories		
13 g carbohydrate		
5 g sugars		
14 g protein		
4 g fat		
0 g saturated fat		
0 g cholesterol		
856 mg sodium		
6 g fiber		
129 IU vitamin D		
1,078 mg potassium		
770 mg calcium		
2 mcg selenium		

1. Preheat the oven to 450°F.

2. Cut tofu lengthwise into 4 slices. Cut each slice into 2 triangles. Place tofu triangles on a plate, and cover with plastic wrap. Top with a second plate and a heavy weight, and let stand for 10 minutes.

3. In a small bowl, whisk together soy sauce, vinegar, vegetable broth, brown sugar Splenda, Dijon mustard, garlic chili sauce, and garlic. Spread ⅓ of mixture in an oblong baking dish.

4. Drain tofu, arrange triangles in the dish, and top with remaining soy sauce mixture. Bake for 10 to 15 minutes or until heated through.

5. Meanwhile, in a large pot fitted with a steamer basket over high heat, bring 1 inch water to a boil. Add bok choy and carrot, cover, and steam for 6 to 8 minutes or until vegetables are tender. Transfer to a plate, drizzle with sesame oil, and sprinkle with salt.

6. Arrange ½ bok choy and 2 tofu triangles on each plate, and serve garnished with scallions and sesame seeds.

 Food for Thought

Sesame oil has a really intense flavor and aroma. It's a great addition to many dishes, but use it sparingly because a little goes a long way.

Kung Pao Tofu

Here's our version of the classic Kung Pao with tofu, peanuts, broccoli florets, and bell peppers—and without the extra fat and calories.

Yield: *8 servings*
Prep time: 10 minutes
Cook time: 14 minutes
Serving size: ½ cup
Each serving has:
146 calories
13 g carbohydrate
2 g sugars
12 g protein
6 g fat
0 g saturated fat
0 g cholesterol
502 mg sodium
4 g fiber
151 IU vitamin D
278 mg potassium
427 mg calcium
1 mcg selenium

2 (14-oz.) pkg. extra-firm tofu

1 tsp. Chinese five-spice powder

1 TB. canola oil

1 cup water

¼ cup low-sodium soy sauce

1 tsp. cornstarch

7 cups broccoli florets

1½ cups bean sprouts

2 small yellow bell peppers, ribs and seeds removed, and diced

2 small red bell peppers, ribs and seeds removed, and diced

2 TB. freshly grated ginger

2 TB. garlic, minced

2 TB. unsalted peanuts

2 TB. whole scallions, chopped

1. Using a paper towel, pat tofu dry and cut into ½-inch cubes. Place in a medium bowl, add ½ teaspoon Chinese five-spice powder, and gently stir to coat.

2. In a large, nonstick skillet over medium-high heat, heat canola oil. Add tofu and cook, stirring every 1 or 2 minutes, for 7 to 9 minutes total or until tofu is golden brown. Transfer to a plate.

3. Meanwhile, in a small bowl, whisk together water, soy sauce, cornstarch, and remaining ½ teaspoon Chinese five-spice powder.

4. Add broccoli, bean sprouts, yellow bell peppers, and red bell peppers to the skillet, and cook, stirring occasionally, for about 4 minutes or until vegetables begin to soften. Add ginger and garlic, and cook, stirring, for about 30 seconds or until fragrant. Reduce heat to low, add soy sauce-cornstarch mixture, and cook, stirring, for about 30 more seconds or until thickened.

5. Return tofu to the pan along with peanuts and scallions, and stir to coat with sauce. Serve as is or over steamed rice.

 Food for Thought

Kung Pao Chicken, on which this dish is based, originated in Schezuan, China. The dish has since been westernized and usually includes chicken or seafood, mixed vegetables, and peanuts.

Vegetarian Paella

This heart-healthy *paella* is full of delicious herbs, vegetables, and rice flavored with a hint of saffron.

3 TB. extra-virgin olive oil

2 medium Vidalia onions, diced

4 cloves garlic, minced

2 small green bell peppers, ribs and seeds removed, and diced

1 small red bell pepper, ribs and seeds removed, and diced

1 small yellow bell pepper, ribs and seeds removed, and diced

4 small vine ripe tomatoes, diced (about 2 cups)

7 cups low-fat, low-sodium vegetable broth

3 cups brown rice

2 tsp. saffron

1 tsp. dried thyme

1 cup water

2 cups broccoli florets

3 cups frozen green peas, thawed

3 TB. chopped fresh parsley

2 TB. chopped fresh basil

½ tsp. kosher salt

¼ tsp. freshly cracked black pepper

Yield: 8 servings
Prep time: 15 minutes
Cook time: 35 minutes
Serving size: ¾ cup
Each serving has:
309 calories
54 g carbohydrate
8 g sugars
8 g protein
7 g fat
1 g saturated fat
0 g cholesterol
365 mg sodium
8 g fiber
0 IU vitamin D
334 mg potassium
50 mg calcium
16 mcg selenium

1. In an extra-wide skillet or stir-fry pan over medium heat, heat olive oil. Add onions and garlic, and sauté for about 5 minutes or until vegetables are translucent.

2. Add green bell peppers, red bell pepper, and yellow bell pepper, and sauté, stirring frequently, for 5 minutes.

3. Add tomatoes, vegetable broth, rice, saffron, thyme, and water. Bring to a simmer, cover, and continue to simmer gently for 15 minutes.

4. Stir in broccoli, peas, and ½ of parsley and basil. Cook for about 3 minutes or until broccoli is cooked through, and season with salt and pepper.

5. Transfer to a large, shallow serving container, or serve straight from the pan. Garnish with remaining parsley and basil.

def•i•ni•tion

Paella is a traditional rice dish that originated in Valencia, Spain, that's usually topped with all sorts of different meats such as seafood and chicken. It has since grown in popularity and is now a staple dish served all over Spain and the world.

Roasted Tomato and Crimini Barley Risotto

Creamy crimini mushroom and roasted tomato risotto pairs with sweet shallots, fresh herbs, and Parmesan cheese.

Yield: 8 servings
Prep time: 15 minutes
Cook time: 1 hour, 26 minutes
Serving size: ½ cup
Each serving has:
270 calories
48 g carbohydrate
4 g sugars
8 g protein
6 g fat
1.5 g saturated fat
4 g cholesterol
545 mg sodium
1 g fiber
9 IU vitamin D
427 mg potassium
105 mg calcium
25 mcg selenium

10 large plum tomatoes, cut in ½

2 TB. extra-virgin olive oil

1 tsp. kosher salt

½ tsp. freshly cracked black pepper

4 cups low-fat, low-sodium vegetable broth

3 cups water

1 pt. crimini mushrooms, quartered

2 shallots, minced

½ cup white wine (optional)

2 cups pearl barley

3 TB. chopped fresh basil

3 TB. chopped fresh parsley

1½ TB. chopped fresh thyme

1 TB. chopped fresh oregano

½ cup grated Parmesan cheese, plus more for garnish

2 TB. silken tofu, puréed

8 whole basil leaves for garnish

1. Preheat the oven to 350°F.

2. Arrange tomatoes in a single layer on a nonstick baking sheet. Drizzle with 1 tablespoon olive oil, and sprinkle with ¼ teaspoon salt and ¼ teaspoon pepper. Toss gently to mix, and rearrange into a single layer. Roast for 25 to 30 minutes or until tomatoes are softened and beginning to brown. Set aside 16 tomato pieces to use for garnish.

3. Meanwhile, in a saucepan over high heat, bring vegetable broth, water, and mushrooms to a boil. Reduce heat to low, and keep at a simmer.

4. In a large, heavy saucepan over medium heat, heat remaining 1 tablespoon olive oil. Add shallots, and sauté for 2 or 3 minutes or until shallots are soft and translucent.

5. Stir in white wine (if using), and cook for 2 or 3 minutes or until most of wine evaporates. Stir in barley, and cook, stirring, for 1 minute. Stir in ½ cup stock mixture, and cook, stirring occasionally, for 5 to 10 minutes or until liquid is completely absorbed.

6. Continue stirring in stock mixture in ½ cup increments, cooking each time until liquid is absorbed before adding more, for 45 to 50 minutes total or until barley is tender. Remove from heat and fold in remaining tomatoes, basil, parsley, thyme, oregano, and Parmesan cheese.

7. Add remaining ¾ teaspoon salt and ¼ teaspoon pepper, and stir to combine.

8. Add puréed tofu and combine.

9. Garnish with reserved roasted tomato wedges, basil leaves, and Parmesan cheese.

Cooking Tip

When making risotto, it's important to add the liquid in equal amounts and stir before adding more liquid. The stirring and the slow additions of liquid help bring out the starches in the barley or rice, and that's what makes the end product so creamy.

Curried Rice, Lentils, and Mixed Veggies

This curried dish with hearty lentils, carrots, snow peas, and broccoli is sure to satisfy your love of Indian cuisine.

Yield: 8 servings
Prep time: 10 minutes
Cook time: 4 or 5 hours
Serving size: ½ cup
Each serving has:
341 calories
71 g carbohydrate
7 g sugars
17 g protein
1.3 g fat
.2 g saturated fat
0 g cholesterol
371 mg sodium
10 g fiber
0 IU vitamin D
1,114 mg potassium
17 mg calcium
9 mcg selenium

2 cups long-grain brown rice

2 TB. curry powder

6½ cups low-fat, low-sodium vegetable broth

½ cup lentils

4 cloves garlic, minced

½ tsp. freshly cracked black pepper

2 medium Vidalia onions, diced

2 small carrots, peeled and sliced into rounds

1 cup whole snow peas

1 cup broccoli florets

1. In a 2½-quart slow cooker, combine rice, curry powder, vegetable broth, lentils, garlic, black pepper, onions, and carrots. Cook on low for 4 or 5 hours.

2. During the last 15 minutes, add snow peas and broccoli, and stir to combine. Serve immediately.

 Food for Thought

> Curry is not one spice, but a combination of spices such as turmeric, cumin, red pepper, and many others.

Roasted Vegetable and Tofu Bowtie Pasta

Oven-roasted vegetables with baked tofu and whole-wheat bowtie pasta mingle with olive oil and fresh herbs.

1 medium eggplant, diced

2 small yellow squash, diced

½ large red onion, diced

2 carrots, peeled and diced

8 button mushrooms, quartered

3 TB. extra-virgin olive oil

1 tsp. chopped fresh oregano

1 tsp. chopped fresh basil

1 tsp. fresh thyme

½ tsp. kosher salt

½ tsp. freshly cracked black pepper

1 (14-oz.) pkg. extra-firm tofu, diced

1¾ cups whole-wheat bowtie pasta

Yield: 8 servings
Prep time: 10 minutes
Cook time: 30 minutes
Serving size: ¾ cup
Each serving has:
302 calories
46 g carbohydrate
5 g sugars
13 g protein
8 g fat
1 g saturated fat
0 g cholesterol
256 mg sodium
5 g fiber
76 IU vitamin D
377 mg potassium
215 mg calcium
.4 mcg selenium

1. Preheat the oven to 400°F.

2. In a large bowl, combine eggplant, squash, onion, carrots, mushrooms, and tofu. Drizzle with olive oil, and toss to coat. Add oregano, basil, thyme, salt, and pepper, and toss again until well coated.

3. Pour vegetables and tofu into a casserole or baking dish, cover with aluminum foil, and bake for 20 to 30 minutes or until vegetables and tofu begin to brown.

4. Meanwhile, fill a large pot with water and bring to a boil over high heat. Add pasta and cook according to the package directions. Drain cooked pasta, and place in a large mixing bowl.

5. Add cooked vegetables to pasta, and toss until well combined. Serve immediately.

Food for Thought

More than 20 different varieties of onions are grown throughout the world. The more common ones are Spanish onions, red onions, and Vidalia onions.

Vegetarian Lasagna

This hearty vegetarian lasagna is layered with eggplant, zucchini, squash, tomato sauce, and mozzarella cheese.

Yield: 8 servings	
Prep time: 30 minutes	
Cook time: 30 minutes	
Serving size: ½ cup	
Each serving has:	
203 calories	
18 g carbohydrate	
10 g sugars	
15 g protein	
9 g fat	
6 g saturated fat	
38 g cholesterol	
637 mg sodium	
5 g fiber	
2 IU vitamin D	
331 mg potassium	
34 mg calcium	
7 mcg selenium	

2 cups broccoli florets

1 small Vidalia onion, chopped (about 1 cup)

1 (15.4-oz.) can low-sodium tomato sauce

1 (15.4-oz.) can low-sodium diced tomatoes, drained

1 small red bell pepper, ribs and seeds removed, and diced (about 1 cup)

2 TB. liquid egg substitute

2 cloves garlic, minced

1½ tsp. chopped fresh basil

1 medium eggplant

2 medium squash

2 medium zucchini

2 cups crumbled feta cheese

¼ cup grated Parmesan cheese

1 cup low-fat shredded mozzarella cheese

1. Preheat the oven to 350°F. Lightly coat a 13×9×2-inch baking dish with cooking spray.

2. In a large bowl, combine broccoli, onion, tomato sauce, canned tomatoes, bell pepper, egg substitute, garlic, and basil. Set aside.

3. Slice eggplant, squash, and zucchini length-wise into ⅛-inch lasagna-noodle slices. Set aside.

4. In a medium bowl, combine feta cheese, Parmesan cheese, and mozzarella cheese.

5. In the prepared baking dish, begin layering, starting with sauce, followed by cheese, alternating with squashes and eggplant slices, and ending with cheese on top.

6. Bake for approximately 30 minutes. Let stand at room temperature 5 minutes before serving.

Cooking Tip

When picking out an eggplant, choose one with tight skin and that has a bright color. Eggplants are pretty mild in flavor and tend to take on the flavor of whatever they cook with. They can be used with or without the skin, and their seeds are entirely edible.

Open-Faced Vegetarian Sloppy Joes

Kids of all ages will love these delicious tofu sloppy joes flavored with a sweet chili tomato sauce.

2 (14-oz.) pkg. firm tofu

1 TB. extra-virgin olive oil

1 large Vidalia onion, *minced*

1 medium green bell pepper, ribs and seeds removed, and diced (1 cup)

3 TB. water

8 TB. ketchup

7 TB. chili sauce

1 tsp. kosher salt

¼ tsp. freshly cracked black pepper

8 slices whole-wheat bread, lightly toasted

Yield: 8 servings
Prep time: 5 minutes
Cook time: 26 minutes
Serving size: ¼ cup plus 1 slice toast
Each serving has:
217 calories
28 g carbohydrate
10 g sugars
15 g protein
6 g fat
.5 g saturated fat
0 g cholesterol
7,662 mg sodium
4 g fiber
172 IU vitamin D
156 mg potassium
468 mg calcium
11 mcg selenium

1. In a medium bowl, and using a fork, mash tofu until a consistency similar to ground beef is reached. Set aside.

2. In a large skillet over medium heat, heat olive oil. Add onion and green bell pepper, and sauté for 5 to 7 minutes or until vegetables are well cooked. Add water.

3. Add tofu and sauté for 15 minutes or until tofu is hot.

4. Add ketchup, chili sauce, salt, and pepper; reduce heat to low, and continue to cook for about 4 minutes or until heated through.

5. Spoon ¼ cup tofu mixture onto each slice of whole-wheat toast, and serve.

def•i•ni•tion

Mincing is just a fancy cooking term for chopping something very fine.

Grilled Veggie Sandwiches with Lemon-Chive Dijonaise

A light lemon and chive dijonaise sauce tops fresh, char-grilled vegetables in these healthful sandwiches.

Yield: *8 servings*
Prep time: 10 minutes
Cook time: 10 minutes
Serving size: 1 sandwich
Each serving has:
98 calories
14 g carbohydrate
4 g sugars
5 g protein
2 g fat
1 g saturated fat
5 g cholesterol
242 mg sodium
2 g fiber
0 IU vitamin D
125 mg potassium
69 mg calcium
12 mcg selenium

¼ cup plain Greek yogurt

5 cloves garlic, minced

3 TB. chopped fresh chives

2 TB. Dijon mustard

1 TB. fresh lemon juice

2 medium red bell peppers, ribs and seeds removed, and sliced (2 cups)

2 small zucchini, sliced into ¼-in. rounds

2 small red onions, sliced into rings (don't separate rings)

1 small yellow squash, sliced into ¼-in. rounds

1 TB. extra-virgin olive oil

8 thin slices whole-wheat bread

¼ cup crumbled feta cheese

1. In a bowl, mix Greek yogurt, garlic, chives, Dijon mustard, and lemon juice. Set aside, covered, in the refrigerator until needed.

2. Preheat the grill to high. Spray the grate with cooking spray.

3. Brush both sides of bell pepper, zucchini, onions, and squash slices with olive oil. Place bell peppers and zucchini in the middle of the grill, and arrange onion and squash slices around them. Cook for about 3 minutes on each side. Bell peppers may take longer. Remove from the grill, and set aside.

4. Spread some yogurt-Dijon mixture on each slice of bread, and sprinkle with feta cheese. Place on the grill cheese side up, cover, and grill for 2 or 3 minutes or until bread is warm and cheese is slightly melted. Watch carefully so bottoms don't burn.

5. Remove bread from the grill, layer with grilled vegetables, and serve.

Cooking Tip

Adding a little vinegar, salt, and pepper to the dijonaise in this recipe turns it into a delicious creamy mustard salad dressing.

Grilled Portobello "Steaks" with Crumbled Feta Cheese

These juicy portobello burgers are char-grilled, seasoned with hints of lemon, and topped with creamy feta cheese.

¼ cup extra-virgin olive oil

¼ cup low-fat, low-sodium vegetable broth

1 TB. fresh lemon juice

1 tsp. Mrs. Dash Lemon Pepper

½ tsp. kosher salt

4 cloves garlic, minced

8 large portobello mushrooms, stems removed and brushed clean

¼ tsp. freshly cracked black pepper

¼ cup crumbled feta cheese

Yield: 8 servings
Prep time: 35 minutes
Cook time: 8 minutes
Serving size: 1 portobello mushroom cap
Each serving has:
81 calories
2 g carbohydrate
.8 g sugars
2 g protein
8 g fat
1.7 g saturated fat
4 g cholesterol
137 mg sodium
.6 g fiber
0 IU vitamin D
145 mg potassium
26 mg calcium
.4 mcg selenium

1. In a large bowl, combine olive oil, vegetable broth, lemon juice, Mrs. Dash Lemon Pepper, kosher salt, and garlic.

2. Add mushroom caps, and submerge in marinade. Cover and marinate for 20 to 30 minutes in the refrigerator.

3. Preheat the grill to medium-high.

4. Remove mushroom caps from marinade, and season with salt and pepper. Discard marinade. Place caps on the grill and cook for 3 or 4 minutes per side or until just tender.

5. Top with feta cheese and serve.

 Food for Thought

What's the difference between a crimini mushroom and a portobello mushroom? Size. When a crimini mushroom reaches about 4 to 6 inches in diameter, it's called a portobello mushroom.

Gnocchi with Spinach and Roasted Tomatoes

Here, hearty potato *gnocchi* teams with fresh spinach and roasted tomatoes and is topped with mozzarella and Parmesan cheeses.

Yield: 8 servings
Prep time: 15 minutes
Cook time: 30 minutes
Serving size: ½ cup
Each serving has:
243 calories
38 g carbohydrate
7 g sugars
13 g protein
4 g fat
1 g saturated fat
8 g cholesterol
520 mg sodium
7 g fiber
9 IU vitamin D
129 mg potassium
218 mg calcium
.4 mcg selenium

1 TB. plus 1 tsp. extra-virgin olive oil

1 (16-oz.) pkg. gnocchi

1 medium Vidalia onion, chopped

4 cloves garlic, minced

½ cup water

6 cups fresh baby spinach

1 (15-oz.) can low-sodium roasted tomatoes, drained

1 TB. Mrs. Dash Italian Seasoning

1 (15-oz.) can white beans, rinsed and drained

2 TB. silken tofu, puréed

¼ tsp. freshly cracked black pepper

½ cup reduced-fat shredded mozzarella cheese

¼ cup grated Parmesan cheese

1. In a large, nonstick skillet over medium heat, heat 1 tablespoon olive oil. Add gnocchi and cook, stirring often, for 5 to 7 minutes or until gnocchi is plumped and starting to brown. Transfer to a bowl and set aside.

2. Add remaining 1 teaspoon oil to the skillet. Add onion and cook, stirring, for 2 minutes. Stir in garlic and water. Cover and cook for 4 to 6 minutes or until onion is soft.

3. Add spinach and cook, stirring, for 1 or 2 minutes or until spinach starts to wilt. Stir in tomatoes, beans, tofu purée, and pepper, and bring to a simmer. Stir in gnocchi and sprinkle with mozzarella and Parmesan cheeses.

4. Cover and cook for about 3 minutes or until cheese is melted and sauce is bubbling. Serve immediately.

def•i•ni•tion

Gnocchi are Italian dumplings. They are a great substitute for pasta in many Italian dishes.

Chapter 20

Surprising Sides

In This Chapter

- ◆ Scrumptious slaws
- ◆ Versatile veggies
- ◆ Polenta, legumes, and more!

Side dishes often play second fiddle to the main course, but that doesn't have to be so! In this chapter, you'll find many quick and easy side dish recipes to complement any number of entrées—or build a meal all on their own. You can easily mix and match any of these delightful sides to create your perfect meal.

What's more, all the recipes in this chapter are healthful, good-for-you sides. If you're looking for delicious, nutritious dishes to serve to friends, family, or simply just enjoy, you've come to the right place.

Apple-Fennel Slaw

This sweet apple and fennel slaw features dried cranberries, apple juice, and a subtle taste of anise. *(Adapted from www.mayoclinic.com.)*

Yield: 8 servings	

Prep time: 2 hours, 25 minutes

Cook time: 10 minutes

Serving size: ¼ cup

Each serving has:

102 calories

18 g carbohydrate

10 g sugars

1 g protein

4 g fat

.5 g saturated fat

0 g cholesterol

50 mg sodium

4 g fiber

0 IU vitamin D

391 mg potassium

41 mg calcium

.4 mcg selenium

2 medium fennel bulbs, thinly sliced

2 large Granny Smith apples, cored and thinly sliced

4 medium carrots, peeled and grated

4 TB. unsweetened dried cranberries

2 TB. extra-virgin olive oil

2 tsp. Splenda

¼ cup apple juice

4 TB. apple cider vinegar

¼ tsp. kosher salt

¼ tsp. freshly cracked black pepper

8 lettuce leaves

1. In a large bowl, combine fennel, apples, carrots, and cranberries. Drizzle olive oil over top, cover, and refrigerate for 15 minutes.

2. In a small saucepan over medium heat, mix together Splenda and apple juice. Cook for about 10 minutes or until reduced to about ⅛ cup. Remove from heat and cool. Stir in cider vinegar.

3. Pour apple juice mixture over fennel-apple slaw, and stir to combine well. Chill for about 2 hours. Serve spooned over lettuce leaves.

Cooking Tip

When using whole fennel, cut the bulb and use it in the dish, and chop the leaves for a nice garnish.

Jicama Slaw

Serve this light, crisp, and sweet jicama slaw as a side to sandwiches or grilled chicken.

1 lb. *jicama*, peeled and shredded

1 large carrot, peeled and shredded

¼ cup red cabbage, shredded

4 TB. fresh lime juice

2 TB. low-fat mayonnaise

1 TB. fresh cilantro, chopped

1 tsp. ground cumin

½ tsp. celery seeds

½ tsp. hot pepper sauce

1 TB. honey

¼ tsp. kosher salt

¼ tsp. freshly cracked black pepper

Yield: 8 servings
Prep time: 1 hour, 20 minutes
Serving size: ¼ cup
Each serving has:
47 calories
9 g carbohydrate
4 g sugars
1 g protein
1 g fat
0 g saturated fat
0 g cholesterol
40 mg sodium
3 g fiber
0 IU vitamin D
129 mg potassium
12 mg calcium
.4 mcg selenium

1. In a large bowl, combine jicama, carrot, cabbage, lime juice, mayonnaise, cilantro, cumin, celery seeds, hot pepper sauce, honey, salt, and pepper.

2. Refrigerate, covered, for 1 hour, stir, and serve.

def•i•ni•tion

Jicama is a member of the legume family but resembles a turnip. It has the texture of a water chestnut and is commonly used in many marinated salads and stir-fries.

Calabacitas

Here, light and healthy zucchini, squash, and pepper ragouts meld with fresh garlic and poblano peppers.

Yield: 8 servings
Prep time: 10 minutes
Cook time: 7 minutes
Serving size: ¼ cup
Each serving has:
56 calories
9 g carbohydrate
3.5 g sugars
2 g protein
2 g fat
.3 g saturated fat
0 g cholesterol
157 mg sodium
2.5 g fiber
0 IU vitamin D
366 mg potassium
23 mg calcium
.5 mcg selenium

1 TB. extra-virgin olive oil

2 small red onions, diced

2 cloves garlic, peeled and minced

1½ poblano peppers, diced

2½ cups zucchini, diced

2½ cups yellow squash, diced

1 red bell pepper, ribs and seeds removed, and diced

½ tsp. kosher salt

2 TB. fresh cilantro, chopped

1. In a large, nonstick skillet over medium heat, heat olive oil. Add onions, garlic, and poblano peppers, and cook, stirring, for about 4 minutes or until vegetables are soft.

2. Add zucchini, squash, red bell pepper, and salt. Cover and cook, stirring once or twice, for about 3 minutes or until vegetables are tender.

3. Remove from heat and stir in cilantro. Serve immediately.

def•i•ni•tion

Calabacita has a number of different meanings, all of which include zucchini. Some definitions state that it's a type of zucchini, and others claim it's a dish made from sautéed pork, zucchini, and squash. In this case, we're going for the sauté of zucchini and squash minus the pork.

Marinated Roasted Red Peppers with Feta Cheese

Here, roasted red peppers marinate in fresh garlic, salt, and pepper alongside delicious basil and feta cheese.

¼ **cup crumbled feta cheese**

4 roasted red peppers, cut in ½ and then into strips

2 cloves garlic, peeled and chopped

1 TB. fresh lemon juice

2 TB. extra-virgin olive oil

¼ **tsp. kosher salt**

½ **tsp. freshly cracked black pepper**

4 TB. fresh basil, chopped

Yield: 8 servings
Prep time: 45 minutes
Serving size: ¼ cup
Each serving has:
51 calories
2 g carbohydrate
1 g sugars
1 g protein
5 g fat
1 g saturated fat
4 g cholesterol
112 mg sodium
.6 g fiber
0 IU vitamin D
5 mg potassium
31 mg calcium
.7 mcg selenium

1. In a medium bowl, combine feta cheese, roasted red peppers, garlic, lemon juice, olive oil, salt, black pepper, and basil.

2. Cover and marinate in the refrigerator for at least 30 minutes. Stir before serving.

Cooking Tip

You can purchase roasted red peppers in your supermarket, but for even better flavor, roast your own peppers over an open flame until all sides are completely black. Leave the charred peppers in a zipper-lock bag until cool enough to handle and then scrape off the charred bits under running water.

Oven-Roasted Brussels Sprouts

Simple and delicious, here yummy fresh brussels sprouts are tossed with fresh garlic, salt, and pepper. *(Adapted from www.allrecipes.com.)*

Yield: 8 servings
Prep time: 10 minutes
Cook time: 50 to 60 minutes
Serving size: ¼ cup
Each serving has:
79 calories
10 g carbohydrate
2.5 g sugars
4 g protein
4 g fat
.5 g saturated fat
0 g cholesterol
319 mg sodium
4 g fiber
0 IU vitamin D
441 mg potassium
48 mg calcium
2 mcg selenium

2 lb. fresh brussels sprouts

2 TB. extra-virgin olive oil

2 cloves garlic, peeled and minced

1 tsp. salt

¾ tsp. freshly cracked black pepper

1. Preheat the oven to 400°F.

2. Trim ends off brussels sprouts, remove any yellow leaves, and cut sprouts in half.

3. Place brussels sprouts, olive oil, garlic, salt, and pepper in a large zipper-lock plastic bag. Seal tightly, and shake to coat. Pour sprouts onto a baking sheet, and place on the center oven rack.

4. Roast for 30 to 45 minutes, shaking pan every 5 to 7 minutes for even browning. Reduce heat if necessary to prevent burning (watch the color on brussels sprouts). Brussels sprouts should be dark brown, almost black, when done.

Cooking Tip

If you're in a hurry, grab some frozen brussels sprouts out of the freezer and toss them in a pan with the olive oil, salt, and pepper. When the sprouts are almost cooked through, add the garlic and finish cooking.

Baked Polenta with Mixed Vegetables and Mozzarella Cheese

Delicious baked polenta is topped with creamy mozzarella cheese, eggplant, bell peppers, and spinach.

2 TB. extra-virgin olive oil

1 medium eggplant, diced

1 small zucchini, finely diced

1 small red bell pepper, ribs and seeds removed, and sliced

1 small yellow bell pepper, ribs and seeds removed, and sliced

½ tsp. kosher salt

½ tsp. freshly cracked black pepper

½ cup water

4 cups baby spinach

2 cups low-sodium marinara sauce

½ cup fresh basil, chopped

14 oz. prepared polenta, sliced lengthwise into 16 thin slices

1½ cups reduced-fat shredded mozzarella

4 whole scallions, chopped

Yield: 8 servings
Prep time: 10 minutes
Cook time: 26 minutes
Serving size: 2 slices topped polenta
Each serving has:
238 calories
34 g carbohydrate
6 g sugars
12 g protein
7 g fat
1 g saturated fat
6 g cholesterol
633 mg sodium
5 g fiber
0 IU vitamin D
209 mg potassium
260 mg calcium
0 mcg selenium

1. Preheat the oven to 450°F. Lightly coat a 9×13-inch baking dish with cooking spray.

2. In a large, nonstick skillet over medium-high heat, heat olive oil. Add eggplant, zucchini, red bell pepper, yellow bell pepper, salt, and pepper, and cook, stirring occasionally, for 4 to 6 minutes or until vegetables are tender and just beginning to brown.

3. Add water and spinach, cover, and cook, stirring once, for about 3 minutes or until spinach is wilted. Stir in marinara sauce and cook for 1 or 2 minutes. Remove from heat and stir in basil.

4. Place polenta slices in a single layer in the prepared baking dish, trimming to fit if necessary. Sprinkle with ¾ cup mozzarella cheese, top with eggplant mixture, and sprinkle with remaining ¾ cup mozzarella cheese. Bake for 12 to 15 minutes or until bubbling and cheese has just melted. Let stand for about 5 minutes.

5. Garnish with chopped scallions, and serve.

 Food for Thought

Polenta is made from ground yellow or white corn, broth, and other flavorings. It's basically a blank canvas that can take on many great flavors.

Mashed Cauliflower

Here, creamy mashed cauliflower combines with rich Parmesan cheese.

Yield: 8 servings
Prep time: 10 minutes
Cook time: 35 minutes
Serving size: ¼ cup
Each serving has:
238 calories
34 g carbohydrate
6 g sugars
12 g protein
7 g fat
1 g saturated fat
6 g cholesterol
633 mg sodium
5 g fiber
0 IU vitamin D
209 mg potassium
260 mg calcium
0 mcg selenium

2 large heads cauliflower, cut into florets

¼ cup low-fat cream cheese

¼ cup silken tofu

4 cloves garlic, peeled and minced

¼ cup grated Parmesan cheese

½ tsp. freshly cracked *white pepper*

1 tsp. kosher salt

¼ tsp. paprika

1. Preheat the oven to 350°F. Lightly coat a 1-quart casserole dish with cooking spray.

2. Bring a large saucepan of salted water to a boil over high heat. Drop cauliflower into boiling water, and cook for about 15 minutes or until cauliflower is fork-tender. Drain well.

3. In a food processor fitted with a chopping blade, add cream cheese and tofu. Add cauliflower and garlic, and blend for 2 or 3 minutes or until creamy.

4. Add Parmesan cheese, season with pepper and salt, and stir.

5. Pour into the prepared casserole dish, top with paprika, and bake for about 20 minutes or until bubbly and hot.

def•i•ni•tion

White pepper is the ripened berry from the pepper plant that's been dried. White pepper is used in many recipes light in color for aesthetic purposes. The flavor of the white and black pepper aren't really that different, so if you only have black on hand, it'll work just fine.

Curried Cauliflower

Here, delicious and colorful curried cauliflower is highlighted by fresh ginger, garlic, and cilantro.

2 tsp. extra-virgin olive oil

2 cups Vidalia onion, thinly sliced

2 TB. fresh ginger peeled and minced

2 TB. curry powder

1 TB. fresh minced garlic

10 cups cauliflower florets (2 medium heads)

1 cup plain Greek yogurt

½ cup fresh cilantro, chopped

1 tsp. fresh lemon juice

1 tsp. kosher salt

½ tsp. freshly cracked black pepper

Yield: 8 servings
Prep time: 5 minutes
Cook time: 24 minutes
Serving size: ¼ cup
Each serving has:
78 calories
12 g carbohydrate
6 g sugars
2 g protein
2 g fat
.5 g saturated fat
2 g cholesterol
357 mg sodium
3 g fiber
0 IU vitamin D
512 mg potassium
92 mg calcium
1.2 mcg selenium

1. In a sauté pan over medium-high heat, heat olive oil. Add onion and ginger, cover, and cook for 3 minutes, stirring frequently.

2. Reduce heat to medium. Add curry powder and garlic, and cook for 30 seconds, stirring constantly.

3. Add cauliflower, Greek yogurt, cilantro, lemon juice, salt, and pepper, and stir well to combine.

4. Bring to a boil, stirring occasionally (yogurt will curdle). Cover, reduce heat to medium-low, and simmer for 20 minutes or until cauliflower is tender. Serve immediately.

Food for Thought

Cruciferous vegetables such as cauliflower and broccoli have been proven to have cancer-fighting properties.

Creole-Style Black-Eyed Peas

These spiced black-eyed peas feature the taste of New Orleans with ginger, cayenne, and garlic.

Yield: 8 servings
Prep time: 5 minutes
Cook time: 3 hours, 20 minutes
Serving size: ¼ cup
Each serving has:
179 calories
33 g carbohydrate
1.3 g sugars
11 g protein
1 g fat
.3 g saturated fat
0 g cholesterol
441 mg sodium
6 g fiber
0 IU vitamin D
779 mg potassium
61 mg calcium
4 mcg selenium

3 cups low-fat, low-sodium vegetable broth

2 cups dried black-eyed peas

1 low-sodium chicken bouillon cube

1 (14.5-oz.) can low-sodium crushed tomatoes

1 large onion, finely chopped

3 tsp. minced garlic

½ tsp. mustard powder

¼ tsp. dry powdered ginger

¼ tsp. cayenne

½ tsp. kosher salt

½ tsp. freshly cracked black pepper

¼ tsp. Splenda

1 bay leaf

½ cup fresh parsley, chopped

1. In a medium saucepan over high heat, add 2 cups vegetable stock and black-eyed peas. Bring to a boil, cook for 2 minutes, cover, remove from heat, and let stand for 1 hour.

2. Drain stock, leaving peas in the saucepan. Add remaining 1 cup vegetable stock, chicken bouillon, tomatoes, onion, garlic, mustard, ginger, cayenne, salt, pepper, Splenda, and bay leaf. Stir and bring to a boil. Cover, reduce heat to medium-high, and simmer for 2 hours, stirring occasionally. Add water as necessary to keep peas covered with liquid.

3. Remove bay leaf, pour peas into a serving bowl, and garnish with parsley. Serve immediately.

Cooking Tip

Black-eyed peas are really beans that have a little black ring around the spot where the bean attaches to the pod that looks like an eye.

oothies, lushies

In This Chapter

- ◆ Sensational smoothies
- ◆ Mouthwatering milkshakes
- ◆ Soothing slushies

Smoothies, shakes, and slushies are a great way to get your protein and fluid, whether you're on the run or not. Many of the recipes in this chapter are very high in protein and can help you meet your daily needs in one glass.

Many of these recipes have about the same base ingredients—tofu, yogurt, etc.—which makes them easily adaptable. For example, you could make a base blend and add different fruits as you like. If you have a juicer, try mixing in some vegetable juices with your fruit to increase the nutrition in your smoothie.

If you get overeager and make too much, don't worry. These sippable nutrition powerhouses are perfect for freezing. When you're running late for work, grab one from the freezer and it'll be ready to drink by lunchtime.

Morning Glory Smoothie

The fresh orange juice and sweet berries in this colorful breakfast smoothie will liven up your day.

Yield: 1 serving
Prep time: 8 minutes
Serving size: 1 smoothie
Each serving has:
234 calories
29 g carbohydrate
8 g sugars
28 g protein
1.3 g fat
0 g saturated fat
0 g cholesterol
305 mg sodium
5 g fiber
146 IU vitamin D
258 mg potassium
552 mg calcium
.4 mcg selenium

¼ **cup fortified orange juice**

1 TB. strawberry protein powder

⅓ **medium banana, peeled and sliced**

¼ **cup frozen mixed berries (blackberries, raspberries, blueberries, etc.)**

¼ **cup silken tofu**

¼ **tsp. Splenda**

¼ **cup ice**

1. In a blender, combine orange juice, protein powder, banana, berries, tofu, Splenda, and ice.

2. Blend for 2 minutes or until smooth.

Cooking Tip

You'll notice this recipe calls for fortified orange juice. Whenever possible, use a fortified juice, yogurt, etc., in your cooking. Because of the malabsorption caused by your surgery, it's always helpful to add some extra vitamins and minerals when you can.

Peanut Butter and Banana Smoothie

Smooth and creamy peanut butter and the fresh taste of bananas and vanilla combine in this tasty smoothie.

⅓ cup frozen banana

1½ TB. reduced-fat creamy peanut butter

4 TB. fortified skim milk

1 TB. vanilla Greek yogurt

¼ cup silken tofu

1 TB. vanilla protein powder

½ cup ice

¼ cup cold water

Yield: 1 serving
Prep time: 8 minutes
Serving size: 1 smoothie
Each serving has:
300 calories
21 g carbohydrate
10 g sugars
34 g protein
10 g fat
2 g saturated fat
2 g cholesterol
524 mg sodium
2 g fiber
86 IU vitamin D
210 mg potassium
275 mg calcium
2 mcg selenium

1. In a blender, combine banana, peanut butter, milk, Greek yogurt, tofu, protein powder, ice, and water.

2. Blend for 2 minutes or until smooth.

 Food for Thought _____

You can get tofu in many different ways: flavored and unflavored, silken, firm, extra firm, etc. For smoothies, silken tofu is best because of its smooth and, well, "silky" texture.

Blueberry-Banana Smoothie

This tasty smoothie is not only high in protein, but also full of flavor, thanks to delicious blueberries and bananas.

Yield: 1 serving
Prep time: 8 minutes
Serving size: 1 smoothie
Each serving has:
156 calories
15 g carbohydrate
9 g sugars
25 g protein
.5 g fat
.1 g saturated fat
1 g cholesterol
294 mg sodium
1.6 g fiber
25 IU vitamin D
237 mg potassium
83 mg calcium
1.6 mcg selenium

4 TB. frozen blueberries

½ cup frozen banana

¾ cup cold water

¼ cup skim milk

1 TB. vanilla protein powder

1 TB. chilled orange juice

¼ cup ice

1. In a blender, combine blueberries, banana, water, milk, protein powder, orange juice, and ice.

2. Purée for 2 minutes or until smooth.

 Food for Thought _____

This recipe would also be delicious with apple juice instead of orange juice.

Piña Colada Smoothie

Take a hiatus from your daily life with this Caribbean pineapple-and-coconut delight—don't worry, it's nonalcoholic so you can drink it at work.

¼ cup chopped pineapple

½ cup cold water

2 TB. skim milk

¼ cup light coconut milk, chilled

¼ cup plain Greek yogurt

1 TB. plain protein powder

½ cup ice

1. In a blender, combine pineapple, water, skim milk, coconut milk, Greek yogurt, protein powder, and ice.

2. Blend for 2 minutes or until smooth.

> ## Cooking Tip
>
> If you're making a smoothie and it's not blending well, try adding a little more liquid.

Yield: 1 serving
Prep time: 8 minutes
Serving size: 1 smoothie
Each serving has:
209 calories
11 g carbohydrate
10 g sugars
26 g protein
8 g fat
7 g saturated fat
4 g cholesterol
309 mg sodium
1 g fiber
0 IU vitamin D
290 mg potassium
125 mg calcium
4 mcg selenium

Frozen Banana Sundae Shake

This decadent banana split milkshake features chocolate and fresh bananas.

Yield: 1 serving
Prep time: 8 minutes
Serving size: 1 shake
Each serving has:
212 calories
26 g carbohydrate
10 g sugars
26 g protein
.7 g fat
.4 g saturated fat
3 g cholesterol
333 mg sodium
1.5 g fiber
25 IU vitamin D
309 mg potassium
139 mg calcium
2.6 mcg selenium

¼ **cup skim milk**

1 TB. vanilla protein powder

⅓ **cup frozen banana**

1 TB. vanilla Greek yogurt

¼ **cup ice**

1 TB. sugar-free chocolate syrup

¾ **cup cold water**

1 TB. light whipped topping

1. In a blender, combine milk, protein powder, banana slices, Greek yogurt, ice, chocolate syrup, and water.

2. Blend for 2 minutes or until smooth.

3. Top with whipped topping before serving.

Cooking Tip _____

When adding berries to a smoothie, it's best to add them frozen to help keep the smoothie ice cold.

Fuzzy Navel Milkshake

In this peaches-and-cream milkshake, creamy Greek yogurt and hints of vanilla add flavor.

¼ cup low-fat, low-sugar vanilla frozen yogurt

¼ cup frozen peach slices

¼ cup orange juice, chilled

1 TB. vanilla Greek yogurt

1 TB. vanilla protein powder

¼ cup ice

¼ cup cold water

1. In a blender, combine frozen yogurt, peaches, orange juice, Greek yogurt, protein powder, ice, and water.

2. Blend for 2 minutes or until smooth.

Cooking Tip

If you'd like to use fresh peaches, peel, remove the pit, and slice before freezing them.

Yield: 1 serving
Prep time: 8 minutes
Serving size: 1 shake
Each serving has:
195 calories
18 g carbohydrate
8 g sugars
26 g protein
3 g fat
2 g saturated fat
12 g cholesterol
312 mg sodium
1 g fiber
0 IU vitamin D
247 mg potassium
110 mg calcium
1 mcg selenium

Mixed-Berry Milkshake

This shake is "berry" delicious, thanks to a mix of your favorite berries, creamy Greek yogurt, and hints of vanilla.

Yield: 8 servings

Prep time: 8 minutes

Serving size: 1 cup

Each serving has:

162 calories

13 g carbohydrate

10 g sugars

26 g protein

1 g fat

.6 g saturated fat

4 g cholesterol

310 mg sodium

1 g fiber

14 IU vitamin D

186 mg potassium

150 mg calcium

2 mcg selenium

---

2 cups vanilla Greek yogurt	5 TB. vanilla protein powder
3 cups water	¼ cup silken tofu
3 cups frozen mixed berries	

1. In a blender, combine Greek yogurt, water, frozen berries, vanilla protein powder, and tofu.

2. Blend for 2 minutes or until smooth.

Cooking Tip

When using tofu in a smoothie, you can also add it in small frozen cubes. Stick with silken tofu though, as it purées best.

Watermelon-Strawberry Slushy

Fresh and light watermelon and strawberries combine in this super-sippable slushy.

6 cups watermelon, rind and seeds removed, and diced

2 TB. fresh lime juice

1 cup whole strawberries, greens removed

2 TB. strawberry protein powder

2 TB. Splenda

1½ cups ice

1 cup cold water

1. In a blender, combine watermelon, lime juice, strawberries, Splenda, ice, and water.

2. Blend for 2 minutes or until smooth.

Food for Thought

There are many different types of watermelons in the world, with colors from pink to yellow and shapes ranging from round to oval.

Yield: 8 servings
Prep time: 8 minutes
Serving size: 1 cup
Each serving has:
59 calories
12 g carbohydrate
10 g sugars
6 g protein
0 g fat
0 g saturated fat
0 g cholesterol
76 mg sodium
1 g fiber
0 IU vitamin D
35 mg potassium
11 mg calcium
0 mcg selenium

Chapter 22

Desserts: How Sweet It Is!

In This Chapter

- ◆ Tantalizing cakes, tarts, and brownies
- ◆ Decadent puddings
- ◆ Fabulous frozen ice creams and sorbets
- ◆ Great granitas

If you're worried that you have to cut out all sweets after your weight loss surgery, take heart. In this chapter, we serve up a number of mouth-watering desserts that are not only delicious, but also healthful for you. All these desserts are low in fat and sugar, thanks to some clever substitutions.

For example, you're going to see a few recipes that use puréed beans to replace some of the butter and shortening—the fat—in the recipe. Beans do contain some fat, but it's good-for-you fat. Also, we used pasteurized egg whites (find these in a carton next to the liquid egg substitutes in the grocery store) in a few of the frozen desserts. Because they're pasteurized, they're considered cooked, so there's no need to worry about consuming raw eggs. (Whole eggs may not be pasteurized, so don't use egg whites from separated eggs.) Also, we used a lot of puréed tofu, which is a good way to get more protein.

Now on to the best part of the meal!

Lemon-Raspberry Cheesecake

Delicious and creamy raspberry and lemon cheesecake star with a sweet vanilla wafer crust.

Yield: 16 servings

Prep time: 3 hours, 50 minutes

Cook time: 50 to 55 minutes

Serving size: 1 slice

Each serving has:

93 calories

10 g carbohydrate

3 g sugars

10 g protein

2 g fat

.4 g saturated fat

4 g cholesterol

285 mg sodium

.2 g fiber

3 IU vitamin D

75 mg potassium

105 mg calcium

2.5 mcg selenium

20 reduced-fat vanilla wafers

1 TB. canola oil

2 cups reduced-fat cottage cheese

1 (8-oz.) pkg. fat-free cream cheese

1 cup plus 2 TB. Splenda

2 TB. cornstarch

¼ cup vanilla protein powder

2 tsp. fresh lemon juice

1½ tsp. vanilla extract

¼ tsp. salt

¾ cup liquid egg substitute

2 TB. lemon zest

2 pt. fresh raspberries

5 fresh mint leaves

1. Preheat the oven to 325°F. Coat a 9-inch springform pan with cooking spray. Wrap the outside of the pan with a double thickness of aluminum foil. Put a kettle of water on to boil for a water bath.

2. In a food processor fitted with a chopping blade, grind vanilla wafers into fine crumbs. Add canola oil, and pulse to blend. Press crumb mixture evenly into the bottom of the prepared springform pan. Wash and dry the food processor bowl.

3. In the food processor, add cottage cheese and process for 2 or 3 minutes or until very smooth and silky, stopping to scrape down the sides once or twice. Add cream cheese, and process for 3 minutes or until smooth.

4. Add 1 cup Splenda, cornstarch, protein powder, lemon juice, vanilla extract, and salt, and process for 2 minutes or until well blended. Add egg substitute and pulse several times just until mixed in. Sprinkle in lemon zest and mix with a rubber spatula. (Do not process.) Scrape filling into crust.

5. Place cheesecake in a shallow roasting pan and pour in enough boiling water to come 1 inch up the outside of the springform pan. Bake for 50 to 55 minutes or until edges are set but center quivers slightly. Turn off the oven. Let cheesecake cool in the oven, with the door slightly open, for 1 hour.

6. Remove the foil from the pan. Cover cheesecake with plastic wrap, and refrigerate for at least 2 hours or until chilled.

7. About 30 minutes before serving, rinse raspberries. Sprinkle with remaining 2 tablespoons Splenda, and toss to coat. Let stand for 20 to 30 minutes or until raspberries are juicy.

8. To serve, place cheesecake on a platter, run a knife around the inside of the springform pan, and remove the pan sides. Top cheesecake with raspberries and their syrup, and garnish with mint leaves.

Food for Thought

It can be difficult to judge when cheesecakes are done cooking. Look for the center to still have a little jiggle. When it's overcooked, it cracks. Keep a close eye on it, and when you see it just start to crack the tiniest bit, it's done.

Rustic Berry Tart

This is one berry delicious and flaky summery tart with fresh blueberries and lemon juice.

Yield: 12 servings
Prep time: 1 hour, 15 minutes
Cook time: 45 to 55 minutes
Serving size: 1 slice
Each serving has:
141 calories
21 g carbohydrate
5 g sugars
6 g protein
4 g fat
.3 g saturated fat
0 g cholesterol
142 mg sodium
3 g fiber
2 IU vitamin D
80 mg potassium
12 mg calcium
6 mcg selenium

½ cup plus 4 TB. whole-wheat flour

½ cup all-purpose flour

1¼ cups vanilla protein powder

1 cup quick-cooking oats

¼ cup plus 4 TB. Splenda

½ tsp. salt

3 TB. vegetable oil, chilled

¼ cup plus 1 TB. water

¼ cup plus 2 TB. liquid egg substitute

3 tsp. freshly squeezed lemon juice

4 cups mixed berries, such as blackberries, raspberries, and blueberries

2 TB. sugar-free berry jam

1. In a medium bowl, whisk together ½ cup whole-wheat flour, all-purpose flour, protein powder, oats, 1 tablespoon Splenda, and salt.

2. Add chilled vegetable oil, and stir until mixture resembles coarse crumbs with a few larger pieces.

3. In a measuring cup, mix together ¼ cup water, ¼ cup egg substitute, and 1 teaspoon lemon juice. Add to flour mixture, stirring with a fork, until dough clumps together. (Add a little water if dough seems too dry.)

4. Turn out dough onto a lightly floured surface, and knead several times. Form dough into a ball, and flatten into a disk. Wrap in plastic wrap and refrigerate for at least 1 hour.

5. Preheat the oven to 425°F. Line a baking sheet with parchment paper or aluminum foil, and lightly coat with cooking spray.

6. In a medium bowl, combine remaining 4 tablespoons whole-wheat flour and ¼ cup Splenda. Set aside.

7. On a lightly floured surface, roll dough into a circle roughly 13 to 14 inches in diameter and about ¼ inch thick. Roll dough circle back over the rolling pin, brush off excess flour, and transfer to the prepared baking sheet.

8. In a large bowl, toss berries with remaining 3 tablespoons Splenda, flour mixture, and remaining 2 teaspoons lemon juice. Spoon into center of crust. Fold edge of dough up and over filling, pleating as necessary.

9. In a small bowl, blend together 2 tablespoons egg substitute and remaining 1 tablespoon water with a fork. Lightly brush over rim of tart.

10. Bake tart for 15 minutes. Reduce oven temperature to 350°F and bake for 30 to 40 minutes or until crust is golden and juices are bubbling. Leaving tart on the parchment (or foil), carefully slide it onto a wire rack. Let cool.

11. Shortly before serving, melt jam in a small saucepan over low heat, and brush over berries. Cut tart into 12 wedges and serve.

 Food for Thought

Berries and other dark colored produce are full of antioxidants which are proven to help protect the body from free radicals which cause cancer.

Angel Food Cake with Greek Yogurt Mousse and Mixed Berries

Light angel food cake pairs with a healthy vanilla yogurt mousse and fresh strawberries, raspberries, blackberries, and blueberries.

Yield: 8 servings
Prep time: 5 minutes
Serving size: 1 slice angel food cake and ¼ cup berries and yogurt mousse
Each serving has:
174 calories
35 g carbohydrate
7 g sugars
6 g protein
1 g fat
.6 g saturated fat
3 g cholesterol
364 mg sodium
1.5 g fiber
0 IU vitamin D
236 mg potassium
170 mg calcium
5 mcg selenium

1 pt. fresh strawberries, sliced

1 pt. fresh raspberries

1 pt. fresh blackberries

1 pt. fresh blueberries

1 (16-oz.) pkg. plain fat-free Greek yogurt

1 tsp. Splenda

1 cup low-fat whipped topping

1 store-bought angel food cake

1. In a medium bowl, mix together strawberries, raspberries, blackberries, blueberries, Greek yogurt, and Splenda, mashing berries slightly to produce some juice.

2. Carefully fold in whipped topping.

3. Slice angel food cake in half horizontally, and pour "mousse" filling in between layers and over top of cake. Serve immediately.

Cooking Tip

You can make your own angel food cake or pound cake for this recipe. If you do, replace the whole eggs with liquid egg substitute and the sugar with Splenda.

Carrot Cake with Cream Cheese Frosting

This carrot cake with delicious walnuts, coconut, and pineapple is topped with a cream cheese frosting you'll love—and with half the fat and calories.

1 (20-oz.) can crushed pineapple

1¾ cups whole-wheat pastry flour

¼ cup vanilla protein powder

2 tsp. baking soda

½ tsp. salt

2 tsp. ground cinnamon

¾ cup liquid egg substitute

1¾ cups Splenda

½ cup vanilla Greek yogurt

¼ cup water

¼ cup canola oil

¼ cup white beans, rinsed, drained, and puréed

2½ tsp. vanilla extract

2 cups carrots, peeled and grated

¼ cup plus 2 tsp. unsweetened coconut flakes

½ cup chopped walnuts

1½ cups fat-free cream cheese

¼ cup confectioners' sugar

1 TB. spray butter or vegetable oil

Yield: 16 servings
Prep time: 25 minutes
Cook time: 40 to 45 minutes
Serving size: 1 slice
Each serving has:
181 calories
23 g carbohydrate
9 g sugars
9 g protein
7 g fat
1 g saturated fat
2 g cholesterol
250 mg sodium
3 g fiber
3 IU vitamin D
189 mg potassium
71 mg calcium
11 mcg selenium

1. Preheat the oven to 350°F. Lightly coat a 9×13-inch baking pan with cooking spray.

2. In a strainer set over a medium bowl, drain pineapple, pressing to extract more juice. Reserve drained pineapple and ¼ cup juice.

3. In another medium bowl, whisk together flour, protein powder, baking soda, salt, and cinnamon.

4. In a large bowl, whisk together egg substitute, 1½ cups Splenda, Greek yogurt, water, canola oil, white bean purée, 1 teaspoon vanilla extract, and ¼ cup reserved pineapple juice until blended. Stir in drained pineapple, carrots, and ¼ cup unsweetened coconut flakes.

5. Add dry ingredients in 3 batches, and mix with a rubber spatula just until blended. Stir in walnuts. Scrape batter into the prepared pan, spreading evenly.

6. Bake for 40 to 45 minutes or until top of cake springs back when touched lightly and a skewer inserted in the center comes out clean. Let cool completely on a wire rack.

7. While cake is cooking, in a medium bowl, and with an electric mixer on low speed, beat cream cheese, confectioners' sugar, remaining ¼ cup Splenda, spray butter, and remaining 1½ teaspoons vanilla extract for 20 seconds or until smooth and creamy. Spread frosting over cooled cake, and sprinkle with coconut flakes.

Cooking Tip

Toasting the coconut flakes is easy and adds a little extra flavor. Simply spread the coconut in a 9×13-inch baking pan and bake in a 350°F oven for 40 to 45 minutes.

Fudgy Chocolate Torte

Rich and fudgy dark, this chocolate cake has a subtle hint of vanilla.

¾ **cup liquid egg substitute**

1¼ **cups Splenda**

2 **tsp. vanilla extract**

½ **cup graham cracker crumbs**

4 **TB. chocolate protein powder**

½ **cup white beans, rinsed, drained, and puréed**

½ **cup sugar-free applesauce**

2 **TB. unsweetened cocoa powder**

¼ **cup semisweet chocolate chunks**

8 **egg whites**

½ **tsp. kosher salt**

Confectioners' sugar

Yield: *8 servings*
Prep time: 25 minutes
Cook time: 40 to 45 minutes
Serving size: 1 slice
Each serving has:
101 calories
14 g carbohydrate
7 g sugars
6 g protein
3 g fat
1 g saturated fat
.2 g cholesterol
252 mg sodium
2 g fiber
5 IU vitamin D
122 mg potassium
17 mg calcium
.7 mcg selenium

1. Preheat the oven to 350°F.

2. In a large bowl, whisk together egg substitute, ¾ cup Splenda, and vanilla extract. Stir in graham cracker crumbs, protein powder, white bean purée, applesauce, cocoa powder, and chocolate.

3. In large, clean bowl and with an electric mixer on medium speed, beat egg whites and salt until frothy. Increase speed to high, and beat until soft peaks form. Add remaining ½ cup Splenda, 1 tablespoon at a time, beating until glossy and stiff peaks form.

4. Using a rubber spatula, stir ¼ of beaten whites into batter. Gently fold in remaining whites. Scrape batter into an ungreased 9-inch springform pan, spreading evenly. Tap pan lightly on the counter to release any air bubbles.

5. Bake for 40 to 45 minutes or until top springs back when touched lightly and a skewer inserted in the center comes out clean. With a knife, loosen edges of torte. Let cool in the pan on a wire rack. (Torte will sink in center.)

6. Remove pan sides and place torte on a serving platter. Dust with confectioners' sugar and serve.

 Food for Thought

To change this chocolate torte into molten chocolate cupcakes, pour the batter into muffin tins and undercook them slightly.

Raspberry Cream Cheese Black Bean Brownies

Yummy rich dark chocolate brownies are topped with raspberries, cream cheese swirls, with hints of vanilla.

Yield: 16 servings
Prep time: 15 minutes
Cook time: 40 minutes
Serving size: 1 square
Each serving has:
44 calories
9 g carbohydrate
.3 g sugars
.6 g protein
.4 g fat
.4 g saturated fat
76 g cholesterol
76 mg sodium
2 g fiber
3 IU vitamin D
103 mg potassium
20 mg calcium
4 mcg selenium

1⅓ cups Splenda

⅓ cup fat-free cream cheese

3 tsp. vanilla extract

1 egg white

2 tsp. plus ½ cup all-purpose flour

¼ cup whole-wheat flour

¼ tsp. baking powder

¼ tsp. baking soda

Pinch kosher salt

⅔ cup unsweetened cocoa powder

¼ cup black beans, rinsed, drained, and puréed

1 TB. skim milk

¾ cup liquid egg substitute

3 TB. reduced-sugar raspberry jam

1. Preheat the oven to 350°F. Lightly coat the bottom of an 8-inch-square baking pan with cooking spray.

2. In a large bowl, and with an electric mixer on medium speed, beat ⅓ cup Splenda, cream cheese, 2 teaspoons vanilla extract, egg white, and 2 teaspoons all-purpose flour for 3 minutes or until well blended. Set aside.

3. In a medium bowl, combine remaining all-purpose flour, whole-wheat flour, baking powder, baking soda, and salt.

4. In another bowl, whisk together remaining 1 cup Splenda, cocoa powder, black bean purée, skim milk, remaining 1 teaspoon vanilla extract, and egg substitute. Add to flour mixture, stirring until just moist.

5. Spread ⅔ of batter in the bottom of the prepared pan. Pour filling over batter, and spread evenly.

6. Carefully drop remaining batter and raspberry jam by spoonfuls over filling. Using a knife, swirl together to marble.

7. Bake for 40 minutes or until a skewer inserted in the center comes out almost clean. Cool on a wire rack, and cut into 16 squares.

Cooking Tip

If raspberry jam isn't your thing, you can substitute other jams, like blackberry jam or strawberry jam.

Fudgy Brownies

You'll dream of these decadent fudgy brownies with toasted walnuts.

½ cup all-purpose flour

¼ cup whole-wheat flour

3 TB. chocolate or vanilla protein powder

⅔ cup confectioners' sugar

3 TB. unsweetened cocoa powder

¾ cup semisweet or bitter-sweet chocolate (50 to 72 percent cacao) chips

1½ TB. canola oil

¼ cup Splenda

1½ TB. light corn syrup

3 TB. lukewarm water

2 tsp. vanilla extract

Pinch kosher salt

¼ cup liquid egg substitute

⅓ cup toasted walnuts, chopped

Yield: 20 servings
Prep time: 35 minutes
Cook time: 20 to 24 minutes
Serving size: 1 brownie
Each serving has:
100 calories
12 g carbohydrate
6 g sugars
4 g protein
5 g fat
1 g saturated fat
0 g cholesterol
25 mg sodium
1 g fiber
1 IU vitamin D
22 mg potassium
4 mg calcium
2 mcg selenium

1. Preheat the oven to 350°F. Line an 8-inch-square baking pan with aluminum foil, letting it overhang on two opposite sides. Lightly coat foil with cooking spray.

2. Into a small bowl, sift together all-purpose flour, whole-wheat flour, protein powder, confectioners' sugar, and cocoa powder. Set aside.

3. In a heavy, medium saucepan over lowest heat, combine ¼ cup chocolate and canola oil. Stir until just melted and smooth, being very careful chocolate does not overheat. Remove from heat and stir in Splenda, vanilla extract, and salt. Stir 3 or 4 minutes or until sugar dissolves. Stir in egg substitute until smoothly incorporated.

4. Gently stir in dry ingredients. Fold in walnuts and remaining chocolate just until well blended. Turn out batter into the prepared pan, spreading evenly.

5. Bake for 20 to 24 minutes or until almost firm in the center and a skewer inserted into the center comes out with some moist batter clinging to it. Let cool on wire rack for approximately 20 minutes.

Cooking Tip

To make cutting brownies (or anything sticky) easier, heat the knife blade in a hot water bath and wipe the blade dry before cutting. Cut and repeat the process as necessary.

Rich Chocolate Pudding

Rich and delicious semisweet chocolate pudding gets it sweetness from Splenda.

Yield: 8 servings
Prep time: 2 hours, 2 minutes
Cook time: 25 minutes
Serving size: ½ cup
Each serving has:
86 calories
14 g carbohydrate
7.5 g sugars
6 g protein
3 g fat
2 g saturated fat
2 g cholesterol
65 mg sodium
4 g fiber
49 IU vitamin D
377 mg potassium
166 mg calcium
4 mcg selenium

1½ cups Splenda

¼ cup unsweetened cocoa powder

⅓ cup cornstarch

4 cups skim milk

¼ cup semisweet chocolate chips

2 tsp. vanilla extract

1. In a small bowl, mix together Splenda and cocoa powder until no cocoa powder lumps remain.

2. In a second small bowl, dissolve cornstarch in 1 cup skim milk.

3. Pour remaining 3 cups milk into a small saucepan, and heat over medium-low heat. After about 15 minutes, when milk is almost to a scalding point, whisk in cocoa powder and Splenda, and pour in cornstarch mixture. Continue to heat, stirring constantly, for about 10 minutes or until mixture is slightly thickened.

4. Remove from heat and stir in semisweet chocolate and vanilla extract.

5. Pour pudding into a bowl and cover with plastic wrap. Refrigerate for about 2 hours or until mixture is completely cold.

 Food for Thought

Why use cocoa powder *and* chocolate in this recipe? Switching out some of the chocolate for cocoa powder reduces the amount of fat and calories in the pudding.

Old-Fashioned Rice Pudding

This tasty old-fashioned rice pudding features dried cranberries, walnuts, and a hint of vanilla.

4⅔ cups light vanilla soy milk

⅔ cup uncooked long-grain rice

¼ cup plus 3 TB. Splenda

½ tsp. kosher salt (optional)

⅔ cup unsweetened dried cranberries

4 TB. walnuts, chopped

1¼ tsp. vanilla extract

1 tsp. ground cinnamon

Yield: 10 servings
Prep time: 2 minutes
Cook time: 70 minutes
Serving size: ½ cup
Each serving has:
141 calories
22 g carbohydrate
9 g sugars
4 g protein
5 g fat
.6 g saturated fat
0 g cholesterol
172 mg sodium
1 g fiber
37 IU vitamin D
118 mg potassium
1,500 mg calcium
.3 mcg selenium

1. Preheat the oven to 325°F. Lightly spray a 9×13-inch baking dish with cooking spray.

2. In a medium saucepan over medium heat, combine soy milk, rice, Splenda, and salt (if using). Bring to a boil, stirring constantly.

3. Pour pudding into the prepared baking dish. Cover and bake for 45 minutes, stirring every 15 minutes.

4. After 45 minutes, remove pudding from the oven and add dried cranberries, walnuts, and vanilla extract. Cover, return to the oven, and bake for 15 more minutes. Remove from the oven and sprinkle with cinnamon. Serve warm or chilled. Store any leftovers in the refrigerator.

Cooking Tip

For a little extra protein, stir in 1 or 2 tablespoons protein powder along with another ¼ cup soy milk in step 2.

Blueberry-Cinnamon Ice Cream

Here, delicious blueberries and cinnamon swirl in creamy ice cream.

Yield: 12 servings
Prep time: 2 hours, 45 minutes
Cook time: 30 minutes
Serving size: ½ cup
Each serving has:
49 calories
6 g carbohydrate
5 g sugars
5 g protein
.5 g fat
.2 g saturated fat
2 g cholesterol
70 mg sodium
.3 g fiber
53 IU vitamin D
167 mg potassium
168 mg calcium
2 mcg selenium

1 vanilla bean

4 cups skim milk

¼ cup liquid egg substitute

½ cup vanilla Greek yogurt

¾ cup silken tofu, puréed

1 cup frozen blueberries

1 tsp. ground cinnamon

1. Cut vanilla bean in half lengthwise, and scrape seeds into a large saucepan. Add scraped pod. Pour milk into the saucepan with vanilla bean. Heat over medium heat for 5 to 10 minutes or until steaming.

2. In a medium bowl, whisk together egg substitute, Greek yogurt, and tofu purée. Gradually pour into hot milk, whisking until blended. Continue to cook over medium heat, stirring with a wooden spoon, for 3 to 5 minutes or until the back of the spoon is lightly coated. Do not bring to a boil or custard will curdle.

3. Strain custard through a fine-mesh sieve into a clean large bowl. Cover and refrigerate for at least 2 hours or until chilled.

4. Whisk mixture and pour into the canister of an ice-cream maker. Freeze for about 40 minutes or according to the manufacturer's directions. During the last 5 minutes of freezing, stir in blueberries and cinnamon. Remove ice cream from ice-cream maker bowl, scoop into a plastic container with a lid, and freeze to firm before serving.

Cooking Tip

This recipe would also make a great plain vanilla ice cream. Just omit the blueberries and cinnamon, or add different kinds of berries like strawberries or blackberries to make different flavors.

Peach Frozen Yogurt

This rich and creamy peach frozen yogurt has hints of vanilla.

3 cups fat-free vanilla Greek yogurt

¾ cups Splenda

1 tsp. *vanilla extract*

2 fresh peaches, peeled and pitted, chopped

Yield: *8 servings*
Prep time: 8 hours, 45 minutes
Serving size: ½ cup
Each serving has:
73 calories
10 g carbohydrate
10 g sugars
5 g protein
2 g fat
1 g saturated fat
6 g cholesterol
64 mg sodium
.5 g fiber
0 IU vitamin D
272 mg potassium
168 mg calcium
3 mcg selenium

1. In a large bowl, combine Greek yogurt, Splenda, and vanilla extract. Pour into ice-cream maker, and freeze for about 40 minutes or according to the manufacturer's instructions.

2. Gently fold in peaches, and freeze overnight in a separate container with a lid.

def•i•ni•tion

Vanilla extract is made by soaking vanilla beans in alcohol. The alcohol remains in the finished product, and believe it or not, vanilla extract, although it smells delicious, tastes awful straight out of the bottle!

Peach Sorbet

This refreshing summer peach sorbet is highlighted by fresh lemon and hints of vanilla.

Yield: 8 servings
Prep time: 1 hour, 45 minutes
Serving size: ¼ cup
Each serving has:
19 calories
2 g carbohydrate
2 g sugars
3 g protein
0 g fat
0 g saturated fat
0 g cholesterol
33 mg sodium
.3 g fiber
0 IU vitamin D
38 mg potassium
1 mg calcium
0 mcg selenium

1 cup fresh peaches, peeled and pitted and chopped

3 TB. Splenda

2 TB. water

2 TB. vanilla protein powder

2 tsp. fresh lemon juice

1 tsp. lemon zest

½ tsp. vanilla extract

1. In a blender, combine peaches, Splenda, water, protein powder, lemon juice, lemon zest, and vanilla extract. Blend on high speed until smooth.

2. Refrigerate 1 hour.

3. Pour mixture into an ice-cream maker, and freeze for about 40 minutes or according to the manufacturer's instructions.

Cooking Tip

This is an easily adaptable recipe for whatever flavor of sorbet you'd like. You can easily change out the peaches for other fruit to mix up the flavor.

Kiwi Sorbet

This sorbet is light and filled with the sweet taste of kiwi.

2 TB. Splenda

1 cup water

11 large *kiwis*, peeled and diced

4 TB. pasteurized egg whites

1 TB. plain protein powder

Yield: 8 servings
Prep time: 45 minutes
Serving size: ½ cup
Each serving has:
81 calories
19 g carbohydrate
10 g sugars
2 g protein
.7 g fat
0 g saturated fat
0 g cholesterol
16 mg sodium
4 g fiber
0 IU vitamin D
394 mg potassium
43 mg calcium
.3 mcg selenium

1. In a blender, combine Splenda, water, kiwis, egg whites, and protein powder. Blend on high speed until smooth.

2. Pour mixture into an ice-cream maker, and freeze for 30 minutes or according to the manufacturer's instructions.

def•i•ni•tion

The **kiwi,** also known as kiwifruit, is a small oval fruit that's fuzzy and brown on the outside. The inside is lime green and has little black seeds that are completely edible.

Ruby Red Grapefruit Sorbet

This tart red grapefruit sorbet is surprisingly pleasing to your taste buds.

Yield: 14 servings
Prep time: 2 hours, 45 minutes
Serving size: ¼ cup
Each serving has:
30 calories
5 g carbohydrate
3 g sugars
2 g protein
0 g fat
0 g saturated fat
0 g cholesterol
27 mg sodium
0 g fiber
0 IU vitamin D
96 mg potassium
5 mg calcium
1 mcg selenium

¼ **cup Splenda**

¼ **tsp. salt**

1 TB. red grapefruit zest

3 cups red grapefruit juice

1 cup sparkling water

2 TB. fresh lemon juice

2 TB. pasteurized egg whites

1 TB. strawberry protein powder

1. In a blender, combine Splenda, salt, grapefruit zest, grapefruit juice, sparkling water, lemon juice, egg whites, and protein powder. Blend on high speed until smooth.

2. Pour mixture into an ice-cream maker and freeze for about 40 minutes or according to the manufacturer's instructions.

3. Freeze for at least 2 hours before serving.

 Food for Thought _____

Grapefruits contain licopene, the antioxidant found in red fruits and vegetables like tomatoes and red grapes, that has been proven to help prevent cancer.

Acai-Pomegranate Granita

This fruity pomegranate and *acai* berry granita features tangy lemon juice.

¼ cup Splenda

4 pomegranate herbal tea bags

3 cups boiling water

½ cup pasteurized egg whites

½ cup plain protein powder

1 cup acai juice

2 TB. fresh lemon juice

Yield: *8 servings*
Prep time: 7 hours
Serving size: ½ cup
Each serving has:
65 calories
3 g carbohydrate
2 g sugars
13 g protein
.3 g fat
0 g saturated fat
0 g cholesterol
160 mg sodium
0 g fiber
0 IU vitamin D
27 mg potassium
1 mg calcium
3 mcg selenium

1. Place Splenda and tea bags in a heatproof bowl.

2. Pour in boiling water, and stir until Splenda has dissolved. Let tea bags steep for about 1 hour or until tea is cooled to room temperature.

3. Remove tea bags and squeeze out liquid.

4. In a blender, combine tea, egg whites, protein powder, acai juice, and lemon juice. Blend on high speed until smooth.

5. Pour mixture into a 9-inch square baking dish. Cover tightly with plastic wrap, and freeze for about 45 minutes or until mixture is icy at the edges of the pan. Whisk to distribute frozen portions evenly. Cover and refreeze for about 45 minutes or until mixture is icy at the edges of the pan and overall texture is slushy. Whisk again to distribute frozen portions evenly. Cover and refreeze for about 3 hours or until frozen solid. Remove from the freezer.

6. Using a fork, scrape granita down the length of the pan, forming icy flakes. Return to the freezer for at least 1 hour. Granita can be made 1 day ahead and kept in the freezer.

def•i•ni•tion

Acai berries are small, round, and dark purple in color, similar to grapes in appearance. They're commonly used to make smoothies, sodas, and other beverages.

"Limoncello" Granita

This tart lemon shaved ice is prefect for hot summer days.

Yield: *8 servings*
Prep time: 6 hours
Cook time: about 2 minutes
Serving size: ½ cup
Each serving has:
20 calories
4 g carbohydrate
2 g sugars
1 g protein
.4 g fat
.2 g saturated fat
1 g cholesterol
16 mg sodium
0 g fiber
0 IU vitamin D
82 mg potassium
44 mg calcium
1 mcg selenium

½ **cup Splenda**

2½ **cups water**

¾ **cup lemon juice**

¾ **cup vanilla Greek yogurt**

¾ **tsp. vanilla extract**

1 **TB. lemon zest**

1. In a small saucepan over medium heat, combine Splenda and water. Bring to a simmer for 1 or 2 minutes or just until sugar dissolves and turns clear. Remove from heat and let cool to room temperature.

2. Stir in lemon juice, Greek yogurt, vanilla extract, and lemon zest.

3. Pour mixture into a 9-inch square baking dish. Cover tightly with plastic wrap, and freeze for about 45 minutes or until mixture is icy at the edges of the pan. Whisk to distribute frozen portions evenly. Cover and refreeze for about 45 minutes or until mixture is icy at the edges of the pan and overall texture is slushy. Whisk again to distribute frozen portions evenly. Cover and refreeze for about 3 hours or until frozen solid. Remove from the freezer.

4. Using a fork, scrape granita down the length of the pan, forming icy flakes. Return to the freezer for at least 1 hour. Granita can be made 1 day ahead and kept in the freezer.

 Food for Thought

Limoncello is a lemon-flavored alcohol originally made in southern Italy by combining lemon rinds, 96 percent alcohol vodka, sugar, and water. The mixture is then allowed to sit until the color turns bright yellow. No alcohol is used in this granita, of course, but the lemon juice and zest add the limoncello flavor.

Cranberry-Pomegranate Granita

This pomegranate and cranberry shaved ice is light and refreshing.

½ cup pasteurized egg whites

½ cup plain protein powder

1 cup pomegranate juice

2 TB. Splenda

1½ cups diet cranberry juice cocktail

1½ cups sparkling water

Yield: 8 servings
Prep time: 6 hours
Serving size: ½ cup
Each serving has:
76 calories
7 g carbohydrate
6 g sugars
13 g protein
0 g fat
0 g saturated fat
0 g cholesterol
159 mg sodium
0 g fiber
0 IU vitamin D
34 mg potassium
10 mg calcium
3 mcg selenium

1. In a blender, combine egg whites, protein powder, pomegranate juice, Splenda, cranberry juice cocktail, and club soda. Blend on high speed until smooth.

2. Pour mixture into a 9-inch square baking dish. Cover tightly with plastic wrap, and freeze for about 45 minutes or until mixture is icy at the edges of the pan. Whisk to distribute frozen portions evenly. Cover and refreeze for about 45 minutes or until mixture is icy at the edges of the pan and overall texture is slushy. Whisk again to distribute frozen portions evenly. Cover and refreeze for about 3 hours or until frozen solid. Remove from the freezer.

3. Using a fork, scrape granita down the length of the pan, forming icy flakes. Return to the freezer for at least 1 hour. Granita can be made 1 day ahead and kept in the freezer.

Cooking Tip

For a little extra flavor, substitute Diet Sprite for the sparkling water.

Honeydew Granita

This refreshingly sweet honeydew shaved ice can be a snack or a dessert.

Yield: 8 servings
Prep time: 6 hours
Serving size: ½ cup
Each serving has:
22 calories
5 g carbohydrate
4 g sugars
1 g protein
0 g fat
0 g saturated fat
0 g cholesterol
89 mg sodium
.4 g fiber
0 IU vitamin D
130 mg potassium
4 mg calcium
1 mcg selenium

½ to 1 small honeydew melon, peeled, seeds removed, and diced (2½ cups)

½ cup sparkling water

¼ cup Splenda

1 TB. pasteurized egg whites

1 TB. fresh lemon juice

½ tsp. ground cinnamon

¼ tsp. salt

1. In a blender, combine honeydew, sparkling water, Splenda, egg whites, lemon juice, cinnamon, and salt. Blend on high speed until smooth.

2. Pour mixture into a 9-inch square baking dish. Cover tightly with plastic wrap, and freeze for about 45 minutes or until mixture is icy at the edges of the pan. Whisk to distribute frozen portions evenly. Cover and refreeze for about 45 minutes or until mixture is icy at the edges of the pan and overall texture is slushy. Whisk again to distribute frozen portions evenly. Cover and refreeze for about 3 hours or until frozen solid. Remove from the freezer.

3. Using a fork, scrape granita down the length of the pan, forming icy flakes. Return to the freezer for at least 1 hour. Granita can be made 1 day ahead and kept in the freezer.

 Cooking Tip

If you're not into cinnamon, you can omit it from the recipe. It will still taste delicious without it.

Watermelon Granita

Sweet and summery, this watermelon shaved ice will be a welcome treat on warm days.

2½ cups seedless watermelon chunks (about 1 small watermelon)

½ cup sparkling water

¼ cup Splenda

1 TB. pasteurized egg whites

1 TB. fresh lime juice

¼ tsp. salt

Yield: 8 servings
Prep time: 6 hours
Serving size: ½ cup
Each serving has:
15 calories
4 g carbohydrate
4 g sugars
.6 g protein
0 g fat
0 g saturated fat
0 g cholesterol
81 mg sodium
.3 g fiber
0 IU vitamin D
8 mg potassium
4 mg calcium
1 mcg selenium

1. In a blender, combine watermelon, sparkling water, Splenda, egg whites, lime juice, and salt. Blend on high speed until smooth.

2. Pour mixture into a 9-inch square baking dish. Cover tightly with plastic wrap, and freeze for about 45 minutes or until mixture is icy at the edges of the pan. Whisk to distribute frozen portions evenly. Cover and refreeze for about 45 minutes or until mixture is icy at the edges of the pan and overall texture is slushy. Whisk again to distribute frozen portions evenly. Cover and refreeze for about 3 hours or until frozen solid. Remove from the freezer.

3. Using a fork, scrape granita down the length of the pan, forming icy flakes. Return to the freezer for at least 1 hour. Granita can be made 1 day ahead and kept in the freezer.

Cooking Tip

If you're serving this granita at a dinner party, try making it using one watermelon with red flesh and a separate batch with yellow-flesh watermelon. Your guests are almost guaranteed to ask for the recipe.

Cinnamon and Almond Espresso Granita

Delicious and "creamy" almond espresso granita pairs with cinnamon swirls.

Yield: 8 servings
Prep time: 35 minutes
Serving size: ½ cup
Each serving has:
25 calories
1 g carbohydrate
0 g sugars
5 g protein
.2 g fat
0 g saturated fat
0 g cholesterol
67 mg sodium
0 g fiber
19 IU vitamin D
27 mg potassium
48 mg calcium
3 mcg selenium

½ cup pasteurized egg whites	½ cup silken tofu
1 TB. vanilla protein powder	1 tsp. ground cinnamon
3 cups brewed decaf espresso	½ tsp. almond extract
⅓ cup Splenda	

1. In a blender, combine egg whites, protein powder, espresso, Splenda, tofu, cinnamon, and almond extract. Blend on high speed until smooth.

2. Pour into an ice-cream maker, and freeze for 30 minutes or according to the manufacturer's instructions.

 Post-Op Pitfall _____

Use almond extract sparingly because it's really strong. You'll know if you use too much because the product will have a *very* sweet almond-y taste.

Glossary

acai berries Small, round, and dark purple in color, similar to grapes in appearance. They're commonly used to make smoothies, sodas, and other beverages.

active dry yeast A common form of yeast that are alive but dormant because of the lack of moisture.

alcohol dehydrogenase A group of enzymes that help your body break down alcohol. They're decreased significantly after gastric bypass.

allspice Named for its flavor echoes of several spices (cinnamon, cloves, nutmeg), allspice is used in many desserts and in rich marinades and stews.

antioxidants Special chemicals that help protect your cells from harmful agents called free radicals.

artichoke hearts The center part of the artichoke flower, often found canned in grocery stores.

arugula A spicy-peppery garden plant with leaves that resemble a dandelion and have a distinctive—and very sharp—flavor.

au gratin The quick broiling of a dish before serving to brown the top ingredients. When used in a recipe name, the term often implies cheese and a creamy sauce.

balsamic vinegar   Vinegar produced primarily in Italy from a specific type of grape and aged in wood barrels. It is heavier, darker, and sweeter than most vinegars.

basil   A flavorful, almost sweet, resinous herb delicious with tomatoes and used in all kinds of Italian or Mediterranean-style dishes.

baste   To keep foods moist during cooking by spooning, brushing, or drizzling with a liquid.

bean thread noodles   Asian-style noodles made from a starch such as mung bean starch and water. Also known as cellophane noodles.

biological value (BV)   A summary of the proportion of the protein your body absorbs from food. It's determined by a test that measures nitrogen, a product of protein metabolism in your body.

body mass index (BMI)   A measure of your weight (in kilograms) over your height (in meters, then squared). BMI is a quick screening tool used to assess whether you have obesity or if you have medical indications for weight loss surgery.

boil   To heat a liquid to a point where water is forced to turn into steam, causing the liquid to bubble. To boil something is to insert it into boiling water. A rapid boil is when a lot of bubbles form on the surface of the liquid.

bok choy (also **Chinese cabbage**)   A member of the cabbage family with thick stems, crisp texture, and fresh flavor. It's perfect for stir-frying.

braise   To cook with the introduction of some liquid, usually over an extended period of time.

broil   To cook in a dry oven under the overhead high-heat element.

broth   *See* stock.

brown   To cook in a skillet, turning, until the food's surface is seared and brown in color, to lock in the juices.

brown rice   Whole-grain rice including the germ with a characteristic pale brown or tan color; more nutritious and flavorful than white rice.

bruschetta (or **crostini**)   Slices of toasted or grilled bread with garlic and olive oil, often with other toppings.

bulgur   A wheat kernel that's been steamed, dried, and crushed and is sold in fine and coarse textures. Because of its high nutritional value, bulgur is often used as a substitute for rice and couscous.

calabacita A type of zucchini; a dish made from sautéed pork, zucchini, and squash.

capers Flavorful buds of a Mediterranean plant, ranging in size from *nonpareil* (about the size of a small pea) to larger, grape-size caper berries produced in Spain.

caramelize To cook sugar over low heat until it develops a sweet caramel flavor. The term is increasingly gaining use to describe cooking vegetables (especially onions) or meat in butter or oil over low heat until they soften, sweeten, and develop a caramel color.

caraway A distinctive spicy seed used for bread, pork, cheese, and cabbage dishes. It is known to reduce stomach upset, which is why it is often paired with, for example, sauerkraut.

carbohydrate A nutritional component found in starches, sugars, fruits, and vegetables that causes a rise in blood glucose levels. Carbohydrates supply energy and many important nutrients, including vitamins, minerals, and antioxidants.

cardamom An intense, sweet-smelling spice, common to Indian cooking, used in baking and coffee.

cayenne A fiery spice made from (hot) chili peppers, especially the cayenne chili, a slender, red, and very hot pepper.

chèvre French for "goat milk cheese," chèvre is a typically creamy-salty soft cheese delicious by itself or paired with fruits or chutney. Chèvres vary in style from mild and creamy to aged, firm, and flavorful.

chickpeas *See* garbanzo beans.

chiffonade The cutting of leafy vegetables and herbs into thin strips by stacking the leaves, largest to smallest, and rolling them tightly, from stem to the tip of the leaf, and cutting across the rolled leaves with a sharp knife to produce fine ribbons.

chili garlic sauce An Asian sauce made from fresh garlic and chili flakes.

chili powder A seasoning blend that includes chili pepper, cumin, garlic, and oregano. Proportions vary among different versions, but they all offer a warm, rich flavor.

chilies (or **chiles**) Any one of many different "hot" peppers, ranging in intensity from the relatively mild ancho pepper to the blisteringly hot habanero.

chives A member of the onion family, chives grow in bunches of long leaves that resemble tall grass or the green tops of onions and offer a light onion flavor.

chop To cut into pieces, usually qualified by an adverb such as "*coarsely* chopped," or by a size measurement such as "chopped into $1/2$-inch pieces." "Finely chopped" is much closer to mince.

cilantro A member of the parsley family and used in Mexican cooking (especially salsa) and some Asian dishes. Use in moderation, as the flavor can overwhelm. The seed of cilantro is the spice coriander.

clove A sweet, strong, almost wintergreen-flavor spice used in baking and with meats such as ham.

coriander A rich, warm, spicy seed with a lemony flavor used in all types of recipes, from African to South American, from entrées to desserts. Coriander is the seeds of the coriander plant. The leaves are called cilantro.

count In terms of seafood or other foods that come in small sizes, the number of that item that compose 1 pound. For example, 31 to 40 count shrimp are large appetizer shrimp often served with cocktail sauce; 51 to 60 count are much smaller.

couscous Granular semolina (durum wheat) that is cooked and used in many Mediterranean and North African dishes.

crème fraîche A thinner, French version of American sour cream.

cumin A fiery, smoky-tasting spice popular in Middle Eastern and Indian dishes. Cumin is a seed; ground cumin seed is the most common form used in cooking.

curry Rich, spicy, Indian-style sauces made with turmeric, cumin, red pepper, and many other spices, and the dishes prepared with them. A curry uses curry powder as its base seasoning.

curry powder A ground blend of rich and flavorful spices used as a basis for curry and many other Indian-influenced dishes. Common ingredients include hot pepper, nutmeg, cumin, cinnamon, pepper, and turmeric. Some curry can also be found in paste form.

devein The removal of the dark vein from the back of a large shrimp with a sharp knife.

dice To cut into small cubes about $1/4$-inch square.

dill A herb perfect for eggs, salmon, cheese dishes, and, of course, vegetables (pickles!).

dredge To cover a piece of food with a dry substance such as flour or corn meal.

dumping syndrome   The sweaty, shaky, very tired feeling some gastric bypass surgery patients get after eating foods high in simple sugar or high in fat. May be related to eating too quickly, and may even occur with protein foods.

falafel   A garbanzo bean patty similar to a fritter, usually fried.

fennel   In seed form, a fragrant, licorice-tasting herb. The bulbs have a much milder flavor and a celerylike crunch and are used as a vegetable in salads or cooked recipes.

flour   Grains ground into a meal. Wheat is perhaps the most common flour. Flour is also made from oats, rye, buckwheat, soybeans, etc. *See also* all-purpose flour; cake flour; whole-wheat flour.

fold   To combine a dense with a light mixture with a circular action from the middle of the bowl.

free radicals   "Radical" molecules, created in your body as part of your natural metabolism, that are unstable and react with the essential molecules, including DNA, fat, and proteins, stealing or giving electrons to other molecules, and changing their chemical structure.

frittata   A skillet-cooked mixture of eggs and other ingredients that's not stirred but is cooked slowly and then either flipped or finished under the broiler.

fry   *See* sauté.

functional foods   Foods that provide nutraceutical-type benefits. For example, eggs fortified with omega-3 fatty acids to help fight or prevent heart disease are a functional food.

garbanzo beans (or **chickpeas**)   A yellow-gold, roundish bean used as the base ingredient in hummus. Chickpeas are high in fiber and low in fat.

generally regarded as safe (GRAS)   A list of foods, beverages, and additives to the diet the U.S. government believes to be safe for the majority of the population to ingest.

ghrelin   A potent hunger hormone that goes down after eating and up before a meal. Ghrelin is lower in the early post-op period in metabolic surgeries like gastric bypass.

ginger   Available in fresh root or dried, ground form, ginger adds a pungent, sweet, and spicy quality to a dish.

gluconeogenesis   The making of glucose (sugar your brain prefers) from protein, which is usually a negative thing because protein should be used for your muscles, etc., and not for sugar. This usually happens when you're not getting enough carbs in your diet.

glutamate   An amino acid or building block of protein, found naturally in protein-containing foods such as cheese, milk, meat, mushrooms, fish, and even vegetables.

glycemic index (GI)   A measure of the blood sugar effects of a single food or beverage. Low-GI foods may be helpful to manage blood sugars/diabetes and may also decrease hunger.

gnocchi   Italian dumplings. They're a great substitute for pasta in many Italian dishes.

grazing   Eating snacks all day long or eating small amounts of different foods all day.

gut   Part of the gastrointestinal tract, especially from the pylorus (at the end of your stomach) including your small and large intestines.

handful   An unscientific measurement; the amount of an ingredient you can hold in your hand.

hearts of palm   Firm, elongated, off-white cylinders from the inside of a palm tree stem tip.

herbes de Provence   A seasoning mix including basil, fennel, marjoram, rosemary, sage, and thyme, common in the south of France.

hoisin sauce   A sweet Asian condiment similar to ketchup made with soybeans, sesame, chili peppers, and sugar.

honeymoon period   The immediate post-op period (around 3 to 6 months) after many weight loss surgery procedures when you don't feel real hunger or have an appetite for food.

hummus   A thick, Middle Eastern spread made of puréed garbanzo beans, lemon juice, olive oil, garlic, and often tahini (sesame seed paste).

incretin effect   A greater insulin response of the pancreas to oral versus intravenous glucose thought to be related to gut hormones, including GLP-1. The improvement in blood sugar control occurs during the first week after gastric bypass surgery, so weight loss may not be the driving mechanism.

indispensible amino acids (IAA)   Amino acids or building blocks of protein you need to get from your diet because your body doesn't make them.

insulin sensitivity   The improved action of insulin, which allows for blood glucose (sugar) uptake into the muscle and fat cells. The cells offer less resistance to allow insulin to enter and do its job with blood sugar uptake.

international units (IUs)   The unit of measure used for vitamin D supplements.

intrinsic factor (IF)   A type of protein made in your stomach that's absorbed in the ileum, the last part of your small intestine. Impairment in production or function of IF may lead to vitamin B_{12} deficiency and result in pernicious anemia.

Italian seasoning   A blend of dried herbs, including basil, oregano, rosemary, and thyme.

jicama   A juicy, crunchy, sweet, large, round Central American vegetable with the texture of a water chestnut commonly used in many marinated salads and stir-fry dishes. If you can't find jicama, try substituting sliced water chestnuts.

julienne   A French word meaning "to slice into very thin pieces."

ketones   By-products of fat breakdown that are released when carbohydrate intake is very low. Keytones help preserve blood glucose.

kiwi (or kiwifruit)   A small oval fruit that's fuzzy and brown on the outside. The fruit inside is lime green and contains edible little black seeds.

kosher salt   A coarse-grained salt made without any additives or iodine.

lentils   Tiny lens-shape pulses used in European, Middle Eastern, and Indian cuisines.

marinate   To soak meat, seafood, or other food in a seasoned sauce, called a marinade, which is high in acid content. The acids break down the muscle of the meat, making it tender and adding flavor.

marjoram   A sweet herb, a cousin of and similar to oregano, popular in Greek, Spanish, and Italian dishes.

meld   To allow flavors to blend and spread over time.

mesclun   Mixed salad greens, usually containing lettuce and assorted greens such as arugula, cress, endive, and others.

metabolic bone disease   An umbrella term for disorders of the bones, including bone weakening that is sometimes seen after weight loss surgery and/or rapid, significant weight loss.

metabolic surgery   Term used to described the chemical changes that occur in the body after surgery like gastric bypass surgery, where new connections between the brain and gastrointestinal tract occur and increase the production of weight-friendly hormones and assist in the remission of certain diseases, such as diabetes.

methylmalonic acid (MMA)   A breakdown product of vitamin B_{12} that can catch up to 50 percent of low levels of this vitamin not detected with a plain blood level test of vitamin B_{12}.

microbiota   Bacteria in your gut (e.g., small intestines) that consist of 100 trillion microorganisms—more cells than found in the human body.

mince   To cut into very small pieces smaller than diced pieces, about $1/8$ inch or smaller.

mindfulness   The art of being present, in the moment.

miso   A fermented, flavorful soybean paste, key in many Japanese dishes. Miso is very salty, so use sparingly.

nutmeg   A sweet, fragrant, musky spice used primarily in baking.

nutraceuticals   Foods, beverages, and supplements in a particular amount that results in their being of medicinal strength or having certain properties to heal or possibly manage disease(s). *See also* functional foods.

obesigenic   A term coined to suggest that in today's society, many things could increase one's chances for overweight or obesity, including availability of fast foods, increased stress, toxic environments, decreased sleep, and a sedentary lifestyle.

oligosaccharides   Carbohydrates containing 3 to 10 simple sugars joined together and are an example of prebiotics. Examples include onions, leeks, garlic, legumes, wheat, asparagus, and other plant foods.

olive oil   A fragrant liquid produced by crushing or pressing olives. Extra-virgin olive oil—the most flavorful and highest quality—is produced from the first pressing of a batch of olives; oil is also produced from later pressings.

omega-3 fats   Heart-healthy fats, found in foods like salmon and sardines, believed to decrease inflammation and heart disease risk.

on the bias   Cut on an angle as opposed to an up-and-down motion. It gives the food a nice presentation, and you have the appearance of getting more food.

oregano   A fragrant, slightly astringent herb used in Greek, Spanish, and Italian dishes.

oxidation   The browning of fruit flesh that happens over time and with exposure to air. Minimize oxidation by rubbing the cut surfaces with a lemon half. Oxidation also affects wine, which is why the taste changes over time after a bottle is opened.

paprika   A rich, red, warm, earthy spice that also lends a rich red color to many dishes.

parathyroid hormone (PTH)   A blood test that's a good measure of the calcium in your body.

parsley   A fresh-tasting green leafy herb, often used as a garnish.

pesto   A thick spread or sauce made with fresh basil leaves, garlic, olive oil, pine nuts, and Parmesan cheese. Some newer versions are made with other herbs.

phenylketonuria (PKU)   A genetic disease in which people cannot breakdown phenylalanlnine, an important amino acid and building block of protein. A special, strict diet is needed, and aspartame must be avoided because it contains phenylalanine.

pica   A disorder sometimes seen with iron deficiency in which people crave, and often eat, inedible items such as dirt, clay, or cornstarch. Excessive ice eating may also be a sign of pica.

pickle   A food, usually a vegetable such as a cucumber, that's been pickled in brine.

pilaf   A rice dish in which the rice is browned in butter or oil and then cooked in a flavorful liquid such as a broth, often with the addition of meats or vegetables. The rice absorbs the broth, resulting in a savory dish.

pita bread   A flat, hollow wheat bread often used for sandwiches or sliced, pizza style, into slices. Terrific soft with dips, or baked or broiled as a vehicle for other ingredients.

poach   To cook a food in simmering liquid, such as water, wine, or broth.

polenta   Cornmeal mush. It is much like grits in a sense, but polenta can be served immediately as a mush, or chilled and cut into shapes and reheated.

portobello mushrooms   A mature and larger form of the smaller crimini mushroom, portobellos are brownish, chewy, and flavorful. Often served as whole caps, grilled, and as thin sautéed slices. *See also* crimini mushrooms.

prebiotics   Indigestible fibers found in some foods that help produce good bacteria (e.g., bananas).

probiotics   Foods or supplements that contain good bacteria believed to increase overall health and possibly help decrease inflammation.

proofing   To allow dough to rise.

prosciutto   Dry, salt-cured ham, that originated in Italy.

protein digestibility corrected amino acid score (PDCAAS)   The measure of the quality and absorption rate of a particular source of protein(s) in the diet.

purée   To reduce a food to a thick, creamy texture, usually using a blender or food processor.

reduce   To boil or simmer a broth or sauce to remove some of the water content, resulting in more concentrated flavor and color.

reserve   To hold a specified ingredient for another use later in the recipe.

risotto   A popular Italian rice dish made by browning Arborio rice in butter or oil and then slowly adding liquid to cook the rice, resulting in a creamy texture.

roast   To cook something uncovered in an oven, usually without additional liquid.

rosemary   A pungent, sweet herb used with chicken, pork, fish, and especially lamb. A little of it goes a long way.

roux   A mixture of butter or another fat and flour, used to thicken sauces and soups.

saffron   A spice made from the stamens of crocus flowers, saffron lends a dramatic yellow color and distinctive flavor to a dish. Use only tiny amounts of this expensive herb.

sage   An herb with a musty yet fruity, lemon-rind scent and "sunny" flavor.

sauté   To pan-cook over lower heat than used for frying.

savory   A popular herb with a fresh, woody taste.

sear   To quickly brown the exterior of a food, especially meat, over high heat to preserve interior moisture.

shallot   A member of the onion family that grows in a bulb somewhat like garlic and has a milder onion flavor. When a recipe calls for shallot, use the entire bulb.

shiitake mushrooms   Large, dark brown mushrooms with a hearty, meaty flavor. Can be used either fresh or dried, grilled, or as a component in other recipes and as a flavoring source for broth.

simmer   To boil gently so the liquid barely bubbles.

SMART goals   Specific, Measurable, Attainable, Realistic, and Timely goals that help improve the successful realization of your desired outcome or goals.

steam To suspend a food over boiling water and allow the heat of the steam (water vapor) to cook the food. A quick cooking method, steaming preserves the flavor and texture of a food.

steep To let sit in hot water, as in steeping tea in hot water for 10 minutes.

stew To slowly cook pieces of food submerged in a liquid. Also, a dish that has been prepared by this method.

stir-fry To cook small pieces of food in a wok or skillet over high heat, moving and turning the food quickly to cook all sides.

stock A flavorful broth made by cooking meats and/or vegetables with seasonings until the liquid absorbs these flavors. This liquid is then strained and the solids discarded. Can be eaten alone or used as a base for soups, stews, etc.

stone-ground mustard Mustard seeds ground with a stone mill to a coarse texture. The flavor is slightly spicier than that of regular mustard.

tahini A paste made from sesame seeds used to flavor many Middle Eastern recipes.

tarragon A sweet, rich-smelling herb perfect with seafood, vegetables (especially asparagus), chicken, and pork.

thyme A minty, zesty herb.

tofu A cheeselike substance made by puréeing soy beans with boiling water. Then that liquid is strained, and a coagulant is added, and curds form (similar to making cheese). Then, the curds are formed into a cube.

turmeric A spicy, pungent yellow root used in many dishes, especially Indian cuisine, for color and flavor. Turmeric is the source of the yellow color in many prepared mustards.

vanilla extract A flavoring made by soaking vanilla beans in alcohol.

vinegar An acidic liquid widely used as dressing and seasoning, often made from fermented grapes, apples, or rice.

walnuts A rich, slightly woody flavored nut.

wasabi Japanese horseradish, a fiery, pungent condiment used with many Japanese-style dishes. Most often sold as a powder; add water to create a paste.

water chestnuts A tuber, popular in many types of Asian-style cooking. The flesh is white, crunchy, and juicy, and the vegetable holds its texture whether cool or hot.

watercress   An aquatic/semi-aquatic plant that has a peppery flavor.

wheat berry   The entire wheat kernel, consisting of the bran, germ, and endosperm. Wheat berries are an excellent source of dietary fiber.

whisk   To rapidly mix, introducing air to the mixture.

white pepper   The ripened berry from the pepper plant that's been dried. White pepper is used in many recipes light in color for aesthetic purposes. The flavor of the white and black pepper aren't really that different, so if you only have black on hand, it'll work just fine.

white vinegar   The most common type of vinegar, produced from grain.

whole-wheat flour   Wheat flour that contains the entire grain.

wild rice   Actually a grass with a rich, nutty flavor, popular as an unusual and nutritious side dish.

wine vinegar   Vinegar produced from red or white wine.

Worcestershire sauce   Originally developed in India and containing tamarind, this spicy sauce is used as a seasoning for many meats and other dishes.

yeast   Tiny fungi that, when mixed with water, sugar, flour, and heat, release carbon dioxide bubbles, which, in turn, cause the bread to rise.

zest   Small slivers of peel, usually from a citrus fruit such as lemon, lime, or orange.

zester   A kitchen tool used to scrape zest off a fruit. A small grater also works well.

Resources

Here we've provided you, dear readers, with all kinds of information to put in your weight loss surgery "tool box" to enhance your chances for life-long weight loss success.

Complementary and Alternative Medicine (CAM)

Mackenzie, Elizabeth, Ph.D., and Birgit Rakel, M.D. *Complementary and Alternative Medicine for Older Adults: Holistic Approaches to Healthy Aging.* New York: Springer Publishing, 2006.

Navarra, Tova. *The Encyclopedia of Complementary and Alternative Medicine.* New York: Facts On File, Inc., 2005.

Depression and Anxiety

Amen, Daniel G., M.D., and Lisa C. Routh, M.D. *Healing Anxiety and Depression.* New York: Berkley Books, 2003.

Bourne, Edmund J., Ph.D. *The Anxiety and Phobia Workbook.* Oakland, CA: New Harbinger Publications, Inc., 1995.

Burns, David D., M.D. *Feeling Good: The New Mood Therapy: The Clinically Proven Drug-Free Treatment for Depression, Revised and Updated.* New York: Quill Publishers, 2000.

———. *Ten Days to Self-Esteem.* New York: HarperCollins, 1993.

Dalai Lama and Nicholas Vreeland, ed. *An Open Heart: Practicing Compassion in Everyday Life.* Boston: Little, Brown and Company, 2001.

Dining Out

Lichten, Joanne, R.D., Ph.D. *Dining Lean: How to Eat Healthy in Your Favorite Restaurants.* Orlando: Nutrifit Publishers, 2000.

———. *How to Stay Healthy and Fit on the Road.* Orlando: Nutrifit Publishers, 2001.

Warshaw, Hope, S. MMSc, R.D. *Eat Out, Eat Right! A Guide to Healthier Restaurant Eating.* Chicago: Surrey Books, 2003.

———. *What to Eat When You're Eating Out.* Alexandria, VA: Small Steps Press, 2006.

Eating Mindfully

Albers, Susan, Psy.D. *Eat, Drink and Be Mindful: How to End Your Struggle with Mindless Eating and Start Savoring Food with Intention and Joy.* Oakland, CA: New Harbinger Publications, Inc., 2009.

———. *Eating Mindfully: How to End the Mindless Eating and Enjoy a Balanced Relationship with Food.* Oakland, CA: New Harbinger Publications, Inc., 2003.

Altman, Donald. *Meal by Meal: 365 Daily Meditations for Finding Balance Through Mindful Eating.* Maui, HI: Inner Ocean Publishing Company, 2004.

Bays, Jan Chosen. *Mindful Eating: A Guide to Rediscovering a Healthy and Joyful Relationship with Food.* Boston and London: Shambala, 2009.

Gerrard, Don. *One Bowl: A Guide to Eating for Body and Spirit.* New York: Marlowe and Company, 2001.

Somov, Pavel Georgievich. *Eating the Moment: 141 Mindful Practices to Overcome Overeating One Meal at a Time.* Oakland, CA: New Harbinger Publications, Inc., 2008.

Tribole, Evelyn, and Elyse Resch. *Intuitive Eating: A Revolutionary Program That Works*. New York: St. Martin's Press, 2003.

Wansink, Brian. *Mindless Eating: Why We Eat More Than We Think*. New York: Bantam Dell, 2007.

Fast-Food/Chain Restaurants

The Fast Food Explorer
www.fatcalories.com

Super Size Me
This film by Morgan Spurlock shows how much of an effect fast food can have on your body.

Free Online Food Logs

The Daily Plate
www.thedailyplate.com

Maintain Fit
www.maintainfit.com

FitDay
www.fitday.com

SparkPeople
www.sparkpeople.com

Meditation

Bodhipaksa. *Still the Minds: Simple Breathing Practices for Inner Peace*. Louisville, CO: Sounds True, Inc., 2002.

Kabat-Zinn, Jon. *Mindfulness for Beginners*. Louisville, CO: Sounds True, Inc., 2006.

Lang, Diana. *Opening to Meditation: A Gentle, Guided Approach* (book and CD). Novato, CA: New World Library, 2004.

Sovik, Rolf. *Moving Inward: The Journey to Meditation*. Honesdale, PA: Himalayan Institute Press, 2005.

Stryker, Rod. *Meditations for Life*. Carbondale, CA: Parayoga (www.parayoga.com), 2005.

———. *Relax into Greatness*. Carbondale, CA: Parayoga (www.parayoga.com), 2003.

Yee, Rodney. *Moving Toward Balance: 8 Weeks of Yoga with Rodney Yee*. Emmaus, PA: Rodale Press, Inc., 2004.

Nutrition Information

NutritionData.com
www.nutritiondata.com

USDA MyPyramid.gov
www.mypyramid.gov

Online Support Groups

Bariatric Eating Message Board
www.bariatriceating.com/BEsupport/messageboard.php

Bariatric Eating Online Support Group
www.bariatriceating.com/BEsupport/supportgroup.php

Daily Strength
www.dailystrength.org/c/Gastric-Bypass-Surgery/forum

Obesity Help
www.obesityhelp.com

Plus-Sized Barbie Blog
plusizedbarbie.blogspot.com

Weight Loss Surgery Kitchen
www.livingafterwls.com/Recipes.html

Organic Foods

Nestle, Marion, Ph.D., M.P.H. *What to Eat.* New York: Farrar, Straus and Giroux, 2007.

Worthington, V. "Nutritional Quality of Organic Versus Conventional Fruits, Vegetables and Grains." *Journal of Alternative and Complementary Medicine* 7(2):161–173, 2001.

ATTRA
attra.ncat.org

The Organic Center
www.organic-center.org/science.nutri.php?action=view&report_id=126

Pedometers

America On the Move
www.americaonthemove.org

Before You Buy a Pedometer
walking.about.com/cs/measure/bb/bybpedometer.htm

Relaxation/Stress Reduction

Benson, Herbert, M.D. *The Relaxation Response, Updated and Expanded Edition.* New York: HarperCollins, 2000.

Borysenko, Joan, Ph.D. *Minding the Body Mending the Mind.* Cambridge, MA: De Capo Press, 2007.

Davis, Martha, Elizabeth Robbins Eshelman, Matthew McKay, and Patrick Fanning. *The Relaxation and Stress Reduction Workbook (New Harbinger Self-Help Workbook).* Oakland, CA: New Harbinger, 2008.

McKay, Matthew, Martha Davis, and Patrick Fanning. *Thoughts and Feelings: Taking Control of Your Moods and Your Life.* Oakland, CA: New Harbinger, 2007.

Self-Support

Breitman, Patti. *How to Say No Without Feeling Guilty.* New York: Broadway Books, 2001.

Chodron, Pema. *Start Where You Are.* Boston: Shambhala Publications, 2001.

Harrell, Keith. *Attitude Is Everything (revised edition).* New York: HarperCollins, 2005.

Jimenez, Lisa, M.Ed. *Conquer Fear!* Mechanicsburg, PA: Executive Books, 2001.

Sources of Protein

All these sites sell sample sizes of protein powders so you can sample to see what you like and what works best for you. Some sell a variety of brands, while others carry only one. Many of these sites also sell vitamins.

Note: Margaret does *not* recommend protein products with collagen (e.g., New Whey Bullet, etc.) due to their low protein quality and low absorption rate.

Bariatric Advantage

www.bariatricadvantage.com/catalog/categoryHandler?cat=Bariatric%20 Advantage%20%3A%20Sampl%20Kits

Nashua Nutrition

www.nashuanutrition.com/store/index.php?target=products&product_id=436

Netrition

www.26.netrition.com/netrition_protein_sampler_pack.html

Unjury Protein Powder

www.unjury.com/ssl/purchasing.php

Vitalady

www.vitalady.com/protein.htm

Websites and Blogs

Some of the blogs listed here are personal blogs, and some are more professional. Not all these bloggers always follow the rules your surgical center may provide you with, and some of these folks may not be the best examples. But you might find their sites to be useful, so we've included them here.

EatingWell
www.eatingwell.com

GoodFoodNearYou
www.goodfoodnearyou.com

Living Well After Weight Loss Surgery
livingafterwls.blogspot.com

Margaret Furtado
www.yahoo.com/health

Melting Mama
www.meltingmama.net

Necessary Mutilation
necessarymutilation.com

ObesityHelp
www.obesityhelp.com

Rebecca Scritchfield
www.rebeccascritchfield.wordpress.com

Weight Loss Surgery Channel
www.weightlosssurgerychannel.com

Weight Loss Surgery Lifestyles
www.wlslifestyles.com

Yoga

A few notes about yoga from Margaret: Some of the following yoga books and/or resources, such as those on power yoga, are more advanced and/or vigorous styles. If you're an absolute yoga beginner, I recommend gentle yoga and/or *The Complete Idiot's Guide* and/or the assistance of a qualified yoga instructor. Check www.yogaalliance.org as well as www.yogafinder.com for classes near you.

Baptiste, Baron. *Journey Into Power, How to Sculpt Your Ideal Body, Free Your True Self, and Transform Your Life with Yoga.* New York: Fireside, 2002.

Budilovsky, Jean, Carolyn Flynn, and Eve Adamson. *The Complete Idiot's Guide to Yoga Illustrated, Fourth Edition.* Indianapolis: Alpha Books, 2006.

Cappy, Peggy. *Yoga for All of Us: A Modified Series of Traditional Poses for Any Age and Ability.* New York: St. Martin's Press, 2006.

Coulter, H. David, *Anatomy of Hatha Yoga, A Manual for Students, Teachers and Practitioners.* Delhi: Motilal Banarsidass Publishers, 2001.

Gates, Rolf. *Meditations from the Mat.* New York: Anchor Books, 2002.

Iyengar, B.K.S. *The Path to Holistic Health.* New York: DK Publishing, 2007.

McCall, Timothy, M.D. *Yoga as Medicine: The Yogic Prescription for Health and Healing.* New York: Bantam Books, 2007.

Index

G

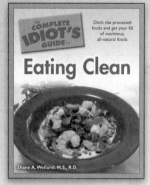
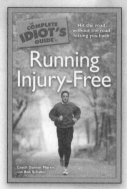
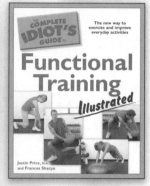
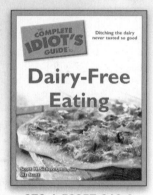
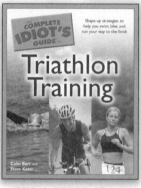
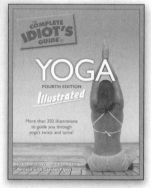
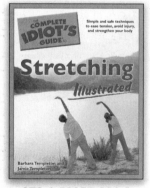
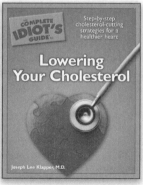
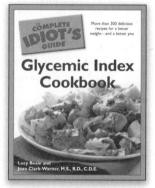